Brain Dead, Brain Absent, Brain Donors

Brain Dead, Brain Absent, Brain Donors

HUMAN SUBJECTS OR HUMAN OBJECTS?

PETER McCULLAGH
John Curtin School of Medical Research
The Australian National University
Canberra
Australia

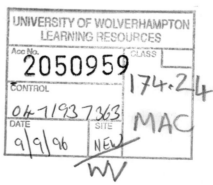
JOHN WILEY & SONS
Chichester · New York · Brisbane · Toronto · Singapore

Copyright © 1993 by John Wiley & Sons Ltd,
Baffins Lane, Chichester,
West Sussex PO19 1UD, England

Other Wiley Editorial Offices

John Wiley & Sons, Inc., 605 Third Avenue,
New York, NY 10158-0012, USA

Jacaranda Wiley Ltd, G.P.O. Box 859, Brisbane,
Queensland 4001, Australia

John Wiley & Sons (Canada) Ltd, 22 Worcester Road,
Rexdale, Ontario M9W 1L1, Canada

John Wiley & Sons (SEA) Pte Ltd, 37 Jalan Pemimpin #05-04,
Block B, Union Industrial Building, Singapore 2057

Library of Congress Cataloguing-in-Publication Data

McCullagh, P. J. (Peter John)
    Brain dead, brain absent, and brain donors : human subjects or
    human objects? / Peter McCullagh.
        p. cm.
    Includes bibliographical references and index.
    ISBN 0 471 93736 3
    1. Brain death. 2. Brain death—Moral and ethical aspects.
    3. Anencephalus. 4. Fetal brain—Transplantation. I. Title.
    [DNLM: 1. Anencephaly. 2. Brain Death. 3. Ethics, Medical.
    4. Organ Procurement. 5. Tissue Donors. WO 690 M478b]
    RA1063.3M4 1992
    174'.2—dc20
    DNLM/DLC
    for Library of Congress   92-49197
                                                                   CIP

British Library Cataloguing in Publication Data

A catalogue record for this book is available from the British Library

ISBN 0 471 93736 3

Typeset in 10/12 point Galliard by
Mathematical Composition Setters Ltd, Salisbury, UK
Printed and bound in Great Britain by
Biddles Ltd, Guildford and King's Lynn

Contents

Acknowledgements

I am indebted to Jim Keaney for many discussions on the significance of the state of brain death and for guidance in the process of revision of Chapters 2 and 3. Elspeth Christiansen read the manuscript and made many suggestions for its improvement. Anabel Walters provided major assistance in the preparation of this book by typing each of the extensive number of drafts through which the manuscript evolved.

Peter McCullagh

1 Introduction

The history of determination of death on the basis of the condition of the brain has been interconnected with the history of organ transplantation. Any explanation of the former requires some familiarity with the latter. The connection, which was established historically, retains considerable contemporary relevance and it is likely that the determination of death and organ transplantation will remain intertwined in the future. Organ transplantation has now been established as a most effective form of treatment for a number of diseases. However, an imbalance between the supply of organs suitable for transplantation and the demand for them has arisen and is increasing.

A number of means to overcome this imbalance have been proposed. All involve some form of reconsideration either of the determination of death or of attitudes towards those in the process of dying. One possibility could be to increase the frequency with which patients who become available as donors within the scope of existing criteria of brain death are actually utilized. A likely difficulty, which already exists but which could be augmented by such a course of action, arises from the wide discrepancy that exists between existing organ procurement practice and the community's understanding of that process. For instance, few individuals outside hospital practice are familiar with what the use of a beating-heart donor entails.

An alternative, which has been actively canvassed to increase donor recruitment, is based upon alteration of the criteria for donor selection. Proposals for such changes necessarily direct attention to the basis for existing and new criteria for identification of organ donors. Expressed somewhat differently, the issue becomes one of deciding when an individual need no longer be regarded as a live human being but can be considered as a resource that is available for the use of others.

The question of determination of when a human subject becomes an object is, I suspect, not one which has commonly been framed in those terms. Traditionally, the transition has been synonymous with the death of an individual and there has been little purpose in attaching an additional form of description to that event. As regards the event of death itself, the point should be made that decisions regarding its nature, whilst they might superficially appear to be responses to medical questions, should rest with the wider community. The selection between the various formulations that have been proposed to define death remains one for society to make. The medical decisions concerning death have to do with its recognition or diagnosis on the basis of attainment of criteria acceptable to society. Refinements in clinical skill and medical technology may provide increasing insight into the biological features of the transition from life to death. They cannot, however, disclose what death is.

There are a number of accompaniments of the biological event of death. A major implication of the transition from subject to object is that an individual can no longer be considered to have the range of interests generally accorded to human beings. In a medical context, a most basic interest to lapse with the transition from subject to object is that of not being used as a means rather than being treated as an end in oneself. Any proposition that medical attendants could use patients in such a way that they could become something other than ends in themselves would be likely to attract universal condemnation on the basis that this infringed the autonomy of the individual. In contrast, use of an individual after death, provided the form of use or its associated circumstances were not outside those acceptable to the community involved, need not be viewed unfavourably. If the form of use offered the prospect of conferring substantial benefit on others, it may indeed be regarded very positively. Using a subject is invariably wrong: using an object is not.

During the last three decades, there has been a substantial change in emphasis in relation to those features which are considered to characterize death. The traditional concept of death revolved around the irreversible cessation of function of the body, manifest by cessation of the propulsion of blood within the circulation by the heart. More recently, death has been conceptualized as irreversible loss of function of the brain. Before the 1960s, the distinction between these two forms of description would have been little more than a hypothetical exercise in terms of medical diagnosis. (It would, nevertheless, have been quite a legitimate exercise in discussing what precisely was to be considered as the defining feature of death, as distinct from other features which invariably led to it, accompanied it or provided a diagnostic indication of its occurrence.) It was only after techniques had been developed for providing resuscitation and ongoing life support to individuals who had sustained brain damage of sufficient severity to result in the permanent loss of the capacity to breath that the distinction acquired practical import. The application of life support systems to individuals in whom irreversible loss of brain functions had caused respiration to cease has resulted in separation between the traditional and the brain-centred manifestations of death.

Apart from advances in life-support technology, which have permitted the maintenance of individuals in whom brain function has been irreversibly lost, the other change which has served to emphasize the issue of conversion of the human subject to an object has been the dramatic increase in efficiency of organ transplantation. This has produced a demand for individuals who meet the criteria for diagnosis of death but who, nevertheless, remain in such a state that their organs are suitable for transplantation. With this incentive to decide when an individual can be regarded as a usable object, together with the realization that the identification of the timing of subject-to-object transition with the traditional recognition of death no longer applied, some reappraisal of the status of patients with extensive and irreversible loss of brain function became inevitable.

Consistency in the manner in which one deals with others would, I believe, be regarded as a necessary feature of any ethical code. This principle has an application considerably wider than that of the doctor–patient relationship. In the case of attitudes and conduct towards individuals who have undergone reification (i.e. a change from subject to object status) it would seem to be necessary that any guiding principles selected should be applicable on all occasions. To have differing guidelines for dealing with individuals deemed to have become objects in different circumstances would appear to be improper. However, as patterns of conduct towards reified individuals in different situations have developed quite independently, and in response to differing needs, inconsistency between them is likely. For this reason, it is necessary that, rather than consider each different clinical situation in isolation, the general implications of possible decisions in one type of situation be considered.

Apart from seeking consistency in approaches to different classes of reified individuals, I believe that it is also necessary that such approaches be adopted only after they have been considered by the general community. The seeming complexity of some of the medical issues and the rapid progress of medical technology can easily lead to decision-making that is retained within the medical community, and often within one specialist group in it. Despite the apparent simplicity and efficiency of confining consideration of the subject in this way, I believe it to be essential that the issue of reification of the individual, the grounds for undertaking it and the subsequent uses to which the human object may be put require the fullest community consideration attainable. This can only occur if sufficient detail about the relevant medical situations is made available to a wider audience and that is an objective of this monograph. This question of maximizing dissemination of information is of importance not only in the context of formulating general community responses, but also in the specific circumstances obtaining, for example, when a family is required to make decisions about the possible use of a member as an organ donor. The *informed* nature of any consent to such usage is essential if it is to be regarded as a valid authorization.

Wide-ranging consideration of guidelines applicable in both existing and potential situations of reification of the individual will require recognition of the implications of decisions taken in one situation for those involved in others. The greatest obstacles to such a generally consistent resolution are likely to be fragmented and *ad hoc* responses to individual issues and the tendency for evolution in medical technology to drive decision-making at a speed inconsistent with adequate marshalling of information and full appreciation of its likely implications. The imperative to do that which has become technically possible, primarily for the reason that it is possible, can subvert more reasoned consideration. When that imperative suggests that a reified individual may be of use in a procedure that is potentially beneficial to another patient, the emotive argument "What a waste *not* to use" is often not far away.

Three situations in which the use of "human objects" has either become established practice in clinical transplantation or is currently the subject of advocacy, will be considered in the following chapters. The objective of the monograph is not only to outline the features and consider the significance associated with each situation, but to identify shared aspects and inconsistencies in practice and to discuss the implications of the different situations for each other. Detailed consideration of each topic will entail some re-tracing of ground already covered in earlier discussion but I believe that this is justified by the advantage of presentation of all aspects of that topic in continuity. Chapters 2 and 3 are concerned with the subject of brain death, with the manner in which the concept has evolved and continues to evolve and with attitudes towards the use of brain-dead individuals. Among the issues to be raised in relation to brain death are the extent to which the general community is accurately informed about the features of brain-dead individuals and the details of their utilization. The question of the adequacy of community understanding of brain death appears to me to be fundamental to any attempt at genuine community involvement in making decisions about the management of these individuals as a class and of any particular patient. An adequate level of information about brain death would seem to be equally important if a community is to have input into the emerging discussion about the possibility of substituting the concept of "cerebral death" for that of "brain death". Finally, widespread consideration of brain death would seem to be indicated by the sharp distinction that is now drawn between use of brain-dead individuals as sources of transplantable organs and as experimental objects. General preparedness to endorse some forms of usage, together with general reticence about others, inevitably raises questions about the extent to which convictions about the status of brain-dead individuals are held.

Chapters 4 and 5 are concerned with the congenital malformation of anencephaly. This condition, which involves massive disruption of the upper part of the brain, has been known since antiquity and is now steadily decreasing in frequency. The diminishing availability of anencephalic infants appears to me to raise the question of whether the prominence recently accorded to debate about their use in transplantation should be attributed to their direct potential usefulness or to the wider implications of any community acquiescence in their utilization. As with brain death, another question concerns the extent to which any community decisions about anencephalics are likely to be *informed* by a reasonably accurate appreciation of the nature of the condition. I believe that it could be argued that the enthusiasm characteristic of the advocacy for usage of anencephalics in transplantation has resulted in the presentation of seriously distorted information about the condition to the community.

Chapter 6 deals with the topic of the use of the foetus as a source of brain tissue for transplantation to individuals with Parkinson's disease. This most recent of the proposals to have been advanced for use of the aborted foetus raises some questions related to the subjects of the preceding chapters, in addition to issues common to other forms of foetal usage. The extent to which formulations of death founded upon irreversible cessation of activity of the brain can sit easily alongside procedures that may entail the removal of viable brain tissue from another category of human subject is debatable. Another question of consistency concerns the contradiction which apparently exists between placing *in vitro* fertilized (IVF) human embryos "off limits" for experimentation from the age of 3 weeks because of the suggested onset of "brain life" at that time, whilst endorsing the removal of brain tissue from conventionally conceived embryos 2 or 3 months older. This contradiction is probably just one aspect of the wider question of the inconsistency inherent in regarding some foetuses at a particular stage of development as subjects for treatment and others at an identical stage as objects for use. This inconsistency is likely to become increasingly sharp as the scope and efficacy of methods of treatment of foetal disease increase.

The final chapter directs attention to shared features, apparent inconsistencies and likely mutual implications of the three examples of reification that have been considered in more detail in the earlier chapters. In doing this, it introduces some proposals for possible responses of the community to the management of the new class of "human objects".

2 Brain Death: its Origins, Evolution and Present Status

"A little boy sitting outside the paediatric intensive care unit looked up as an older child was wheeled out on a cart surrounded by a group of nurses and physicians. The chest of the prospective donor was moving up and down with respirations produced by a ventilator. 'That's my brother,' said the little boy. 'He's dead and they're taking him to surgery'."[1]

The aim of this chapter is to provide some background to current understanding and application of the "brain death" concept. Apart from tracing the evolution of the concept itself during the two decades since 1970, it examines issues which have influenced that process. Additionally, it identifies some observations that have been made on brain-dead patients but which, I believe, are not adequately accounted for by the concept. The acceptance of brain death, and its widespread use in clinical practice, has led to some unresolved discrepancies in attitudes among both the medical and wider communities, which will be considered in both this and the following chapter. Chapter 3 will also deal with some of the issues which may influence further evolution of understanding of brain death and the types of use to which brain-dead patients may be put. The principal topics to be considered in it will include future relationships between the concepts of brain death and cerebral death, the entry of brain-dead subjects into experimentation and some possible solutions that have been proposed to cope with an increasing shortage of organ donors.

THE HISTORICAL ORIGINS OF BRAIN DEATH

Some familiarity with the history of application of the brain-death concept is likely to be of assistance both in understanding its present status and in anticipating the direction of future developments. In retrospect, it becomes evident that quite diverse reasons for the validity of the brain-death concept have been presented at different times, and even at the same time by individuals from differing backgrounds. These divergences in understanding of what is meant by the term have, in some instances, been compounded by semantic confusion. However, it is also necessary, in any attempt to reconstruct the development of the brain-death concept, to take account of the influence of transplantation practice. Technological refinement of transplantation practice has generated changing demands in relation to the condition of organs. Extension of the range of organs that may be transplanted has also had an impact. Finally, it is appropriate to recognize that there has been an increasing degree of divergence between medical specialists and the community at large in the understanding of what "brain death" means, and organ harvesting from brain-dead individuals entails.

The notion of brain death was not, in the first instance, a contrivance to facilitate the identification of subjects who would be suitable donors of transplantable organs. Except in the special case of neonates, which will be considered in Chapter 4, the idea of brain death and guidelines for its recognition were developed originally as a means to assist in making decisions to discontinue treatment of terminally- or irretrievably-ill patients. Traditionally, such decisions have always been made for the reason that further treatment could offer no benefit to the patient and might actually be burdensome. The recognition of a state termed "brain death" was intended to supplement, certainly not to replace, this approach to discontinuation of treatment centred upon the interests of the patient.

The requirement for a new set of criteria to identify death became an inevitable consequence of refinements in medical technology, which permitted the artificial maintenance of respiration and, consequently, of cardiac contraction in patients who had sustained brain damage so severe as to interrupt spontaneous respiration irreversibly. The extent to which designation of patients as "brain dead" came also progressively to fulfil requirements other than those directly associated with discontinuation of futile treatment will be considered in this chapter. However, it should be emphasized at the outset that, acting solely on medical as distinct from medico-legal grounds, physicians experienced in intensive resuscitation ought rarely need to pass through all the stages of a formal diagnosis of brain death in order to decide whether a patient should continue to be maintained on a life-support system. In practice, this judgement could usually be made primarily on the basis of whether further treatment was likely to be of benefit to the patient.

Whilst the definition of the state of brain death occurred independently of the process of identifying prospective organ donors, attitudes towards both brain death and the management of individuals diagnosed as brain dead have been influenced inevitably by the concurrent development of transplant surgery. For example, one influence on the management of brain dead subjects with potential for organ harvesting, which soon becomes apparent if one reviews practice since the introduction of brain-death definitions in the mid-1960s, relates to the procedures to be adopted when donor and recipient are geographically separated. When clinical transplantation was first developing, the axiom was established that donor management could not be modified to serve the interests of the recipient. This was reflected in the practice, adopted by some of the original transplant teams, of transferring the recipient to the hospital that was caring for the donor. The rationale underlying this manoeuvre was to reduce the period during which organs to be transplanted remained deprived of oxygen (because blood circulation had ceased) at body temperature. Strategies to minimize this "warm ischaemia time", during which deterioration in organ condition can rapidly occur, have been a crucial feature of transplantation programmes. Whereas the recipient may originally have been taken to the donor, more recent practice, when the isolated organ is unsuitable for transporting, has involved the transfer of the donor to the recipient. (As will be indicated in Chapter 5, in its most extreme form this has sometimes entailed the ferrying of moribund, anencephalic infants across a continent.) The axiom that management of the prospective organ donor should not be modified in the interests of a recipient continues to be observed up to the time of diagnosis of brain death. However, from that time, management is very specifically modified in the interest of the recipient. This may include the continuation of existing intensive life-support measures and the institution of new ones, and the management of complications such as cardiac arrest by vigorous resuscitation.

As already indicated, the purpose of a diagnosis of brain death, when this was first introduced into practice, was to release patients from the imposition of further treatment which offered them no possible benefit. In practical terms, this judgement was sometimes made by deciding whether the form of treatment contemplated was "ordinary" or "extraordinary". Extraordinary measures would encompass those in which the discomfort or inconvenience imposed upon the patient appeared to be disproportionate to any likely benefit *to the patient*. As the original intention of recognizing brain death was to spare patients from treatment that was likely to be futile and burdensome, it appears paradoxical that a diagnosis of brain death has, more recently, become a guarantee that a full range of such treatment *will* be imposed, provided the individual is suitable as an organ source and accessible to facilities for transplantation. Whilst many of the changes in approach to the brain dead, which have been responsible for the development of this paradox, have been gradual, albeit significant, there have been some radical modifications of previous practice. Undoubtedly, the most striking of these has been the adoption of the practice of undertaking organ removal from beating-heart donors rather than waiting upon the cessation of effective pumping of blood by the heart as was an invariable feature of the original protocols.

THE RECOGNITION OF BRAIN DEATH

> " [We] have been trained to believe that until this last cardiac contraction, while there's life, there's hope. All this changed dramatically with the first successful human cardiac transplantation on December 3, 1967".[2]

This contemporary response to the introduction of cardiac transplantation brings out the point that this procedure had a major impact on attitudes towards death. This was manifest in two distinct ways. The first was, effectively, to separate cessation of cardiac function from death. It was demonstrated that life need not cease with the cessation of an individual's heart. Cardiac action and life could thereafter be regarded as separable entities. In consequence, retention of cardiac function could be argued no longer necessarily to be equivalent to retention of life. The second means of influence of the introduction of heart transplantation on attitudes towards death was the requirement that was thereby introduced for the use of beating-heart donors. This aspect will be considered in the following chapter.

Definition of brain death

"[U]nlike the traditional moment of death, upon which layman and physician have always agreed, the end point chosen for certification of brain death is a matter of opinion not obvious to everyone."[2]

In considering the difficulties arising in relation to decisions about brain death, an American neurologist continued:

"Because the concept of brain death involves social, legal and theological issues which physicians have not specifically been trained to consider, some suggest that we trust those who have been to weigh the implications for us. Similar requests were made of the physicists who first concerned themselves with broad implications of nuclear fission. The results have been disastrous."[2]

The events of the following two decades suggest that physicians have determined the direction of evolution of practice in relation to brain death, but that the weighing of implications has lagged behind.

The formal definition of brain death varies between jurisdictions. Furthermore, both the definition and, in particular, the interpretations placed on it, have undergone substantial modification since the subject was first addressed in the 1960s. Some of the most influential statements on brain death have contained ambiguities. For example, the earliest of the major statements, the report of an *ad hoc* committee of the Harvard Medical School, has attracted repeated comment on account of the ambiguity evident in its objectives. The opening sentence of this report:

"Our primary purpose is to define irreversible coma as a new criterion for death."

continues to produce uncertainty about the committee's intentions.[3] Statements in other parts of the report imply that the members of the committee wished to establish the identity of "brain death" with death and this is the interpretation that has been placed on it since that time. Another ambiguity in the report is apparent in the comment, in relation to brain-dead individuals, that "the burden is great on individuals who suffer permanent loss of intellect". A number of commentaries on this report have queried the suggestion that an already dead patient could bear a burden.[4]

The "Harvard criteria" established in 1968 by this committee have shaped subsequent attitudes and practice in regard to diagnosis of brain death, at least in the United States of America. A notable influence of the report of the committee has been the establishment of a requirement for evidence of cessation of function of the *entire* brain. For instance, the USA President's commission for the study of ethical problems in medicine and biomedical and behavioural research, affirmed in 1981 that "an individual with irreversible cessation of all functions of the entire brain, including the brain stem, is dead".[5] However, in amplifying (and effectively qualifying) this definition, the report indicated that the expression "functions of the entire brain" referred only to those functions that could be clinically assessed, i.e. demonstration of loss of functions using laboratory tests was not a mandatory requirement. The omission of such tests represented a substantial variation from the earlier "Harvard criteria". These had specified a requirement for a reproducible, flat electroencephalogram (EEG). (The electroencephalogram is a record of the electrical activity of the brain. Its significance in relation to brain death and the information that it may provide about the nature of this state will be considered on pp. 40–43.) Linking diagnosis of death to the loss of functions that can be clinically observed implied that the only diagnostic measures to be employed would be physical examination and the relatively simple tests usually undertaken in the course of it. The introduction of this linkage inevitably ensured that, if subsequent extensions of understanding of brain function were achieved by laboratory techniques, then this might lead to divergences between assessments of brain status undertaken by clinical means alone and those based on newer technological approaches. Whilst clinical diagnosis of brain death is based upon positive findings in the course of examination of the patient, diagnostic features that reflect the absence of measurable functions will remain subject to reappraisal with changes in the technology available to measure those functions.

In contrast with the concept of loss of function of the whole brain that is implied by the criteria accepted in the United States of America, the British definition of brain death has been based exclusively on loss of function of the brain stem. The conference of Medical Royal Colleges stated in 1976 that:

> "It is agreed that permanent functional death of the brain stem constitutes brain death."[6]

(Presumably, the expression "functional death" was intended to have a meaning equivalent to the phrase "irreversible cessation of function", subsequently used by the USA President's Commission. Nevertheless, while it may provide a convenient shorthand means of expressing this meaning, it is open to the construction that "death" may refer to different states, with the variety of death depending on the chosen manifestation, for instance functional or structural.) The criteria for brain death enumerated then were considered to be "sufficient to distinguish between those patients who retain the functional capacity to have a chance of even partial recovery and those in whom no such possibility exists". In effect, "death" became shorthand for "irreversible". I infer from the British definition that its specification of the brain stem, rather than the whole brain, was based on the *predictive* value of its permanent loss of function (namely that cessation of all brain function was then an inevitable consequence), rather than on any proposition that the brain stem was functionally the central part of the whole brain. However, in an addendum to the original statement, released 3 years later, the conference moved to adopt the position that:

> "Brain death represents the stage at which a patient becomes truly dead, because by then all functions of the brain have permanently and irreversibly ceased".[7]

Comparison of the 1976 and 1979 statements indicates that the 1979 release effectively upgraded the interpretation of the clinical criteria recommended in 1976 from being a diagnosis of irreversibility to become a diagnosis of death.

The original differences between UK and USA definitions of brain death have persisted. In commenting upon the UK criteria, an American physician Julius Korein, a member of the USA President's Commission remarked:

> "I believe that the criteria for diagnosis of brain death should be considered as an issue independent of the problems related to organ transplantation. The British code, however, links the diagnosis of brain death irretrievably with transplantation."[8]

Apart from differences between sets of criteria for diagnosing brain death in different localities, variations have developed in some of the measurements specified for diagnosis. One example of a measurement usually specified in diagnostic criteria is the blood concentration of carbon dioxide. (Increase in the concentration of carbon dioxide in the blood provides a stimulus to that part of the brain stem responsible for control of respiration. Failure of the brain stem to respond to an adequate stimulus by initiating respiration is considered to indicate its inactivation.) In discussing the substantial differences between brain death as defined in the USA and UK (and, incidentally, noting that Canada differed from both of these countries in its requirement for "irreversible global brain dysfunction") two Canadian clinicians drew attention to the variation existing in the specified concentrations of blood carbon dioxide required in different countries if loss of a patient's respiratory drive is to be adequately certified. They commented that, as organ retrieval programmes extended internationally, a consensus on criteria for brain death was imperative:

> "Clinical criteria make it possible to be brain dead in one country and not in another."[9]

The difficulties inherent in the interpretation of some accounts of brain death in the medical literature have been further compounded by the inappropriate use of descriptive terms. For example, use of "cerebral" as the adjective derived from "brain" has led to confusion between brain death and the distinct condition of "cerebral death", which has been proposed by some neurologists to replace it. In "cerebral death" the brain stem remains intact and functional. Consequently, although the patient is irreversibly unconscious, spontaneous breathing occurs (in some instances for many years) and the patient does not require maintenance on a ventilator and other intensive life-support measures.

The basis for selection of the brain as the organ the cessation of function in which connotes death

As discussed above, the idea of "brain death" as an expression of death emerged in response to the recognition of patients with irreversible brain damage of such an extent that suspension of ventilatory support would result in permanent cessation of respiration and, as a consequence, of cardiac contraction. The actual cessation of function of heart and lungs was traditionally regarded as indicative of death. The criteria for recognition of "brain death" emerged as a result of retrospective analysis of the clinical features of brain-injured patients, whose subsequent clinical course confirmed that irreversible loss of brain function had occurred. The manner in which those criteria have evolved will be considered later. However, it is relevant at this stage to observe that, whilst there has been considerable discussion about the requirements for diagnosis of "death of the brain", there has been much less discussion of the question of *why the brain was selected* as the organ, the failure of which may be identified with death, despite the continuing function of other organs. Although the legitimacy of selecting the brain in this role has been questioned only infrequently, there does not appear to be a single, generally accepted explanation for its selection. A wide range of reasons that are not mutually exclusive have been proposed by different commentators at different times. A list of possible reasons, which is certainly not exhaustive, would include:

- following irreversible cessation of brain function, all other organ systems will inevitably cease to function
- unlike other organ systems, brain function, once lost, is irreplaceable
- irreversible loss of brain function is synonymous with permanent loss of consciousness
- loss of sentience is a feature of loss of brain function
- the integrative function of the brain is lost if the brain ceases to function
- recognition of death on the basis of loss of brain function is doing no more than recognizing overtly the reason underlying the traditional diagnosis of death following cessation of the blood circulation.

Conviction in equating irreversible cessation of brain function with death has often been based on the belief that cessation of function of all the other organ systems will inevitably follow as a consequence even though life support is maintained. While this belief appears to be correct, it has become clear that the interval between brain death and cardiac arrest may be much longer than anticipated. The point will be made later on pp. 35–39 that the likely time of cessation of function of other organs in patients maintained on a respirator after irreversible cessation of brain function is not necessarily as early as has sometimes been argued. Nevertheless, the inevitability that other organ systems will at some time cease to function as a consequence of the occurrence of brain death is undoubted. However, if one argues, on the basis of this, that "brain dead" is equivalent to "dead", one is effectively substituting a forecast of the patient's future course for the actual present state. Unless one is prepared consistently to adopt the position that a hopeless outlook justifies the presumption that that outlook has already been fulfilled, this argument would seem to have substantial limitations.

The irreplaceability of the brain and hence of brain function has been advanced as a reason for regarding "brain death" and "death" as identical. Modern transplantation practice repeatedly demonstrates that other organs, such as the heart, lungs and liver, can be replaced in the event of their failure and, at the same time, emphasizes the irreplaceability of the brain. Whilst the technology to replace heart and lung function, either by organ transplantation or by the use of prosthetic devices, has been steadily developing, comparable substitution, at least in the case of higher brain functions, does not appear to be in prospect. Whereas the cessation of *spontaneous* cardiac function was unquestionably regarded as death when the possibility of replacing that function did not exist, it is unlikely that anyone would now regard as dead an individual in whom cardiac function had completely ceased, but in whom a prosthetic device had assumed this responsibility (perhaps pending the procurement of a heart suitable for transplantation).

In a notable essay prophetically titled "Against the stream: comments on the definition and redefinition of death" written in 1970 during the early days of the brain-death concept, Hans Jonas made the point that the older definitions of death did not dismiss artificially induced and sustained cardiorespiratory functioning as not being life.[10] He posed the question of the attitude that would be adopted towards an individual in whom brain-stem functions had irreversibly ceased but in whom it was possible to replace these artificially by means of an external agency. He opined that such artificial means might be invoked and that the individual would not be considered "dead" on account of the non-spontaneity of these functions: "we would... not be finicky about the resulting function lacking spontaneity". I suggest that, two decades later, the central issue is *not* whether artificial replacement of brain-stem functioning in an individual lacking this (and so complying with the UK definition of brain death) is ever likely to be feasible (it might be). Nor is it the question of whether it would be in the interests of a patient to utilize such technology, were it to become available. Rather, it remains the question of whether irreversible loss of *spontaneous* function is adequate to warrant a diagnosis of death when it involves the brain stem but not when it affects another organ, such as the heart, functioning of which is essential for life.

A particularly straightforward exposition of the argument that its irreplaceability singles out the brain as the organ, the loss of which equates with death, was presented by Dr Norman Shumway, arguably the single most significant contributor to development of heart transplantation. He gave testimony at the trial in 1974 of a person responsible for shooting another in the head. The defence claimed that the victim had died, not as a result of being shot but because of the removal of his heart by Dr Shumway. In response to this, the surgeon testified that:

> "I'm saying anyone whose brain is dead is dead. It is the one determinant that would be universally applicable, because the brain is the one organ *that can't be transplanted*" (my italics).[11]

The irreversible loss of consciousness entailed has been claimed by some authors as the reason for identifying loss of brain function with death. (As will be considered in Chapter 3, irreversible loss of consciousness can occur without complete loss of brain function. The occurrence of such loss of consciousness, even in the presence of continuing brain-stem function, has been adopted also as the basis of claims for equation of "cerebral death" or "persistent vegetative state" with death.) In presenting a case for irreversible loss of consciousness as the reason why cessation of brain function has been equated with death, Gervais wrote:

> "I hope to establish that we declare death because of permanent unconsciousness... The reason for declaring death in the case of brain death is that the respirator cannot support upper brain activity, and the patient is therefore permanently unconscious."[12]

Gervais sought to establish less demanding criteria for cessation of brain function, than those that are currently accepted, namely loss only of "higher" functions with retention of brain-stem-mediated activities, such as respiration. This argument was presented as grounds for adoption of a "cerebral death" standard. Nevertheless, I believe that the permanent loss of consciousness associated with "brain death" has already been a most influential factor in facilitating its acceptance as total death. Arguments for equivalence of permanent loss of consciousness with total death may have indirectly drawn strength from the general acceptance of the corollary that the retention of consciousness *excludes* a diagnosis of death. I have little doubt that the impact of loss of consciousness on acceptance of brain death has been considerable.

One possible objection to acceptance of permanent loss of consciousness as an infallible indication of cessation of brain function, let alone of death, could be that such a position fails to take any account of the possibility of continuation of subconscious activity in a damaged brain. The anatomical location of sub-conscious activity as it occurs in the intact, normal brain remains undefined. No reliable instrumental means have been developed to permit observation of sub-conscious activity in a subject's intact brain. The normal functions of many parts of the brain remain unknown. Similarly, it is not possible to identify electrical activity from many parts of the normal brain and, consequently, it is impossible to be confident about whether those parts remain intact or have been destroyed in the brain-dead individual.

Very little is known concerning the parts of the brain involved in subconscious activity and no means are available to an observer to document this activity in another individual. There have been some suggestions that electrical activity, which might be attributable to subconscious brain function, might persist after some instances of brain injury. For example, it has been reported that the EEG in a patient in whom the brain stem had been destroyed but the cerebral hemispheres remained partially intact suggested that "if there was cognition at all it would probably have been in the realm of dream type rather than waking reality".[13]

Whilst it is not feasible to gain access to the subjective experiences of an indi-vidual unable to communicate them, lack of the capacity to communicate with others cannot, of itself, be taken to confirm lack of any capacity to experience. A neurologist writing on the subject of the reality of death experience developed the argument that as the "final common mechanism" responsible for death of the brain (unless it is directly destroyed by trauma) is oxygen deprivation, some inferences might be drawn from experimental study of this subject:

"During terminal anoxia—which inevitably happens—neurons start degenerating in the brain in different locations at various speeds, depending upon their individual need for oxygen. During this period of oxygen deprivation, certain structures of the brain, such as the hippocampus, may show epileptic seizure activity."[14]

As most of this form of activity fails to propagate to distant parts of the brain (the hippocampus is located deep within the cerebral hemisphere), it would not be detectable by electrodes placed on the scalp as in the clinical situation. In attempting to speculate on the possible subjective accompaniments of such terminal brain activity, Rodin suggested:

"As anoxia persists, delusions and hallucinations occur until, finally, complete unconsciousness supervenes."[14]

Some basis for these suggestions is available from numerous accounts given by patients who had experienced a period of anoxia of the brain following circula-tory arrest, which had been successfully reversed. Patients in this situation had *not* been dead. Nevertheless their experiences may represent the closest observations to the occurrence of death that are likely to become available.

Whatever the nature of the experiences of an individual during terminal anoxia of the brain, it would be expected that these would be of brief duration. However, the point has been raised by Rodin that the institution of life-support measures might result in the extension of these processes beyond that of a transient episode. The nature of the experiences suggested by him as possible subjective accompaniments of the electrical activity observed in the brain during terminal anoxia has been the subject of comment by others:

> "If we are to define unconsciousness as the complete loss of awareness of environment and self, then man cannot directly experience unconsciousness. Furthermore, unconsciousness cannot consistently be documented using present scientific techniques. Thus, the widespread belief that total unconsciousness is the last event becomes more a theoretical possibility than a scientific truth... '[N]o one has shown through objective scientific research that unconsciousness is indeed the final stage of dying. In fact, many near death survivors have described visual and auditory experiences which have appeared to begin *after* the onset of unconsciousness but *before* the institution of life-saving measures." [15]

Should the possibility that undetectable subconscious activity may persist in a brain-damaged individual who nevertheless has irreversibly lost consciousness and satisfies the criteria for brain death be of any concern? I believe that any persistence of subconscious activity, in a brain-dead individual, could be of considerable importance. This would be accorded on the same grounds that significance has been accorded consciousness by some commentators in identifying the brain as the crucial organ in defining death. Consciousness appears to have acquired much of its importance because of its prerequisite role for expression of the human potential for rationality. I suspect that an equally valid case could be made that subconscious mental activity on abstract themes is likely to be an exclusive feature of human beings. If this were so, the possibility of continuation of such undetectable activity in a permanently unconscious subject could be seen as a contraindication to diagnosing total loss of higher functions. As will be discussed on pp. 28–32 the persistence of function in some parts of the brain, the role of which is unknown, is no longer regarded as invalidating a diagnosis of brain death.

The extent to which loss of sentience, in particular of any capacity to appreciate pain, following irreversible loss of brain function has contributed to acceptance of the brain as the prime organ in recognizing death is difficult to gauge. The argument that individuals in a state which renders them incapable of experiencing pain should be available for use, has been advanced as a basis for intervention, for example, for the purpose of removing organs for transplantation. This reasoning has been applied in the case of anencephalic infants (to be considered in Chapters 4 and 5) and presumptions of non-sentience also feature in arguments for intervention on the foetus at an early stage after its removal from the uterus (Chapter 6). However, whilst the loss of sentience may be one of the consequences of death, as is the loss of consciousness, neither form of deprivation can be held directly to establish that the brain is the organ in which loss of function *equates* with death.

In considering the nature of brain death and its possible relationship to death, Jonas nominated the relevance to this issue of the loss of sentience by brain-dead subjects. It is possible that recognition that any retention of consciousness unequivocally excludes a diagnosis of death may lead some to believe that loss of consciousness, therefore, indicates death. In discussing the issue of possible sensitivity to pain on the part of "brain dead" subjects (one of the likely accompaniments of any partial retention of consciousness) Jonas wrote:

> "But I wish to emphasize that the question of possible suffering (easily brushed aside by a sufficient show of reassuring expert consensus) is merely a subsidiary and not the real point of my argument; this to reiterate, turns on the indeterminacy of the boundaries between *life and death*, not between sensitivity and insensitivity."[16]

An alternative to this philosophical point of view from a neurologist closely involved in the development of brain-death criteria queried:

> "Is there more than atavistic mysticism in the essentially untestable supposition of residual sentience in the isolated forebrain, or in cell aggregates elsewhere in the cortex or deeper structures?"[17]

In circumstances where observation is incapable of differentiating between the alternatives, the issue to be addressed may be that of where the burden of disproving the other position should rest.

Any positive argument identifying the brain as the crucial organ in defining death requires the establishment not only of positive claims for this identification, such as the irreversible loss of consciousness, but also sound reasons why continuing function of other organs, such as the heart, does not impede the diagnosis. The point, already mentioned, that cessation of the function of other organs may be anticipated as a consequence of cessation of brain function, could be one of these. Another possible approach was used by Gervais in arguing that persistent cardiac function in patients manifesting *cerebral* death (that is, as will be described in Chapter 3, irreversible loss of consciousness accompanied by persistent spontaneous respiration) need not be significant. Taking account of the argument of Jonas, discussed above, that *non-spontaneity* of cardiac function in a patient in whom this was being maintained artificially would not allow death to be diagnosed if other systems continue to function, Gervais postulated:

> "We must show that spontaneity of heart and lung functioning is no longer to be regarded as a sign of life. The point of Jonas's argument is that nonspontaneity is not an issue."[18]

I do not agree that spontaneous cardiac function can be ignored in diagnosing death on the basis that non-spontaneous cardiac function can be adequate to exclude a diagnosis of death. When this point is considered in isolation, the certainty that death is imminent (as, for example, in a "conventional brain-dead" subject about to be disconnected from a ventilator), does not appear to provide adequate grounds, on its own, for considering that death has already occurred as long as normal cardiac function continues.

Loss of the integrative function of the brain, concurrently with cessation of brain function, has been advanced as the basis, in its own right, for equating brain death with death. This does not appear to have been one of the original reasons presented for designation of the brain as the critical organ in death but it has perhaps become the most frequently cited reason. I take the expression "integrative function", when used in relation to the brain to refer to the influences which the brain and other neurological structures, such as the autonomic nervous system, exert on many other organ systems and on control of the stability of bodily properties, such as temperature and fluid balance. Arguments based on loss of its integrative function as the reason for the centrality of loss of brain function appear to have achieved prominence secondarily as the procurement of transplantable organs from brain-dead subjects became an issue. In particular, they seem to have been advanced in response to observations of the type to be dealt with on pp. 39–52 which imply that *complete* loss of brain function has frequently not occurred in brain-dead patients. The thrust of such responses has been that, if the brain is exclusively responsible for integration of function of the other organ systems, then damage to the brain sufficient to destroy that integrative capacity represents death of the organism, irrespective of whether independent function of other organ systems persists.

In presenting the case for validity of the brain-death concept on the basis of loss of the brain's integrative function, Lamb concedes that:

"Other organs are essential for life to continue, for example, without a viable liver or skin tissue, life would be impossible."[19]

He then frames the question:

"Does this suggest a degree of arbitrariness in assigning greater significance to brain functions?"[19]

The answer provided identifies its integrative role as the basis for primacy of the brain:

"The centrality accorded to the brain is not due merely to its irreplaceability: it is bound up with its role as supreme regulator and co-ordinator."[19]

All of the preceding arguments for the centrality of loss of brain function in recognizing death have relied substantially upon propositions that had little if any currency before the introduction of the brain-death concept. However, the argument has also been presented that the brain-death concept is no more than a representation of the conventional concept of death. Thus some commentators have made the point that diagnosis of death because of discontinuation of brain function has been the real basis of traditional diagnosis in response to cessation of cardiac action. In considering this subject, Gervais noted the position of earlier writers that diagnosis of death directly on the basis of loss of brain function represents no more than an alternative to indirect approaches to the same goal. She frames this argument as follows:

> "We have declared people dead based on the traditional criteria because we have known that when the heart stops, all possibility of brain life is lost. Now, in cases where machines impair our understanding of the heart's status and we are able to measure the status of the brain more directly, we can apply our tests to the brain itself."[20]

As Gervais was arguing for the legitimacy of irreversible loss of consciousness, · rather than of brain-stem function, as the basis for brain death she found the argument for identity of "traditional" and "brain death" modes of diagnosis of death unpersuasive. My reservation about the argument as spelt out above arises from doubts that the motive it imputes for traditional diagnosis of death was indeed foremost in the minds of those making that diagnosis. I am not convinced that cessation of cardiac function, for example, has been traditionally regarded as signifying death because of its consequences for brain function, rather than on account of its intrinsic importance.

The half-dozen explanations for the centrality of brain function noted above, and various combinations of them, have all been presented by authors arguing the case for acceptance of either the "conventional" notion of brain death or for the classification of "cerebral death" as death. A rare dissenting proposal was formulated by Jonas when questioning the underlying motivation for the development of the brain-death concept. Jonas indicted the attitude prevailing towards death:

> "The cowardice of modern secular society which shrinks from death as an unmitigated evil needs the assurance (or fiction) that he is already dead when the decision (i.e. to discontinue resuscitation) is to be made. The responsibility of a value-laden decision is replaced by the mechanics of a value-free routine."[21]

Perhaps not surprisingly, subsequent writers approaching the subject from the perspective of the linkage between brain death and organ procurement have paid little attention to Jonas' view.

The meaning conveyed by the term "brain death"

Some ambiguities exist in relation to the *meanings* attached to the term brain death, as distinct from the reasoning underlying its derivation. On one interpretation, the term could be considered to describe death of the patient as manifest by, or as a result of, loss of brain function. Alternatively, the term could be read primarily to imply death of a particular organ, the brain, with whatever consequences for the patient follow from that. If this second interpretation is adopted, a question arises about the fraction of the brain that must be inactivated before the organ is adjudged as dead.

A second source of potential ambiguity that is introduced with use of the term "brain death" relates to whether this term is intended to be an accurate description of the nature of a patient's present condition or no more than a concise term for identifying a specific group of clinical features with a reliably defined outcome. In view of the technical difficulty in establishing the state of the brain at the time of diagnosis by independent means, I suspect that the term is increasingly used primarily to identify a clinical condition which will have a particular outcome. Nevertheless, when used in this way it is inevitable that the term will incidentally suggest considerable detail about the pathological mechanism responsible for the patient's condition.

Two attributes that are likely to be automatically associated with brain death in the minds of those using the term are its irreversibility and the question of the existence and the nature of any structural changes in the organ that are responsible for the clinical features. Examination of these aspects may provide a starting point from which to trace some of the possible variations in perception of the condition.

Irreversibility is necessarily an essential feature of any condition that is classified as death, whether it relates to a cell, an organ or a whole organism. Consequently, it assumes a central position in any attempt to define brain death. Nevertheless, it is a feature shared by many conditions apart from death. It would not, of itself, for example, distinguish brain death from many other forms of brain damage of lesser severity. Arguments about the legitimacy of brain death as a manifestation of death have often centred on its irreversibility. As will be discussed subsequently on pp. 34–35 this may often *not* have been the relevant question. I believe that the serious challenges that have been raised to the brain-death concept are generally concerned with its nature rather than its reversibility. Nevertheless, the answers often appear to have been more concerned with reversibility than with nature.

Irreversibility in relation to any brain-dead subject is patently a characteristic that can only be inferred in that patient from the experience of other cases presenting similar features. Its positive confirmation in any case will only be achieved when cardiac function has ceased without any recovery of brain function having occurred. Disproof of irreversibility, in any individual at some future time, would effectively vitiate a diagnosis of brain death made in relation to that patient at the present time. Apart from the risk that consideration of irreversibility may divert attention from other characteristics that should be mandatory if one seeks to establish a state of brain death, the other important aspect of irreversibility, I suggest, relates to whether one equates the time at which it is first recognised with the time of attainment of the ultimate outcome. Is the "point of no return" at which the patient's condition becomes irreversible to be regarded as synonymous with death? This question will receive attention later pp. 33–34.

The frequent restriction of discussions of brain death, especially in the last decade, to functional evidence for its occurrence inevitably draws attention to the question of whether the existence of any structural or anatomical equivalent of that functional loss is envisaged. Can brain death exist as a valid entity if envisaged solely in terms of a functional loss or is it necessary that the state also includes a corresponding, reproducible and demonstrable structural change? While it may be possible to consider a philosophical proposition that permanent loss of a specified range of functions is the death of the individual, I find it difficult to envisage a state of physiological loss that is not a manifestation of underlying structural changes.

There is, of course, ample precedent for accepted states of functional abnormality in *living* patients for which a corresponding and underlying structural state has not been detected. Most psychiatric diseases fall into this category. Nevertheless, I believe that many physicians would expect that an, as yet undetected, anatomical correlate (perhaps restricted to a subcellular or molecular level) underlies these psychiatric conditions. The questions that arise in relation to brain death are whether a reliable anatomical correlate *exists* and whether it can be *detected*.

If one considers the means by which the nature of brain death was inferred, it is apparent that this did not follow the path of step-by-step correlation of proven pathological changes with concurrent clinical features and an associated prognosis. On the contrary, it appears to have been inferred as much by changes in attitude towards phenomena that had become clinically familiar, with resulting reassessment of them. In reviewing the history of development of the brain-death concept, Black recalled that:

> "In 1968, an opinion poll of neurologists and electroencephalographers found that 'nearly all neurologists thought that a new definition of death to include brain death was of importance and that this concept was not premature'."[22]

The original descriptions of the brain-death concept were framed in terms of clinical changes and forecasts of the later outcome, and not in terms of pathological changes underlying the clinical signs. Whilst the existence of characteristic structural changes at the time that brain death is diagnosed may have been assumed originally, the idea that the state of brain death is a manifestation of structural destruction of the brain has more recently often been actively discarded. For example, the suggestion by Green and Wikler[23] that brain death represented the *ruining of the substrate* for conscious processes rather than the *loss of those conscious processes* alone was vigorously attacked by Gervais.[24]

Whilst it is universally acknowledged that the recognition of the brain-dead state is directly attributable to the introduction and refinement of life-support technology, it may be less widely appreciated that the use of life-support systems is very likely to have altered the time-scale over which the changes characteristic of death occur in the brain. One group of neurologists discussing the diagnosis of brain death on clinical grounds alone considered that:

> "While there are not difficulties in this respect when patients are not on artificial life support systems, the situation becomes problematic once such measures have been instituted. They allow the extension of the process of dying over days, weeks or months with various dissociations between clinical and electroencephalographic states."[13]

It was suggested that most cases with suspected brain death show various mixtures of cerebral hemisphere and brain-stem damage.

A succession of discordant observations has been reported in relation to brain death in recent years. These have dealt with the detection of clinical signs suggestive of retention of activity in some parts of the brain of brain-dead individuals (see pp. 39–40). As a result of these observations, I believe that it has now become quite difficult to support the contention that complete destruction of the brain has occurred in many individuals by the time of diagnosis of brain death. On the contrary, it seems that the time may be approaching when any definition of brain death that was to be couched in terms of anatomical loss would have to nominate destruction of a specified proportion of the brain beyond which brain death, by definition, existed. As will be discussed at a later stage (pp. 48–52), validation of any structural changes in brain death by means of post-mortem anatomical examination remains extremely difficult. It requires differentiation of pathological changes that occurred *before* cessation of the individual's circulation (i.e. after brain death has been diagnosed but whilst the heart continued beating) from the deterioration that occurs very rapidly *after* "conventional" death (when cardiac arrest occurs). If brain death is conceptualized in the first instance, as structural damage (detectable or otherwise), this leads to the further question of whether confidence that this has already occurred should be regarded as a prerequisite to diagnosis *in the individual case*.

A related question, which was raised in a 1976 review of the legal aspects of the Harvard *ad hoc* committee report concerned the conclusion, implicit in the report, that the absence of clinically perceptible signs of life could justifiably be equated with absence of life itself.[25] A more vigorous attack on this conclusion was mounted by Byrne and his colleagues in a 1979 article. This specifically took issue with the concept of brain death, both in its content and its title, "Brain death—an opposing viewpoint". Its principal contention was that cessation of brain function cannot be regarded as synonymous with destruction of the brain. In presenting this viewpoint, Byrne *et al.* (1979) suggested that the prevalent idea of brain death confounded what functions with its functioning.[26] They issued a challenge for those who supported the concept of brain death to substitute "complete destruction" for "irreversible cessation of total function" in defining it. This proposal elicited considerable criticism, especially from some of those who had contributed to development of the brain death concept.

One response to the opposing viewpoint of Byrne *et al.* expressly stated the conviction of its writers that total and irreversible cessation of brain function is equivalent to total destruction of the brain "and hence tantamount to functional or physiological decapitation". This was as clear a statement as any that a specific anatomical basis for clinically observed brain death was believed to exist.[27] The analogy with decapitation, which Veitch and Tendler drew in this article, is still frequently used to explain, and to defend from questioning, the existence of brain death. Decapitation, having strong structural connotations, is a condition that most persons can both visualize and equate with death. I believe that it represents a prime example of the introduction of a spurious analogy and will consider this later (see p. 39).

Reservations about the nature of brain death, from a different perspective, were expressed by a 1982 editorial in the *Journal of the American Medical Association*.[28] In commenting upon a report of the management of two pregnant, brain-dead women, attention was directed to the inherent difficulty in accepting the proposition that life could be prolonged in a dead body. The authors, a physician and an ethicist, commented that the linguistic inconsistencies raised by the report "reveal a deep—and in our view, justified—ambivalence about conventional wisdom on the definition of death, particularly the brain-death standard". They believed that:

> "The death of the brain seems not to serve as a boundary; it is a tragic, ultimately fatal loss, but not death itself. Bodily death occurs later, when integrated function ceases."[28]

Whilst a number of medical personnel may have shared the ambivalence, few have gone so far as to question the identification of brain death with bodily death.

Another question, namely whether brain death is a new kind or concept of death, or merely represents a grouping of criteria of "conventional" death, was raised at a symposium conducted in 1978 by the New York Academy of Sciences. The speaker responsible, Richard Roelofs, concluded that brain death was no more than a criterion of death ("a state of affairs, typically some bodily condition of the patient which suffices to justify the judgement that the patient is dead"). He specifically raised:

> "the question about the epistemic connection between having a ruined brain and being dead: that is, we may be asking whether the fact that a patient has a ruined brain is a good and sufficient reason for saying that the patient is dead. Notice that we might very well agree to employ brain death in this way, as a criterion of death, even if we did not agree that brain death is a kind of death."[29]

This proposition evoked the editorial response that most contributors to the symposium were in disagreement with it.

Leaving aside the issue of whether "brain death" is to be regarded as a criterion or a concept, another question which arises in relation to it may be phrased: "Is 'brain dead' dead enough for automatic use of the subject in ways that would be appropriate for a 'conventionally dead' individual?" I believe that the question remains unanswered, probably unasked, as to whether brain death should be regarded as a state the entry into which renders a subject equivalent in all respects to a conventionally dead patient. Both conventional death and brain death would be universally considered to contraindicate any further treatment on the grounds that this would be futile for the patient. However, there have been indications that most communities do not automatically accept that brain dead-subjects may be treated in all respects as are the conventionally dead. Differentiation between appropriate and inappropriate management of brain dead patients occurs uncommonly when discontinuation of support and organ removal are compared but almost universally when the comparison is between usage in transplantation and experimentation. An example of the first form of differentiation was provided by a 1984 report commissioned by the Swedish government. This recommended that destruction of an individual's brain as a result of interruption of blood supply could be diagnosed on clinical grounds alone, unless removal of organs for transplantation was contemplated, in which case radiological examination to confirm that blood flow had ceased would be required.[30] The possible risk of this recommendation, identified by a British commentator, was that it might alarm the public "by suggesting that doctors have to be more certain about death in some settings than others".[31] The very marked differentiation that is usually drawn between use as an organ source and as an experimental subject will be considered in detail in Chapter 3. In passing from the meanings attached to the expression "brain death", it could be noted that its retention and entrenchment over a quarter of a century suggests that sufficient differences are still perceived to prevent its being encompassed within the general term "death".

CRITERIA FOR BRAIN DEATH

The basis for brain-death criteria

Criteria to identify brain death could be designed either to exclude signs of persistent life or to detect signs which conclusively indicate death. There has been considerable growth in understanding of the relative prognostic significance of a variety of neurological signs in patients sustaining severe brain injury. Most of these signs, and the tests employed to evoke them, have been derived empirically. Their reliability in forecasting has been confirmed by prospective study of groups of patients meeting selected criteria. In general, they provide excellent indications of the irreversibility of the patient's condition. However, as already stressed, irreversibility is only one of the features of brain death. Criteria that reliably indicate irreversibility of loss of detectable brain function need not necessarily prove that brain death has *already* occurred. Data collected for one purpose are unlikely to provide an accurate answer to a different question. A substantial difference can exist between the accuracy with which a specific array of clinical features can be identified and the precision with which the nature of the underlying pathological condition can be inferred from them. When the task becomes that of determining whether brain death has already occurred, the reliability of the criteria used in identifying irreversibility may become largely irrelevant. In the absence of direct intervention to biopsy the patient's brain, there is no way of independently confirming brain death at the time of its diagnosis. Consequently, the criteria may be in use not only to determine whether an individual patient is in the inferred state, but also that such a state actually exists. It has been suggested that criteria based on brain-stem functioning are often considered to be useful, not because they refer to what death really is but, primarily, because they permit the making of reliable diagnoses.[32]

A substantial arbitrary component exists in the specification of the criteria to be used to diagnose, *and therefore also to characterize, brain death*. Veatch recommended that:

> "we shall have to follow safer-course policies of using measures to declare death only in cases in which we are convinced that some necessary physical basis for life is missing, even if that means that some dead patients will be treated as alive."[33]

Arbitrary considerations may determine the manner in which more objective measurements of phenomena are utilized in appraisal of brain death. Irrespective of the inherent rigour of a particular test, subjectivity in its application to any situation will influence the outcome.

Before leaving discussion of the background to brain-death criteria, the point should be made that there has been considerable tendency to circularity of argument in its derivation and substantiation. In the absence of independent means to verify a diagnosis of brain death at the time it is made, an attempt is required to "backdate" pathological features observed at post-mortem examination considerably later. Reflecting this difficulty in correlating pathological characteristics with the clinical features at the time of diagnosis of brain death, Black remarked that an opinion poll of neuropathologists was undertaken in 1973 "to point out the unresolved issues regarding the neuropathological features of the dying brain."[22]

The results of the 1973 study of the pathology of brain death will be considered on pp. 48–52 but it is relevant to consideration of the nature of the process used to establish the entity to refer briefly to the latter aspect now. One paper, in reporting the outcome of the study, commented:

> "Because of renewed public and scientific interest in the concept of brain death and its diagnostic criteria, an opinion survey was undertaken polling the membership of the American Association of Neuropathologists regarding the definition, gross

and microscopical features, and pathogenesis of the syndrome popularly designated the 'respirator brain'."[34]

In another paper, entitled "A critique of the respirator brain", the researchers responsible for the survey indicated that the data gathered during it were reported not to recommend a set of "democratically determined criteria for respirator brain", but to point out the unresolved issues. They also posed the question, "How reliable is consensus in the elucidation of scientific truth?"[35]

Legal incentives for the development of brain-death criteria

Impetus for the refinement of the concept of brain death and for the selection of criteria to recognize it was not provided exclusively on medical grounds. One influence responsible for the early promotion of the brain-death concept in the USA was the perception that to terminate resuscitative measures, such as artificial respiration, if death had not been diagnosed might leave a physician open to legal action. Consequently, a need arose not only for formulation of brain-death criteria, but for their recognition in law.

Discontinuation of treatment for the reason that it could afford no benefit to the recipient would clearly be an appropriate course in many clinical situations *irrespective* of whether brain death had occurred. It is clear that some advocates of acceptance of the brain-death concept have failed to appreciate that a diagnosis of brain death is commonly superfluous, on medical grounds, in taking a decision to cease resuscitative measures. An example of this attitude, for instance, is provided by Lamb:

"The physician has a primary duty to maintain life. Once he is satisfied beyond doubt that the patient is dead, he has no moral duty to ventilate a cadaver."[36]

Another statement of the same contention, but with an altered emphasis, was:

"Once death has been diagnosed in accordance with accepted medical criteria, the pronouncement of death and the discontinuation of life-support systems are mandatory."[37]

Whilst the statement itself may seem so obvious as to query the necessity for its expression, or its reproduction here, I believe that it is worth re-emphasizing and refuting, the implication which it carries that discontinuation of life-support cannot be mandatory, in the interests of the patient, without a pronouncement of death. A more realistic summation of the situation would be "once a physician is satisfied beyond doubt that any resuscitation will no longer be of benefit to a patient he has no duty to prolong life support." The fear of litigation may impose liabilities that morality does not. For example, a perceived requirement for legal indemnity when certifying brain death has probably contributed to the emphasis, frequently placed in the United States, on securing a permanent EEG record of the absence of electrical activity in the brain.

Apart from conferring legal indemnity on a physician discontinuing therapy on a brain-dead subject, legislative recognition of this state has had the effect of facilitating the laying of a charge of homicide against anyone responsible for rendering another person brain dead. Such charges were successfully sustained in 1978 by states in the USA, both possessing and lacking formal legal recognition of brain death.[38]

Perhaps the statutory recognition of brain death will serve to fulfil other functions. One stream of legal advice has suggested the withholding of death directives from attending physicians in order to achieve tax savings by delaying the moment of death.

> "If the client reached his condition near year-end, with creative tax advice and prior planning, the client could in effect, permit others to select for him the tax year in which he died."[39]

Witness the prescience of the adage concerning taxes and death.

It is also conceivable that some currently advocated changes to homicide laws could exert a major impact on the criteria for determining brain death. Thus, there have been calls for legislative amendments to permit the imposition of more severe sentences, perhaps comparable with those applicable to homicide, for causing "neocortical death" or a persistent vegetative state. These calls have been coupled with others for reduction in the penalties to be imposed upon those responsible for "releasing" patients from a persistent vegetative state by expediting the cessation of heart and lung function.

The evolution of brain-death criteria and of the concept they define

The understanding of what the term "brain death" is meant to convey has changed since its introduction, as also have the criteria for its diagnosis. I believe that this change in understanding reflects both the presence of a substantial arbitrary component in matching the concept to clinical reality, as well as a progressive increase in the extent to which residual brain function has been detected in brain-dead subjects. One source of arbitrary decisions in translating the concept into evaluation of patients was mentioned by Veatch:

> "We must come to grips with the possibility, indeed the probability, that we shall never be able to make precise physiologic measures of the irreversible loss of mental processes."[33]

He was referring to the situation of the patient who has lost cognition but still has intact cardiorespiratory function (reflecting continuing brain-stem function). However, the precise physiological status of cerebral function is similarly indeterminate in the classical brain-dead patient in whom respiration is artificially maintained. More intensive examination of brain-dead patients maintained on artificial ventilator support has suggested that there may be retention of a number of brain functions that was not previously unsuspected. This subject will be discussed on pp. 39–40.

The occurrence of geographically determined variations in protocols for diagnosis of brain death has already been mentioned. An especially noticeable difference has arisen in relation to (apnea) tests for the loss of spontaneous respiration. It has already been pointed out that numerical variations in some of the details specified for the conduct of tests to demonstrate whether an individual has lost the capacity to breathe spontaneously, can result in that individual being legally dead in one jurisdiction but not in another.[9] The basis of apnea (lack of breathing) tests is to decide whether the patient resumes spontaneous respiration in response to an increase in the level of carbon dioxide in the blood sufficient to stimulate the respiratory centre in the intact brain to react. The arbitrary nature of the conditions selected for conduct of this test is reflected in the designation of different sets of criteria, in particular of different blood levels of carbon dioxide, as adequate to test for the irreversible inactivation of the respiratory centre. It was observed in one commentary on this subject that "no single standardized method of apnea testing has gained wide acceptance."[40] Reflecting this situation, the physicians at one Dutch clinic reported that, when they applied the procedures specified in the current, authoritative USA guidelines, it was impossible to produce an increase in blood carbon dioxide levels sufficiently great to be able to guarantee from the lack of response that spontaneous respiration had ceased.[41]

The original notions of brain death included phrases such as "loss of all brain function" or, with the possible suggestion of a structural equivalent to this loss, "total brain death". However, by 1978, neither of these concepts remained as an essential part of the brain dead state. A leading article in the *New England Journal of Medicine*, at that time concluded that:

> "It makes no practical difference if some hundreds of thousands of the many millions of brain cells are still functional, and it is certainly impractical at present to test the function of all brain-cell clusters."[42]

I believe that this change in attitude carries more substantial implications for brain death as a *concept* than it acknowledges in terms of the practicality of brain death *criteria*. In effect, it recognizes that brain death is to be regarded as differing from other outcomes of brain injury primarily in a *quantitative* sense. Thus, brain death may not differ qualitatively from, for example, the persistent vegetative state. It would, however, differ qualitatively from the traditional concept of death in which the brain in its entirety is dead. *The New England Journal of Medicine* article could legitimately invite the question, "What percentage of brain cells could remain alive without altering the patient's status from that of being brain dead?" This appears to me to represent a significant change from the original notion of brain death.

Brain death, as originally understood, appeared to be as absolute as the conventional understanding of death itself. I suspect that much of the community support that has been gained for the use of brain-dead subjects as a means of ensuing the ready procurement of organs for transplantation was based on this absolute perception. The re-appraisal of brain death entailed in retreating from an absolutist position could prompt questions relating to the percentage survival of neurons required before a patient is not diagnosed as "brain dead", albeit irreversibly disabled and destined for early death. Is the significance of partial survival of different structures within the brain to be weighted in relation to the extent of knowledge of the function that they mediate? Alternatively, should the significance of inability to detect a particular function be adjusted to take account of the practicality of detection of that function? How is the *understanding* of brain death (as distinct from the *criteria* around which that understanding has been structured) to accommodate new information which suggests that there is residual activity in regions of the brain not previously accessible to testing? Will the likelihood of a given individual being accepted as brain dead decrease in inverse proportion to the extent of diagnostic sophistication available in the relevant hospital?

The change to acceptance of brain death as being a state that is not inconsistent with retention of some detectable brain functions has been noted by a number of writers. For example, several anaesthetists and intensive care specialists have concluded that:

> "It is, however, not the purpose of the current criteria for the diagnosis of brain-stem death to identify total cessation of function of all brainstem neurons, but rather to define the degree of loss of function at which irreversible brainstem damage has occurred ...It is the point of no return."[43]

This appears to me to represent an explicit confounding of present status and outlook. Such a position has been commonly presented in discussion of brain death and, together with the widespread impression that this state entails the *total* loss of function of the organ, appears to have played a major, and not adequately recognized, part in the acceptance of brain death in the general community.

Reference has already been made to the manner in which changes in understanding of the nature of "brain death" have been mirrored by changes of its definition by various authorities. Commenting critically upon this aspect, as it was exemplified in successive pronouncements on the subject by the conference of Medical Royal Colleges, an anaesthetist wrote to the *British Medical Journal* as follows:

> "The criteria for brain-stem death were introduced in 1976 'to establish diagnostic criteria of such rigour that on their fulfilment, the mechanical ventilator can be

switched off in the secure knowledge that there is no possible chance of recovery', but not that the patient is already dead. This refinement was introduced in the 1979 memorandum in response to the need to obtain vital organs from 'beating-heart donors'."[44]

This letter contains two assertions, the first of which is the point discussed above, namely that the criteria for brain death (and, hence, the condition that they serve to identify) have undergone substantial change. The second assertion is that these changes in criteria have been motivated by an imperative to supply organs for transplantation.

It is very doubtful that the beliefs of the general community in relation to the nature of brain death have kept pace with changes in medical conceptualization of the state. One British commentator summarized the situation as he saw it in 1985:

"The seeds of these misconceptions were sown some time ago by the collective authors of the American Uniform Determination of Death Act in which death is equated with the 'irreversible cessation of all functions of the entire brain, including the brain stem'. A currently uninformed public will sooner or later discover how misleading this simple formulation is... In the usual clinical context of brain death there is no certain way of ascertaining that major areas of the brain such as the cerebellum, the basal ganglia or the thalami have irreversibly ceased to function. A clinical diagnosis of 'whole brain death' is in this sense a fiction'."[31]

I suggest that the aspect of these comments by Dr Pallis which should be of most concern is his reference to "a currently uninformed public". The importance of *informed* consent as a prerequisite to participation by an individual in organ donation from himself or in organ removal from another has been recognized in the majority of communities, which remain unprepared to intervene on the bodies of brain-dead individuals without family permission. It is generally expected that both consent given in relation to self by an individual in good health who signs some form of donor card and consent to use of a brain-dead relative will only be accepted as valid after accurate explanation of what brain death and organ removal entail. However, if most members of the community are uninformed, the value of any consent is questionable.

In the light of Pallis' comments about the uninformed state of the community, it is interesting that, in the same article, he expressed surprise at a recommendation from a Swedish committee that could potentially allow the extent of an individual's consent to be adjusted to his or her state of information:

"It suggests that the Swedish Transplant Act should allow potential donors to issue prohibitions (binding on both next of kin and medical personnel) against the removal of their organs 'prior to the discontinuation of circulatory support'."[31]

Pallis expressed concern about the possibility that the recommendation could impair efforts "to convince people that the brain dead are truly dead."[31]

Considerable success has undoubtedly been achieved in generating public interest in and support for transplantation programmes. However, it is not clear whether this support has been accompanied by comparable acceptance of the brain-death concept. For example, a commentary written in 1971 on the changes in the definition of death that were occurring then, drew attention to the experience that "second-hand benefits are, without embarrassment, admitted to be a major (if not *the* major) reason for updating the criteria for pronouncing a man dead."[45] The writer continued:

> "It can only be regarded as unsavory and dangerous, both for medicine and for the community at large, to permit the determination of one person's death to to be contaminated by a consideration of the needs of others. Having said this, however, I hasten to add that the redefiners also think that their criteria do happen to fit the fact of death."[45]

In the period when beating-heart, brain-dead subjects were first coming into use, it seems likely that acceptance of brain death was far from uniform among medical personnel. A 1973 article in *Pediatrics* reported that 46% of physicians, 42% of freshman medical students and 60% of lay people did not consider brain death an adequate definition of cessation of life. The authors considered that, at that time, "the classic concept of death is ingrained".[46] Considerable confusion has clearly been generated in the course of modifying community perceptions about brain death. Typical of this confusion was the statement of a judge in Florida:

> "This lady is dead and has been dead and she is kept alive artificially."[47]

Even on the most favourable interpretation, such a statement would suggest considerable confusion in the mind of the judge at both conceptual and semantic levels.

THE ROLE OF SOME CONFOUNDING ISSUES IN ESTABLISHING AND REINFORCING THE CONCEPT OF BRAIN DEATH

Several topics which have frequently been introduced into discussion of the meaning of brain death, the reliability of its diagnosis and the subsequent use of brain-dead subjects will be considered now. The inter-relationship between patients' future medical course and their present condition, and the extent to which management is determined by the former in the case of the brain dead, may have wider implications for use of other classes of subjects and will receive emphasis. In the case of the possibility, which has occasionally been raised, that an individual accurately diagnosed as brain dead could recover, the point to be emphasized will be the irrelevance of this issue for consideration of the use of the brain dead. A third topic, namely the interval that can be expected to elapse between the occurrence of brain death and cessation of contraction of the heart, has had, I believe, a substantial influence on the acceptance of the brain-dead state and merits examination for that reason. Finally, presentation of the idea of brain death, especially in the context of community education, has made extensive use of an analogue of brain death that I consider does not withstand analysis. I have chosen to group these four topics together because each of them has been introduced into discussions of brain death in ways that have been potentially misleading. Although none of them now occupies as prominent a part in discussion of brain death, as it did during development of the concept, the results of their earlier consideration have been incorporated into the general perception of the state.

The non-equivalence of prognosis and current status

Whilst the future outlook of any patient is very likely to be influenced by his or her current medical condition, the two states are quite distinct. The current condition of a brain-dead individual is likely to be that of continued retention of integrity and function in all organ systems, apart from the central nervous system. There is also likely to be persisting function in some, presently unmeasurable, proportion of the brain. The forecast for the patient is of rapid cessation of all functioning by organ systems when the respirator is disconnected. It is entirely reasonable that a management strategy be formulated after consideration of this prognosis. However, in the case of some medical conditions there has been a recent tendency to substitute management programmes that would only become appropriate when that prognosis has been realized. I do not believe that this substitution is reasonable. The changes that have been progressively introduced in the management of brain-dead subjects exemplify this form of substitution. Prognostic implications for the brain-dead patient are frequently found to be so persuasive that measures which assume their fulfilment are implemented despite the obvious presence of clinical features that indicate that they have yet to be fulfilled.

The feature of the brain-dead patient's condition that is most conducive to equating (incorrectly, I believe) current status with prognosis, is its irreversibility. There is no doubt that the various sets of criteria, correctly applied, can provide accurate assessment of both the present condition (irreversible loss of clinically detectable brain function) and of the course of that condition (cessation of function in all organ systems is inevitable). However, it is unlikely that it will be possible to adduce evidence to establish that the brain has *already* become completely and irreversibly non-functional. As pointed out earlier, other states of brain damage in which the brain clearly remains alive, such as persistent vegetative states, are as reliably irreversible as is the state of brain death.

Another aspect of the tendency to equate the current status and the future course and resultant management of irreversibly comatose patients may be reflected in the attitude that formal diagnosis of brain death is required if one is not to initiate, or is to discontinue, life support. This attitude, alluded to on pp. 27–28 which completely overlooks the point that there is no obligation to provide resuscitation that is not in the patient's interest, is entrenched in some writing on brain death.[36] Jonas' inference that the assurance of a secure diagnosis incorporating the word "dead" was sought may have been close to the mark.[21] Another instance of equating current status and forecast course, this time in the case of patients in a persistent vegetative state, has been their subsequent treatment as dead subjects.[39]

Assertions that current status cannot validly be described in terms of prognosis run the risk of misrepresentation as claims for the prognostic unreliability of the criteria used to identify brain death. Discussion of this subject sometimes fails to differentiate between two issues: namely, the reliability with which irreversibility can be predicted in patients meeting brain-death criteria, and that with which their current status can be unequivocally identified. Consequently, questioning of exactly what pathological condition exists at the time that brain-death criteria are satisfied, may elicit the (irrelevant) response that recovery from brain death has never been observed.

Recovery from brain death: a non-issue

To what extent does demonstration that the prognosis implied by a diagnosis of brain death is invariably accurate establish the validity of the brain death concept? To the extent that the existence of brain death as a factual state and the reliability of measures used to diagnose it have been challenged on the grounds of subsequent recovery of consciousness in patients satisfying brain-death criteria, the absence of any reliable reports of such recovery strongly supports both existence of the state and reliability of the diagnostic measures. An argument has sometimes been presented to the effect that, if recovery has been observed following a diagnosis of brain death, the concept itself is spurious. A notable example of claims for recovery from brain death occurred in a BBC *Panorama* programme in 1980. The programme dealt with the cases of a number of patients who had recovered after extended periods of unconsciousness. However, as pointed out in many medical criticisms of the programme, none of the patients whose cases were examined had ever met the criteria required for a diagnosis of brain death.[48] The importance of the community perception of brain death as an irreversible, absolute state that can be accurately diagnosed was reflected in the response to the *Panorama* programme, namely a sharp fall in the ensuing monthly score of British organ transplants.[49] There do not appear to have been any adequately authenticated incidents in which subjects meeting all the criteria of brain death have recovered. However, in the course of justifiably criticizing and dismissing arguments for instances of recovery from brain death, most commentators appear to have proceeded to draw the unwarranted conclusion that the failure of such claims in itself validates the proposition that patients diagnosed as brain dead *are dead at the time at which this diagnosis is made*. One exception to this general conclusion was forthcoming in a letter to the *Lancet* from Drs Wainwright-Evans and Lum, in the wake of the *Panorama* programme. They wrote that:

> "The greater problem—also implicit in the question asked—is whether 'properly tested and found virtually certain to die within a few days' should be equated with 'dead'."[50]

I believe that acceptance of the proposition that invariable failure of recovery to occur following diagnosis of brain death "proves" that "brain death equates with death" is another variant of confounding prognosis and current status.

Apart from the contention that "failure to recover" may be legitimately equated with "already dead", a related argument that has often been employed to validate the status of patients diagnosed as brain dead has centred on the rapidity with which total death invariably succeeded brain death. This proposition also requires re-examination.

Interval elapsing between brain death and cardiac arrest: another non-issue

> "Despite all efforts to maintain the donor's circulation, irreversible cardiac arrest usually occurs within 48 to 72 hours of brain death in adults, although it may take as long as 10 days in children. Indeed acceptance of the concept of brain death depended upon this close temporal association between brain death and cardiac arrest."[51]

This assessment of the historical role of the interval likely to separate a diagnosis of brain death from the occurrence of cardiac arrest was made as recently as 1989.

Death has traditionally been diagnosed on the basis of cessation of respiration and of cardiac contraction. With the refinement of resuscitative techniques, the argument that contraction of the heart would invariably cease soon after diagnosis of brain death, irrespective of any attempts to defer it by intensive resuscitation, was advanced as a major proof that brain death was indeed what it was claimed to be. Assuming for a moment, that the invariability of the close sequence claimed for the two events is factual, what are the implications of this association for the claim that brain death equates with traditional death? Is it reasonable to draw inferences about the similarity of the nature of the two events from their relative timing? If it is, the question could become one of deciding on the maximum interval that could elapse between brain death and cardiac arrest in the individual patient without weakening the proposition that the two events are closely related components of a single sequence. A second, more pragmatic, question might be concerned with the reasons for close linkage. Does it necessarily reflect a single underlying biological process or could it be explained on the basis of recognition by the attending clinicians that vigorous attempts to maintain cardiorespiratory function following diagnosis of brain death would be unjustified and improper?

An explicit statement of the argument, which holds that the temporal proximity of cardiac arrest to brain death indicates the close relationship of the latter to traditional death, was provided by two London neurologists. Participating in the discussion of brain death triggered by the *Panorama* television programme, they wrote:

> "To diagnose brainstem death is therefore to predict early cessation of heartbeat; and to diagnose cessation of heartbeat is to predict imminent death of all body cells (and thus total brain death). It is these correlations which form the basis for our confidence in identifying brainstem death as the essential component of 'total brain death', and so far no one has produced any exceptions to this chain of events."[52]

The certainty with which the occurrence of cardiac arrest soon after brain death was anticipated was also indicated in a 1978 review of the history of the concept of brain death by Korein:

> "No investigator contributing to this volume has presented evidence that irreversible cardiac arrest may be postponed more than a week (exclusive of that in infants and children), and most often these final irreversible changes occur prior to 48 and even 24 hours after brain death."[53]

A Swedish contributor to the same volume observed that patients meeting the criteria of brain death could not be maintained for a significant period:

> "The mean period of continuing activity of the heart is only three to five days."[54]

In his major article on brain death, also published in the *New England Journal of Medicine* in 1978, Black cited six studies in which the length of the interval between diagnosis of brain death and the occurrence of cardiac arrest was recorded. The longest interval recorded was 14 days, but cardiac arrest occurred much earlier in most patients.[55] An emphatic statement to the same end was provided by Jennett and Hessett in 1981:

> "There is abundant evidence that once brain death has been confirmed the heart always stops within 14 days (usually much sooner) even though ventilation is maintained."[56]

However, despite this apparent consensus, a report was published shortly afterwards, by Parisi *et al.*,[57] which effectively called into question the inevitability of rapid transit from brain death to cardiac arrest. To the extent that occurrence of a rapid transition is considered to provide significant grounds for the identity of brain death with traditional death, the report of Parisi *et al.* certainly complicated this interpretation:

> "It is widely held that in patients with brain death who are receiving continued ventilation and full medical care, spontaneous cessation of the heartbeat will ensue within a period of hours or a few days. In this report, we describe a middle-aged man in whom a number of generally accepted sets of clinical criteria for brain death were met, and in whom cardiac activity ceased only after ventilatory support was discontinued over two months later."[57]

Apparently, the basis for this instance of maintenance of support for 68 days after brain death was the inability of the attending clinicians to obtain family consent for its cessation. Eventual disconnection of the respirator required a court order. In keeping with these circumstances, the major conclusion drawn from this case by the authors of the report was that statutory criteria for determination of death were essential in order to avoid similar incidents.

Perhaps not surprisingly, Parisi's paper evoked a number of responses. These ranged from criticism of the accuracy of the diagnosis of brain death,[58] to reports of other cases of prolonged maintenance of cardiac function after brain death.[59,60] A possibility, not explored in the correspondence, was that if the diagnosis by Parisi and his colleagues had been incorrect, then their mistake could have been repeated in other clinics and the accepted brain death criteria would be called into question. Discontinuation of life-support measures in the case of other irreversibly comatose, but *not* brain-dead, patients should not present any problems. However, the use of non-brain-dead, beating-heart subjects as sources of organs for transplantation would present many problems. I believe that this prospect would be raised by any situation in which the accuracy of diagnosis of brain death in an established clinic is questioned. A third correspondent wrote in response to the Parisi report:

> "My God, what took them so long to turn off ventilatory support?"[61]

The possibility of prolonged persistence of cardiac function after brain death has been discussed, and its realization also reported, in relation to pregnant subjects. An early report of maintenance of a brain-dead woman in order to "gain time and thereby reduce the degree of prematurity of the infant" adopted the assumption that there was likely to be a limited period, perhaps of 2 weeks, over which this could be achieved. Discussion was directed to possible benefits accruing to the foetus from such an extension of intra-uterine life.[62] The ethical aspects of maintaining respirator support of pregnant, brain-dead women were the subject of a later discussion.[63] Use of the brain-dead subject as an "incubator" for the purpose of achieving greater maturity has some similarities with the employment of brain-dead subjects in experimentation and will be examined in that context later. However, my present interest in this issue arises from reports of continuation of cardiac function in pregnant subjects for periods in excess of 2 months after brain death. Such information inevitably casts doubts on the hypothesis that cardiac arrest always follows soon after brain death, even if full medical support is provided.

A subsequent report described in detail the maintenance of a brain-dead pregnant woman from 22 to 31 weeks gestation, at which time a viable infant was delivered and survived.[64] The accuracy of diagnosis of brain death in this case appears to have been beyond dispute (once again, if it was contended that the condition could be mistakenly diagnosed in a major hospital, there would be a clear implication that non-brain-dead subjects would have been included among beating-heart organ donors on some occasions). In discussing the case, the clinicians responsible for maintenance of the patient identified the expense of the exercise as a major ethical consideration. However, they also commented upon the length of circulatory survival that had been achieved after brain death and contrasted this with what had traditionally been believed to be possible. They suggested:

> "It is possible that this lack of prolonged somatic survival (referring to the conventionally expected short period between brain death and cardiac arrest) is due as much to the prognostic futility of maintaining cardiorespiratory support in a brain-dead patient as it is to any inherent technical difficulty in maintaining such support."[64]

This seems to me to be a very reasonable proposition. It is not immediately apparent that there is any way in which extended maintenance of patients in whom brain death had already been diagnosed could be justified in the interests of the patient. To undertake the maintenance of a series of such patients in order to ascertain the duration of survival that could be achieved with adequate resuscitation would be emphatically to enter the realm of experimentation. Attempts to publish the results of such an experiment would, one predicts, attract opprobrium, not commendation.

The conclusion now appears inescapable that, contrary to earlier assumptions, cardiac arrest need not invariably follow within a short time of brain death. Demonstration that the earlier widely accepted contention, that cardiac arrest inevitably follows soon after brain death, is incorrect has some implications for attitudes towards the brain-death concept. To the extent that acceptance of the brain-death concept as an accurate reflection of the clinical situation was achieved *because* of the presumed nexus with cardiac arrest, that acceptance may require qualification. The probability that cardiac arrest will closely follow brain death, unless extraordinary resuscitative measures are employed, should be seen as no more than a prognostic feature and certainly not as an indication of the nature of brain death. As stressed previously, prognosis may legitimately guide the clinician in selecting a management program for a patient but it should never be treated as an assessment of current status. Most importantly, observations of prolonged continuation of cardiac action following brain death indicate that previous propositions, which purported to equate "brain death" with "total death" on the grounds that the two are not separable in time to any extent, are invalid.

Analogues of brain death

In seeking to explain the nature of brain death, especially to lay audiences, much use has been made of the analogy of the freshly decapitated subject in whom circulation and ventilation are being artificially maintained. I believe that this a a singularly misleading, indeed a dishonest, comparison to draw. Whereas the decapitated subject in receipt of cardiorespiratory support is totally lacking in any input to, or activity in, any part of the brain, this certainly is not the case with brain-dead subjects. The extent of persistence of other brain activities that remain undetectable with existing technology may eventually prove to be considerable. Furthermore, it is quite spurious to imply that similar degrees of certainty attach to inferences about the state of the brain in a severed head and in a brain-dead patient.

A more reasonable analogy with the decapitated subject, with regard to brain status, would be the individual in whose case, following diagnosis of brain death, the respirator had been disconnected with resultant cardiac arrest. After an interval of complete cessation of blood circulation, having ensured destruction of the brain, if cardiac action was artificially restarted and the subject again connected to the respirator, the status could more closely approximate that of the decapitated corpse. To the extent that the "decapitated subject" analogy has been employed to facilitate acceptance of brain death, that acceptance should again be qualified.

CLINICAL OBSERVATIONS IN CONFLICT WITH THE BRAIN-DEATH CONCEPT: RESPONSES TO THEM

Since the development and widespread application of criteria for making the diagnosis of brain death, there have been many accounts of the features of subjects who satisfy those criteria. In a number of instances, the features reported in brain-dead subjects have proved to be inconsistent, to varying degrees, with the original conception of brain death. While it is my intention to discuss some examples of these inconsistencies, the significant feature to which I wish first to draw attention is *not* the discordant observations themselves, but the nature of the responses which they have elicited from those reporting them. The regular response when publishing an inconsistent finding has been *not* to question the extent to which the original notion diverges from reality but either to categorize the new finding as not relevant or to modify the meaning which the writer attaches to the term "brain death". This progressive modification of the meaning of the term is not entirely unexpected if one recalls the history of its origin as a shorthand expression for a state the existence of which was inferred exclusively on the basis of loss of function measurable with then existing technology. I do not believe that the distinction between the *nature* of the state that the term "brain death" was intended to represent and its prognosis and manifestations was clearly drawn at the outset by most commentators.

The observations to be discussed include several which imply the possibility of some persistence of activity in the upper parts of the brain (as suggested by electroencephalogram, blood flow and pituitary gland function) and others related to retention of brain-stem functions (regulation of blood pressure, control of oesophageal muscular activity and electrical responses by the brain to sounds). The other subject to be considered is the nature of the structural abnormalities of the brain that have been observed microscopically to correlate with the clinical diagnosis of brain death. All of the observations to be cited have been available in the medical literature for a considerable period and, hence, a general awareness of them by medical personnel concerned with the use of brain-dead subjects could reasonably be assumed.

The electroencephalogram (EEG) in brain-dead patients

An electroencephalogram (EEG) consists of records of electrical activity of the brain as measured by the application of electrodes to a variety of positions on the head. In some neurological disorders, it can provide information of value in the diagnosis and subsequent management of the individual patient; it can also be a useful technique for research into brain function, for example, in relation to brain activity during sleep. The mechanisms of production of the EEG and the precise parts of the brain responsible for the production of its various components are not completely understood. It is likely that activity is more readily detectable from some parts of the cerebral hemispheres than from others. Furthermore, the EEG has little capacity to monitor activity in the brain stem and cerebellum. Consequently, the technique is of little use in diagnosing abnormalities confined to the brain stem. There appears to have been a universal expectation at the time at which the brain death concept was formulated that EEG activity would invariably have ceased in brain-dead subjects. A similar general impression has persisted, perhaps simplistically, in the intervening period. However, as information about brain-dead subjects has accumulated, it has become abundantly clear that this assumption is frequently incorrect.

Considerable confusion appears to have been introduced into the medical literature dealing with use of the EEG in brain-dead subjects by failure to differentiate clearly between its distinct applications, namely its uses as a research tool, a diagnostic aid in brain disease and a means of assessment of the prognosis of individual patients. As regards this latter application, further confusion has been engendered by inadequate distinction between usage in response solely to clinical requirements and that with a medico-legal motivation.

The belief that the EEG was of considerable value in the management of brain-dead individuals seems to have been especially prevalent in the USA. However, it was increasingly recognized subsequently that, provided the clinical criteria of brain death had been fulfilled, any EEG activity likely to be detected would have little bearing on the outcome of the case. This point, that retention of EEG activity in these patients did not have any favourable prognostic connotations, was effectively made in a retrospective review of the case histories of a large series of brain-dead patients, published in 1979. This reported that none of those patients, satisfying the clinical criteria for brain death but nevertheless retaining some form of EEG activity, survived for longer than 96 h. It was concluded that:

"although the EEG may have identified patients with persistent neuronal activity, it was not a predictor of improved outcome once cerebral and brain-stem function was clinically absent."[65]

A French study, reported in 1970, showed that:

"when apneic coma and absent brain stem reflexes occurred in a context of structural brain disease minor residual electroencephalographic activity was common but never persisted. In the vast majority of cases no electroencephalogram could be recorded after 48 hours."[17]

Of a series of 1000 patients without EEG activity and 147 with detectable activity, all of whom met the criteria for irreversible cessation of brain-stem function, all experienced cardiac arrest within a few days.[17] The prevailing difference between the USA and the UK in attitudes towards use of the EEG was attributed in 1979 "to the climate of public opinion, especially in relation to medico-legal matters and litigation."[66] An alternative explanation, sometimes expressed, is that EEG measurement was uncommon in the UK because adequate EEG equipment was not widely available.

Whereas use of EEG in patients clinically diagnosed as brain dead is of no prognostic value, it has contributed to research into the nature of the condition defined by the accepted clinical criteria. I have alluded above to the strength of establishment of the concept of brain death and its durability in the face of subsequent conflicting observations. The manner in which existing convictions about the nature of the brain-dead state accommodated what might have been seen as contradictory data provided by the use of the EEG is probably the best example of this. Numerous reports of the persistence of EEG activity in patients satisfying the criteria for brain death appeared in the first decade of their application to diagnosis of the condition. (Temporary absence of EEG activity in patients who are *not* brain dead has also been observed. There have been reports of the reappearance of EEG activity after periods of absence exceeding a week.[67] From such cases it has been concluded both that lack of EEG activity does not reliably indicate brain death and that its return does not necessarily indicate any potential for recovery. Reappearance of the EEG implies only a change in function of the central nervous system.)

Reports of persistent EEG have evoked an almost uniform response. Some early examples of this were documented in a volume on brain death published in 1976. One report, appended in a footnote, concerned seven children in whom EEG activity persisted from the time of diagnosis of brain death until cardiac arrest occurred (an interval of from 2 to 32 days). The response to this report was that "it may represent another limitation on the use of EEG on young children and infants in the problem of diagnosing brain death."[54]

"I do not believe there could be residual sentience above a dead brain stem."[17]

This evaluation of the significance of persistent EEG activity in patients meeting brain-death criteria led its author to call on those not in agreement:

"to face up to the scenario of a patient with a dead brain stem, doomed to asystole (cardiac arrest) within a few days, yet showing remnants of electroencephalographic activity—which they equate with residual sentience. Can they conceive of a greater hell than an isolated sentience, aware of its precarious existence, and with no means of expression?"[17]

This appears to me to be a compelling argument for discontinuing life-support measures in such patients. If so, it should be an equally persuasive argument for not *prolonging* the use of life support for other purposes, such as use as an organ donor. At best, residual EEG activity could be equated with the *possibility* of persistence of some residual activity, not with the realization of that possibility.

A report from a Chicago hospital revealed that approximately one fifth of a series of patients clinically diagnosed as brain dead continued to manifest EEG activity for an average further period of 36 h. In two patients, EEG activity resembling that observed during normal sleep remained detectable 168 h after the diagnosis of brain death. The authors interpreted this observation as evidence for the proposition that "brain death" has occurred once a critical number of neurons have been irreversibly damaged.[68] They also noted that a recent survey of American neurologists and neurosurgeons had revealed that 65% of responding specialists considered an isoelectric EEG necessary before brain death could be declared. A similar construction had already been placed on an earlier report of the persistence of EEG activity in children in whom clinical criteria of brain death had been met and cerebral blood flow could not be demonstrated. The interpretation of this observation, namely that the concept should not be jeopardized by observations inconsistent with it, was conveyed by the title to the article, "Failure of electroencephalography to diagnose brain death in comatose children."[69]

Two implicit attitudes appear to have been influential in determining responses to any observation of persistent EEG activity in brain-dead patients.

The first has been that a persistent EEG is without prognostic implications.[70] This belief, which has been established on the basis of considerable clinical experience, is often coupled with the assumption, that, because "conventional" death is not only inevitable, but probably imminent, brain death *has already occurred*. The second attitude holds that termination of supportive treatment may only be considered *when brain death has been diagnosed*. As previously indicated, I believe this to be an invalid constraint. The Chicago study, referred to above, acknowledged this possible impact of retention of EEG activity on patient management in the following terms:

> "The presence of EEG activity, despite clinical examinations entirely consistent with irreversible brain death, resulted in continuation of supportive care and delayed the final declaration of death for hours, days and, in one case, weeks, without altering the final fatal outcome."[68]

If persistent EEG were to be accepted as incompatible with the occurrence of brain death, it is likely that clinicians who are influenced by this second attitude would feel that a necessity for undue prolongation of fruitless resuscitation had been imposed upon them by the persistent EEG. An alternative response to reports of persistence of EEG (and, indeed, of the other functions to be discussed) in brain-dead patients, could be to reconsider the *nature* of the condition identified by the diagnostic criteria for brain death. In commenting upon the possible response of clinicians concerned with the persistence of EEG activity in a patient meeting criteria for irreversible loss of brain-stem function, the British neurologist to whom reference was made in the penultimate paragraph queried, "Would they anaesthetise such a preparation? Or just sedate it?"[17] Perhaps the answer would be, once again, to discontinue life support?

As already noted, attitudes towards the use of the EEG in brain-dead subjects vary with geographic location. In accounting for use of the EEG in the USA, it has been suggested that American physicians "have to protect the young people who are educated with them against the malevolent ravages of opportunistic lawyers." It was proposed that the practice of medicine in the USA occurs "in a climate where physicians have been brought to court as potential murderers for having killed an already dead patient." Consequently, they are likely to resort to use of the EEG "to save a great deal of later polemical accusation."[17] Another major reason for divergence between USA and UK attitudes to the EEG derives from the different pathological states envisaged by the definitions of brain death as applied in the two countries. Whereas USA practice requires cessation of function in *all* parts of the brain, the UK equivalent is concerned only with death of the brain stem. The condition of the cerebral cortex in the British patient is irrelevant to a diagnosis of brain death. As the major part of EEG activity is believed to derive from the cerebral hemispheres, this technique has, by definition, nothing to contribute to diagnosis of brain-stem death. Attitudes towards the concept of brain death and the EEG technology have evolved together, with each influencing the other.

Brain blood flow in brain-dead subjects

Measurement of blood flow within the brain by radiographic examination following the introduction of either radio-opaque contrast media or radio-isotopes into the bloodstream has been undertaken in the investigation of brain-dead patients. In general, blood flow to the cerebral hemispheres has been found to be either very markedly reduced or undetectable within the limits of sensitivity of the test. [71] Measurements of brain blood flow have been used occasionally as a means of confirming that patients with the clinical features of brain death are dead. This has especially been the case in children. Whilst examination of blood flow does not appear to add much to management of the individual case, it has occasionally suggested that the established assumptions about the state of brain tissue in patients diagnosed as brain dead may not be universally applicable. For example, a 1987 report of a case from the Johns Hopkins Hospital in Baltimore raised this question in its title, "Is brain death really cessation of all intracranial function?" [72] In this report, Fackler and Rogers described the retention of some cerebral circulation 2 days after the development of clinical features adequate for diagnosis of brain death. They also recalled a number of earlier reports of similar outcomes. As was the case with persistent EEG activity, there was no suggestion that retention of partial brain blood flow carried any implication of a better prognosis. Indeed, Fackler and Rogers made the point that any decision to persist with resuscitation on the basis of retention of brain blood flow would be unjustifiable. Nevertheless, they commented:

> "The purpose of our report is not to invalidate the concept of brain death. Rather, this case illustrates that physicians can no longer remain comfortable declaring brain death 'knowing' that all the brain is dead." [72]

As was the case with discordant EEG observations, evidence of retention of some brain blood flow should certainly not contraindicate discontinuation of resuscitation. Whether it should be similarly dismissed in considering the use of the patient as an organ source is, I suggest, a separate issue. However, it appears rarely to have been considered as such.

Retention of pituitary function in brain-dead subjects

In discussing their case of persistent brain blood flow in a brain-dead subject, Fackler and Rogers commented that:

> "Further evidence of intracranial function despite brain death comes from limited studies of neuroendocrine function." [72]

They recalled an earlier report of patients in whom persistent function of the pituitary gland was observed despite lack of demonstrable brain blood flow.

The pituitary gland is attached to the brain at the base of the cerebral hemispheres. One of its functions is to produce a range of hormones that are released into the bloodstream and are then distributed throughout the body to regulate the activity of a group of other glands. One part of the pituitary gland produces a hormone that acts upon the kidney to concentrate urine. In its absence, a condition termed "diabetes insipidus", characterized by the production of large quantities of dilute urine, soon appears. All of the pituitary hormones can be measured in the circulating blood by means of very sensitive tests and so it may be feasible to determine the extent of any remaining pituitary function with greater precision than is possible in the case of the brain itself. Pituitary gland blood supply is provided by small branches from the arteries which supply the hypothalamic region of the brain to which the gland is attached. For this reason, it has been inferred that destruction of the brain and the cessation of intracranial blood flow, which accompanies and produces brain death, should result in cessation of function of the pituitary gland. Accordingly, a number of studies have been undertaken with the objective of developing techniques for measurement of pituitary hormone levels in the peripheral bloodstream as a guide to cessation of pituitary gland function in the brain dead. However, as mentioned above, pituitary function has frequently been found to persist after brain death. For example, a group of researchers at the Royal Postgraduate Medical School in London was concerned by "the controversy over the lack of objective tests to support the clinical diagnosis of brain death."[73] They examined the practicability of using cessation of pituitary function, as reflected in blood hormone levels, as an objective sign of brain death. However, they found that blood levels of pituitary hormones remained unchanged in five patients during the 24 h following diagnosis of brain death. It was concluded that "hormonal evaluation of such patients is of no value in confirming the diagnosis." It is also notable that diabetes insipidus develops in only a (minority) proportion of individuals meeting the criteria for diagnosis as brain dead.

Presumptions that pituitary function should have ceased in brain-dead subjects who are being maintained as a source of transplantable organs, have led to suggestions that administration of hormones to replace those no longer produced by these patients' pituitary gland might improve the condition of the organs to be harvested. This form of hormonal replacement therapy is a new concept in the perioperative management of the beating-heart cadaveric donor. However, clinical trial of this proposal has failed to support the hypothesis that pituitary deficiency was a regular consequence of brain death, i.e. evidence is lacking both for consistent lowering of blood levels of pituitary hormones in brain-dead individuals and for improvement in the condition of brain-dead patients following supplementary treatment with pituitary hormones.[74,75] Whereas the rationale for measurement of pituitary hormone levels in brain-dead patients had been to provide tests to confirm the occurrence of brain death, the unexpected result of observation does not appear to have stimulated attempts to re-evaluate the nature of the brain-dead state.

Response of blood pressure in brain-dead patients undergoing surgery

The level of pressure in the blood circulation of a normal subject is subject to control by a regulatory set of nerves referred to as the autonomic nervous system. Impulses transmitted via this system are responsible for the alterations in blood pressure normally observed in response to various types of external stimuli applied to the body. The generally accepted explanation of the functioning of the autonomic nervous system infers that its central control mechanisms are located in the brain stem. Consequently, the description in 1985 of a series of brain-dead patients, in all of whom changes in blood pressure resembling those to be expected in non-brain-dead subjects were evoked by surgical incision in the course of organ removal, was unexpected. In seeking an explanation for the occurrence of "significant hemodynamic responses to painful stimuli in cadaver organ donors",[43] the authors of this report concluded that these responses were probably attributable to some residual brain-stem function. They emphasized that the current (1985) criteria for diagnosis of brain death were not intended "to identify total cessation of function of all brain stem neurons", but rather to detect the occurrence of irreversible brain-stem damage. Furthermore, they predicted that:

> "The recognition of partial brain stem function, other than that currently identified by the clinical brain death criteria, may be expected as increasingly sophisticated technology is used to examine brain stem function."[43]

Once again, as occurred with the publication of discordant observations concerning brain blood flow and pituitary function in brain-dead patients, the reaction of these clinicians to observation of blood pressure changes in response to painful stimuli was to emphasize the *prognostic* aspects of brain death and to pay less attention to the implications of the new observations for the original concept. In particular, it was emphasized that the new observations did not invalidate the criteria for *diagnosis* of brain death. However, the comment was made that:

> "These hemodynamic changes may frequently produce uneasiness in the medical and nursing staff."[43]

In the light of this, it was recommended that:

> "Although these responses may suggest partial lower medullary function, the medical personnel caring for the donor should be reassured that such a response does not invalidate the diagnosis of brain death."[43]

That is, hypothesis should take precedence over observation.

Oesophageal muscle contraction in brain-dead subjects

A further suggestion of persistence of function in some of the brain-stem nuclei of brain-dead patients was provided by studies, published in 1987, of muscular activity in the lower part of the oesophagus.[76] Spontaneous oesophageal muscular contraction is believed to be dependent upon activity of the brain stem. However, a report from two British anaesthetists described the persistence of spontaneous oesophageal muscular contractions in brain-dead subjects.[76] As was the case with the blood pressure responses described above, the operation of local reflexes that had been established at a very early stage after injury and did not require any brain-stem function, was considered to be an unlikely explanation. The authors noted that:

"Irrespective of the mechanism by which spontaneous lower oesophageal contractions are generated, we cannot accept the suggestion... that measuring such contractions provides a means of predicting, or even confirming, the presence of brain stem death;"[76]

In responding to this report, another clinician offered two possible explanations for the observations of retained function in brain-dead subjects. The first explanation was that spontaneous lower oesophageal contraction is an intrinsic response of the oesophagus "for which there is no evidence, all the evidence pointing in the opposite direction."[77] The other explanation invoked "some residual function in the oesophageal motility centre (in the brain stem) for which the current clinical tests of brain stem function are insufficiently sensitive."[77] The comment of another anaesthetist on the subject was to the effect that "the brain stem activity reported may not represent life in all its fullness, but neither does it equate with death."[44]

Reappearance of brain-stem reflexes

There have been claims for the reappearance of brain-stem responses following auditory stimulation of a brain-dead subject. Electrical impulses can normally be recorded from the brain in response to the application of sound to a subject's ear. This response, although measured from the cerebrum, is processed initially in the brain stem. Consequently, electrical responses to acoustic stimuli would not be expected in a brain-dead subject. Reappearance of such responses have, nevertheless, been reported following a period of absence.[78] While an alternative explanation for the temporary disappearance of this sign in a patient who was not brain dead was subsequently presented,[79] the original authors held to their explanation that its temporary loss, on account of *reversible* loss of function of the appropriate region of the brain stem, was a reality.[80] The outcome was that, whilst loss of an auditory brain-stem response was considered to imply a very poor prognosis, it was suggested that it could not be used in isolation as a criterion of brain death. The demonstration, even on a single occasion, that loss of a specific brain-stem function was not irreversible was sufficient to exclude it as a criterion. The possibility of whether recovery of some brain-stem functions can occur after their loss due to temporary interruption of blood or oxygen supply remains questionable. Nevertheless, it should not be ignored out of hand given the emphasis placed on irreversible loss of brain-stem function in formulation of the concept of brain death. The possible significance of the retention of electrical responses to sound in brain-dead patients was discussed at an early stage of development of the brain death concept:

> "Furthermore auditory potentials can sometimes be evoked in otherwise isopotential electroencephalograms. Obviously, these would not occur if some brain tissue were not alive. Yet, in themselves, such potentials are not always considered evidence of brain viability."[2]

Microscopic examination of the brain of brain-dead subjects

The approach generally accepted to discover and to validate correlations between the pathological changes that underlie a particular disease process in any organ and the clinical features that result from these changes is to compare the microscopic structure of the affected organ with the symptoms produced by its dysfunction. Such a clinicopathological correlation may be achieved by examination of the entire organ removed from the body at the time of post-mortem examination, of tissue samples removed during life by biopsy procedures or by a combination of these approaches. The assumption implicit in the first approach is that the tissue, as obtained and examined post-mortem, accurately reflects its structure at the earlier time when the clinical abnormalities were recorded. The soundness of this assumption will depend upon the extent to which the structure of the organ remains unaltered between the time of cessation of blood circulation, which occurs at the time of conventional death, and the permanent fixation of the tissue in preparation for microscopic examination.

A distinctive feature of brain tissue is that post-mortem changes, over and above any pathological features already present at the time of circulatory cessation, occur with extreme rapidity. An equally distinctive feature is that changes occurring as a result of deprivation of blood and/or oxygen supply (that would usually be the final mechanism leading to brain death) may bear a strong resemblance to those that regularly occur post-mortem, i.e. *after* cessation of circulation as part of conventional death. A good illustration of the difficulty which can be presented by the need to distinguish post-mortem and earlier changes is provided by the solution adopted by some Swedish researchers eager to ensure that their studies of the fine structure and function of brain cells were not invalidated because post-mortem changes had intervened before the tissue could be examined microscopically. Their response to this impasse was to take tissue from the brain of the freshly aborted foetus within minutes of its removal from the uterus.[81] Short of biopsy of the brain, a procedure that is rarely undertaken, apart from in the diagnosis of viral encephalitis, it is not feasible to obtain tissue completely unaffected by post-mortem changes. This rapid deterioration of the fine structure of the brain following conventional death has not proved to be a major impediment to investigation and diagnosis of most pathological conditions of the brain as the abnormalities that are being examined can be readily differentiated by their appearance from post-mortem changes. However, the confounding effect of post-mortem changes on the fine structure of the cells of the brain may present a major obstacle to validation of brain death on microscopic grounds because of the general similarity between the two types of change.

The scientific report that has come to be regarded as definitive in establishing brain death as a genuine entity on microscopic grounds was published in 1971 by Mohandas and Chou.[82] The aim of their investigation was summarized:

> "What we are attempting to define and establish beyond reasonable doubt is the state of irreversible damage to the brain stem."[82]

In the introduction to their report, Mohandas and Chou indicated that the two reasons which necessitated definition of irreversible damage were reduction of burden on patient, family and hospital and provision of organs for transplantation. No distinction was drawn between the requirements necessary for these two purposes. In commenting upon their study, Molinari acknowledged the prognostic value of the clinical features that they nominated:

> "These criteria imply that the prediction of death or a fatal prognosis is tantamount to brain death."[83]

However, he also expressed some reservations about whether the study had actually established a reliable correlation between clinical features and subsequent pathological findings:

> "Since pathologic findings did not always confirm brain death, even in patients meeting the more stringent Harvard criteria, the end-point or proof of validity of these criteria remains ill-defined. Prediction of a fatal outcome is not a valid criterion for accuracy of standards designed to determine that death has already occurred."[83]

The difficulty in determining whether structural changes that are discovered microscopically at post-mortem examination are an accurate reflection of what had already occurred at the time of diagnosis of brain death arises because of the extreme susceptibility of brain tissue to anoxia, referred to above. These changes, if they had not occurred at the time of diagnosis, may have occurred before or after the time of cardiac arrest and "conventional" death. The development of an inflammatory response to dead or damaged neurons requires the persistence of blood circulation after the initial damage has occurred. Consequently, the presence of microscopic features suggestive of an inflammatory response provides an indication that the accompanying changes in neurons are not post-mortem effects. Inflammatory responses to dead brain cells would be unlikely to be observed if circulatory cessation had followed within an hour of brain death. On the other hand, the presence of inflammatory changes in association with degeneration of brain cells in an individual whose cardiac function had persisted for some days after brain death implies that destruction of neurons had occurred *before* circulation ceased. It would not necessarily indicate the placement in time between diagnosis of brain death and occurrence of cardiac arrest, at which irreversible damage to the cells of the brain had occurred. It could be speculated, but certainly not established, that destruction had occurred by the time of clinical brain-death diagnosis.

The difficulty inherent in establishing any precise correlation between the onset of those clinical signs that are generally interpreted as denoting brain death and the timing of occurrence of the pathological changes in brain structure that constitute the entity of "respirator brain" have been recognized in most studies of this subject. The comprehensive, multi-centre study of the subject, which was mentioned in discussing the basis of brain-death criteria on pp. 26–27, noted that there was little inflammatory or cellular reaction evident in respirator brains.[35] It was observed that:

> "Certain changes are almost indistinguishable from the postmortem alterations resulting from delayed fixation or after storage of the cadaver at temperatures over 90°F... Even the most experienced neuropathologists have difficulty in differentiating the changes when both anoxic and autolytic factors operate to varying degrees in different parts of the brain."[35]

(Autolysis is the process of self-digestion that occurs when tissues break down after death.) This report provided some insight into the process by which establishment of the pathological equivalent of the clinical state of brain death was achieved:

> "Although initially some of the centre neuropathologists did not give credence to the concept, they agreed, after some indoctrination by the consultants, to accept the criteria listed in Table 3 as the basis for classifying the central nervous system findings in terms of respirator and nonrespirator brains."[35]

As already mentioned, the pathological criteria for diagnosis of "respirator brain" were established on the basis of a questionnaire circulated among neuropathologists. Moseley *et al.* noted that "a few respondents explicitly refused to participate citing skepticism as to the value of consensus in scientific endeavour."[34] One notable feature of the clinicopathological correlation between neurological and post-mortem structural features in the multi-centre trial conducted under the auspices of the National Institute of Neurological

Diseases and Stroke, was the occurrence of a group of patients in whom the implications of these two forms of assessment were discordant. In some of these cases, EEG activity, persisting close to the time of cardiac arrest, was accompanied by post-mortem features conforming with the criteria developed as distinctive of respirator brain. The authors commented in relation to these cases, "They are a motley group, whether considered from clinical, EEG or neuropathological angles."[35] The frequency of such cases with incongruous features can be gauged from the authors' observation that "almost half of the respirator brain cases had biological activity in the last EEG recorded."[35] Some of these EEG recordings were taken only shortly before cardiac arrest occurred. On the other hand, only 40% of the brains from patients who died after respirator dependency showed the changes that were considered to be "typical" of respirator brain.

The existence of the "motley group" of patients referred to above might lead one to question the extent to which there exists a uniform, structural equivalent to the clinical state of brain death. In commenting upon the multi-centre study of the pathological changes, Molinari observed:

"but one of the major and most disturbing findings was that detailed autopsy studies of the brain did not always show signs of autolysis and other features of death of the brain preceding the actual terminal events."[83]

He concluded that:

"Since pathological findings did not always confirm brain death, even in patients meeting the more stringent Harvard criteria, the end-point or proof of validity of these criteria remains ill-defined."[83]

The authors of the reports on the study appear to have been well aware of this point:

"The skeptics suggest that the morphological changes in these specimens merely indicate that the brain ceased to be viable *during* the period of artificial respiration and point to the similarity between the pathological changes seen in respirator brain and those observed in autolytic brains after delayed post mortem refrigeration."[34]

As reliable correlation between morbid anatomy and clinical features is generally considered to be an essential foundation for the accurate characterization of any newly described disease state, the circularity of argument and the arbitrary nature of the selection of objective pathological criteria to characterize the structural abnormalities associated with brain death provide some cause for concern.

"In attempting to assess the validity of clinical signs in the diagnosis of brain death, the most difficult problem at present is the recognition of an alternate and incontrovertible end point against which all criteria may be compared. Standard neuropathological examinations have not met this requirement."[84]

This I believe, remains as accurate an assessment as it was when written in 1978.

SUMMARY

To recapitulate the content of this chapter, review of the historical origins of brain death indicates that, whilst the concept was initially developed solely in the interests of the affected patient, its subsequent evolution has been heavily influenced by the concurrent emergence of clinical transplantation. Development of the concept has not followed an identical course in all locations and, consequently, there is not a uniform agreement on precisely what the state of brain death entails.

Ongoing investigation of patients meeting the criteria of brain death has resulted in an evolution in medical understanding of the nature of the state. Whilst the original concept was framed in terms of destruction of the brain and the equivalent envisaged to this was total and irreversible loss of function, brain death is now more likely to be thought of as the irreversible loss of critical functions. There is more than one opinion as to which functions are to be regarded as critical.

The following chapter will examine the manner in which the concept of what characterizes brain death is currently the subject of debate. The manner in which brain-dead subjects are used at present will be considered as also will possible changes in that usage. The influence that identification of individuals as brain dead can have on others and the relevance of this to the future of transplantation programmes will then be discussed.

REFERENCES

1. Youngner, S. J., Allen, M., Bartlett, E. T., Cascorbi, H. F., Hau, T., Jackson, D. L., Mahowald, M. B. and Martin, B. J. (1985) Psychosocial and ethical implications of organ retrieval. *New England Journal of Medicine*, **313**, 321–324.
2. Toole, J. F. (1971) The neurologist and the concept of brain death. *Perspectives in Biology and Medicine*, **14**, 599–607.
3. Beecher, H. K. (1968) A definition of irreversible coma. Report of the *ad hoc* committee of the Harvard Medical School to examine the definition of brain death. *Journal of the American Medical Association*, **205**, 337–340.
4. Skegg, P. D. G. (1974) Irreversibly comatose individuals: "alive" or "dead". *Cambridge Law Journal*, **33**, 130–144.
5. Lynn, J. Guidelines for the determination of death. Report of the medical consultants on the diagnosis of death to the President's Commission for the study of ethical problems in medicine and biomedical and behavioural research (1981) *Journal of the American Medical Association*, **246**, 2184–2186.

6. Conference of Medical Royal Colleges and their Faculties in the United Kingdom (1976) Diagnosis of brain death. *British Medical Journal*, **2**, 1187–1188.
7. Conference of Medical Royal Colleges and their Faculties in the United Kingdom (1979) Diagnosis of death. *British Medical Journal*, **1**, 332.
8. Korein, J. (1980) Diagnosis of brain death. *British Medical Journal*, **281**, 1424.
9. Levin, S. D. and Whyte, R. K. (1988) Brain death sans frontières. *New England Journal of Medicine*, **318**, 852.
10. Jonas, H. (1974) Against the stream: comments on the definition of death. In *Philosophical Essays. From Ancient Creed to Technological Man*, pp. 132–140. Prentice Hall, Englewood Cliffs.
11. Lamb, D. *Death, Brain Dead and Ethics*, (1985), Croom Helm, London, p. 75, quoted from Gaylin, W. Harvesting the dead, in *Harper's Magazine*, 1974.
12. Gervais, K. G. (1986) *Redefining Death*, p. 32. Yale University Press, New Haven.
13. Rodin, E., Tahir, S., Austin, D. and Andaya, L. (1985) Brainsteam death. *Clinical Electroencephalography*, **16**, 63–71.
14. Rodin, E. A. (1980) The reality of death experiences. A personal perspective. *The Journal of Nervous and Mental Disease*, **168**, 259–263.
15. Sabom, M. B. (1980) Commentary on 'the reality of death experiences' by Ernst Rodin. *The Journal of Nervous and Mental Disease*, **168**, 266–267.
16. *Op. cit.* Ref. 10, p. 130.
17. Pallis, C. (1983) ABC of brain stem death. The arguments about the EEG. *British Medical Journal*, **286**, 284–287.
18. *Op. cit.* Ref. 12, p. 165.
19. *Op. cit.* Ref. 11, p. 37.
20. *Op. cit.* Ref. 12, p. 35.
21. *Op. cit.* Ref. 10, p. 139.
22. Black, P. M. (1978) Brain death (second of two parts). *New England Journal of Medicine*, **299**, 393–401.
23. Green, M. B. and Wikler, D. (1980) Brain death and personal identity. *Philosophy and Public Affairs*, **9**, 105–133.
24. *Op. cit.* Gervais, K. G. (1986) (Ref. 12), p. 135.
25. van Till, H. A. H. (1976) Diagnosis of death in comatose patients under resuscitation treatment: a critical review of the Harvard Report. *American Journal of Law and Medicine*, **2**, 1–40.
26. Byrne, P. A., O'Reilly, S. and Quary, P. M. (1979) Brain death—an opposing viewpoint. *Journal of the American Medical Association*, **242**, 1985–1990.
27. Veith, F. J. and Tendler, M. D. (1980) In response to an opposing viewpoint on brain death. *Journal of the American Medical Association*, **243**, 1808–1809.
28. Siegler, M. and Wikler, D. (1982) Brain death and live birth. *Journal of the American Medical Association*, **248**, 1101–1102.
29. Roelofs, R. (1978) Some preliminary remarks on brain death. *Annals of the New York Academy of Sciences*, **315**, 39–44.
30. Report of the Swedish Committee on Defining Death (1984) The Concept of Death. Summary. Swedish ministry of Health and Social Affairs, Stockholm.
31. Pallis, C. (1985) Defining death. *British Medical Journal*, **291**, 666–667.
32. Wikler, D. (1990) Brain-related criteria for the beginning and end of life. *Transplantation Proceedings*, **22**, 989–990.
33. Veatch, R. M. (1978) The definition of death: ethical, philosophical and policy confusions. *Annals of the New York Academy of Sciences*, **315**, 307–321.
34. Moseley, J. I., Molinari, G. F. and Walker, A. E. (1976) Respirator brain. Report of a survey and review of current concepts. *Archives of Pathology*, **100**, 61–64.
35. Walker, A. E., Diamond, E. L. and Moseley, J. (1975) The neuropathological

findings in irreversible coma. A critique of the respirator brain. *Journal of Neuropathology and Experimental Neurology*, **34**, 295–323.

36. *Op. cit.* Ref. 11, p. 98.
37. Cranford, R. E. and Smith, D. R. (1987) Consciousness: the most critical moral (constitutional) standard for human personhood. *American Journal of Law and Medicine*, **13**, 233–248.
38. Curran, W. J. (1978) Settling the medicolegal issues concerning brain-death statutes: matters of legal ethics and judicial precedent. *New England Journal of Medicine*, **299**, 31–32.
39. Smith D. R. (1986) Legal recognition of neocortical death. *Cornell Law Review*, **71**, 850–888.
40. Belsh, J. M., Blatt, R. and Schiffman, P. L. (1986) Apnea testing in brain death. *Archives of Internal Medicine*, **146**, 2385–2388.
41. Van Donselaar, C. A., Meerwaldt, J. D. and Van Gijn, J. (1986) Apnea testing to confirm brain death in clinical practice. *Journal of Neurology, Neurosurgery and Psychiatry*, **49**, 1071–1073.
42. Sweet, W. H. (1978) Brain death. *New England Journal of Medicine*, **299**, 410–412.
43. Wetzel, R. C., Setzer, N., Stiff, J. L. and Rogers, M. C. (1985) Hemodynamic responses in brain dead organ donor patients. *Anesthesia and Analgesia*, **64**, 125–128.
44. Hill, D. J. (1987) Lower oesophageal contractility as an indicator of brain death in paralysed and mechanically ventilated patients with head injury. *British Medical Journal*, **294**, 1488.
45. Kass, L. R. (1971) Death as an event: a commentary on Robert Morison. *Science*, **173**, 698–702.
46. Delmonico, F. L. and Randolph, J. G. (1973) Death: a concept in transition. *Pediatrics*, **51**, 234–239.
47. Life-support ended, a woman dies. *New York Times*, December 5, 1976.
48. Luksza, A. R., Atherton, S. T., Jones, E. S., Dawes, P., Daniels, J. A. and Bisasur, P. (1980) Transplants—are the donors really dead? *British Medical Journal*, **281**, 1140.
49. Bradley, B. A. and Brooman, P. M. (1980) *Panorama's* lost transplants. *Lancet*, **ii**, 1258–1259.
50. Wainwright-Evans, D. and Lum, L. C. (1980) Brain death. *Lancet*, **2**, 1022.
51. Soifer, B. E. and Gelb, A. W. (1989) The multiple organ donor: identification and management. *Annals of Internal Medicine*, **110**, 814–823.
52. Legg, N. J. and Prior, P. F. (1980) Brain death. *Lancet*, **2**, 1378.
53. Korein, J. (1978) The problem of brain death: development and history. *Annals of the New York Academy of Sciences*, **315**, 19–38.
54. Ingvar, D. H. and Brun, A. (1978) Survival after severe cerebral anoxia with destruction of the cerebral cortex: the apallic syndrome. *Annals of the New York Academy of Sciences*, **315**, 184–214.
55. Black, P. M. (1978) Brain death (first part). *New England Journal of Medicine*, **299**, 338–344.
56. Jennett, B. and Hessett, C. (1981) Brain death in Britain as reflected in renal donors. *British Medical Journal*, **283**, 359–362.
57. Parisi, J. E., Kim, R. C., Collins, G. H. and Hilfinger, M. F. (1982) Brain death with prolonged somatic survival. *New England Journal of Medicine*, **306**, 14–16.
58. Nagle, C. E. (1982) Brain death with prolonged somatic survival. *New England Journal of Medicine*, **306**, 1361.

59. Fabro, F. (1982) Brain death with prolonged somatic survival. *New England Journal of Medicine*, **306**, 1361.
60. Klein, R. C. (1982) Brain death with prolonged somatic survival. *New England Journal of Medicine*, **306**, 1362.
61. Harris, R. (1982) Brain death with prolonged somatic survival. *New England Journal of Medicine*, **306**, 1362.
62. Dillon, W. P. (1982) Life support and maternal brain death during pregnancy. *Journal of the American Medical Association*, **248**, 1089–1091.
63. Loewy, E. H. (1987) The pregnant brain dead and the fetus: must we always try to wrest life from death? *American Journal of Obstetrics and Gynecology*, **157**, 1097–1101.
64. Field, D. R., Gates, E. A., Creasy, R. K., Jonsen, A. R. and Lares, R. K. (1988) Maternal brain death during pregnancy. Medical and ethical issues. *Journal of the American Medical Association*, **260**, 816–822.
65. Powner, D. J. and Fromm, G. H. (1979) The electroencephalogram in the determination of brain death. *New England Journal of Medicine*, **300**, 502.
66. Scott, D. F. and Prior, P. F. (1979) Prediction of brain damage by electoencephalography. *New England Journal of Medicine*, **300**, 1219.
67. Juguilor, A. C. C. and Reilly, E. L. (1982) Development of EEG activity after ten days of electrocerebral inactivity. A case report in a premature neonate— hydranencephaly or massive ventricular enlargement. *Clinical Electroencephalography*, **13**, 233–240.
68. Grigg, M. M., Kelly, M. A., Celesia, G. G., Ghobrial, M. W. and Ross, E. R. (1987) Electroencephalographic activity after brain death. *Archives of Neurology*, **44**, 948–954.
69. Ashwal, S. and Schneider, S. (1979) Failure of electroencephalography to diagnose brain death in comatose children. *Annals of Neurology*, **6**, 512–517.
70. Hughes, J. R. (1978) Limitations of the EEG in coma and brain death. *Annals of the New York Academy of Sciences*, **315**, 121–135.
71. Korein, J., Braunstein, P., George, A., Wichter, M., Kricheff, I., Lieberman, A. and Pearson, J. (1977) Brain death: I Angiographic correlation with the radioisotopic bolus technique for evaluation of critical deficit of cerebral blood flow. *Annals of Neurology*, **2**, 195–205.
72. Fackler, J. C. and Rogers, M. C. (1987) Is brain death really cessation of all intracranial function? *Journal of Pediatrics*, **110**, 84–86.
73. Hall, G. M., Mashiter, K., Lumley, J. and Robson, J. G. (1980) Hypothalamic— pituitary function in the "brain-dead" patient. *Lancet*, **2**, 1259.
74. Schrader, H., Krogness, K., Aakvaag, A., Sortland, O. and Purivs, K. (1980) Changes of pituitary hormones in brain death. *Acta Neurochirurgica*, **52**, 239–248.
75. Robertson, K. M., Hramiak, I. M. and Gelb, A. W. (1989) Endocrine changes and haemodynamic stability after brain death. *Transplantation Proceedings*, **21**, 1197–1198.
76. Aitkenhead, A. R. and Thomas, D. I. (1987) Lower oesophageal contractility as an indicator of brain death in paralysed and mechanically ventilated patients with head injury. *British Medical Journal*, **294**, 1287.
77. Sinclair, M. E. (1987) Lower oesophageal contractility as an indicator of brain death in paralysed and mechanically ventilated patients with head injury. *British Medical Journal*, **294**, 1488.
78. Taylor, M. J., Houston, B. D. and Lowry, N. J. (1983) Recovery of auditory brainstem responses after a severe hypoxic ischemic insult. *New England Journal of Medicine*, **309**, 1169–1170.

79. Owen, J. H. and Lai, C. W. (1984) Auditory brain-stem responses after hypoxic brain damage. *New England Journal of Medicine*, **310**, 991–992.
80. Taylor, M. J., Houston, B. D. and Lowry, N. J. (1984) Auditory brain-stem responses after hypoxic brain damage. *New England Journal of Medicine*, **310**, 992.
81. Nobin, A. and Bjorklund, A. (1973) Topography of the monoamine neuron systems in the human brain as revealed in fetuses. *Acta Physiologica Scandinavia*, (Suppl. 388) 4.
82. Mohandas, A. and Chou, S. N. (1971) Brain death: a clinical and pathological study. *Journal of Neurosurgery*, **35**, 211–217.
83. Molinari, G. F. (1978) Review of clinical criteria of brain death. *Annals of the New York Academy of Sciences*, **315**, 62–69.
84. Allen, N., Burkholder, J. and Comiscioni, J. (1978) Clinical criteria of brain death. *Annals of the New York Academy of Sciences*, **315**, 70–95.

3 Brain Death: Future Trends and Applications

As emphasized in Chapter 2, scientific understanding of the nature of the state termed "brain death" has changed considerably in the last 20 years. It is highly likely that contemporary understanding of brain death by neurologists, who have researched the subject, differs considerably from impressions of the subject held by the general community. Some of the reservations that have been expressed, as information about the state accumulated, in relation to questions such as whether "brain death" corresponds reliably with destruction of the brain and hence whether it is valid to equate it with "death" were discussed in Chapter 2. At the present time, there appears to be considerable pressure for reconsideration of what is meant by the term "brain death". At the same time that the term has been criticized by some for falling short of "death", there are calls from others for the adoption of less stringent criteria for its definition and recognition, In particular, it has been argued that the condition termed "cerebral death" should be regarded as equivalent to brain death.

RELATIONSHIP OF CEREBRAL DEATH TO BRAIN DEATH

Cerebral or neocortical death and brain death are both terms intended to describe clinically defined states. As was the case with brain death, the term cerebral death was coined to categorize a specific set of clinical features and a prognosis differing from that of brain death. This condition, which is more often referred to as "persistent vegetative state", is also considered to correspond with consistent pathological changes, distinguishable from those of brain death, in the structure of the central nervous system. "Brain death", as described in Chapter 2, implies either the irreversible cessation of function of both the brain stem and higher parts of the brain, including the cerebral hemispheres (in the USA), or of the brain stem alone, with consequent early cessation of function in other parts of the brain (in the UK). On the other hand, "cerebral death" implies destruction of the cerebral hemispheres but retention of structural integrity and function (including spontaneous respiration) of the brain stem.

Patients falling within the classification of cerebral death may present in two clinical forms: a persistent vegetative state or coma. Patients in a persistent vegetative state

> "have an eyes-open unconsciousness. They are awake but unaware. The eyes are
> open at times, during periods of normal wakefulness, and they have physiologic
> sleep/wake cycles which are readily apparent to observers. The damage in these
> patients is to the higher centres of the brain...the lower centres of the brain and
> brain stem are relatively intact."[1]

The general neurological assessment of patients in a persistent vegetative state is
that they have lost "all conscious awareness, including the capacity to experience
pain and suffering." Nevertheless, many of these patients display activity in
response to stimuli:

> "Nearly all regain sleep–wake cycles; many display the facial appearance of interest;
> and some even show emotional fluctuations with occasional infant-like tearing or
> smiling in response to non-verbal stimuli. Although none follow moving objects
> consistently, some occasionally move the eyes slowly towards visual stimuli. Others
> blink inconsistently to visual threat, startle or close the eyes in response to sudden
> noises, or demonstrate reflex groping or sucking."[2]

The responsiveness of patients in a persistent vegetative state may vary over a
period of time. The explanation presented to explain these behavioural patterns
is that they are entirely reflex in origin.

The persistent vegetative state is a consequence more often of a catastrophic
drop in blood pressure (as after myocardial infarction) than of trauma. It has
become more common as the standard of intensive resuscitation available to
patients during the first few days after its onset, when brain-stem function may
also be impaired, has improved. Many patients who are subsequently diagnosed
as being in the persistent vegetative state have required ventilator support for the
first few days until brain-stem function returns.

> "In contrast to the vegetative state, coma (the other clinical manifestation of
> cerebral death) is an eyes-closed unconsciousness. In these patients, there is
> extensive damage to the brain stem."[1]

These patients usually encounter respiratory complications leading to their death
within weeks or months. With the exception of rare cases of patients in a persistent vegetative state who have regained consciousness, sometimes after
prolonged intervals, both brain and cerebral death have been observed to be
irreversible. Undoubtedly it is this feature that has prompted the inclusion of
"death" in their description. However, whilst cardiac arrest with circulatory
cessation is often regarded as an early and inevitable sequel of brain death,
respiration and circulation may continue for prolonged periods in some patients
who have sustained cerebral death.

Since the time when the term "brain death" was first used, there have been
instances of linguistic confusion with the term "cerebral death". There have also

been persistent suggestions that a diagnosis of cerebral death should be accepted as equivalent to brain death for purposes of withdrawal of treatment, donor recruitment and legal certification of death. The case for replacement of brain death by cerebral death has generally been supported by the argument that irreversible loss of cognition provides a more appropriate sign of the end of human life than does loss of respiration. This case has been advanced by Gervais in a monograph appropriately entitled *Redefining Death*:

> "I hope to show that the neocortical death criterion rest on the same conceptual foundation as the brain death criterion, and hence is justified by the same argument."[3]

If "brain death" and "cerebral death" are interpreted literally as categorizing lesions of precisely the extent that these terms were intended to imply, the difference between the *notions* of what the two states entail is both clear cut and considerable. However, in view of the series of findings, already discussed on pp. 39–52 which suggest that there can be retention of activity in both the cerebral hemispheres and the brain stem of some patients satisfying the clinical criteria of brain death, the concept of loss of a crucial proportion of brain function and/or integrative functions, *rather than that of total loss*, has been proposed for this state. Consequently, I believe that the magnitude of the distinction between brain death, as it is now recognized, and cerebral death, as it is theoretically defined, may be less than was originally considered. It is unarguable that a state which patently does not correspond with complete destruction of the brain is now accepted as "brain death", i.e. the term used to identify the condition may no longer be an accurate description of its nature. Consequently, it could also be argued that the difference between this state and neocortical death becomes more of a quantitative matter of the proportion of the brain retaining some function rather than the qualitative difference which the two terms are often intended to convey.

Calls for the adoption of cerebral-death criteria to define brain death can be found in the literature from soon after the introduction of the latter term. For instance, a 1975 report of the British Transplantation Society, which considered the shortage of organs suitable for transplantation at that time, included the observation that:

> "Sir Michael Woodruff favoured a more radical approach to changing the law. On the question of cerebral death, he saw no objection to the diagnosis of death based on irreversible cessation of cerebral function provided the great majority of ordinary people were aware, and accepted, that doctors were using the word 'death' in this way."[4]

That the great majority of the people are unlikely to understand either the nature of "cerebral death" or that of the state to which the term "brain death" currently applies could be an occasion for some concern about the informed nature of any acceptance provided in relation to the use of these patients.

Another early call for adoption of a cerebral-death standard was based on the premise that the survival of the neocortex is "a precondition of what is distinctively human". It was argued that, unless treatment of patients in whom only the brain stem is functioning could be shown to benefit them, then "withdrawal of treatment can be justified, and an acceptance of only a neocortical definition of brain death may be indicated".[5] Whilst failure of treatment to afford benefit would appear to be very reasonable grounds for its withdrawal, it is not at all clear to me why it should also automatically provide grounds for a diagnosis of brain death. Unlike the Woodruff statement, which was explicitly directed towards increasing organ supply, it was not clear from the context of this communication whether "withdrawal of treatment" was to be construed as a warrant for "continuation of treatment until an organ recipient was prepared".

An event which was concerned with *cerebral* death, although it commonly initiated discussion of brain death, was the case of Karen Ann Quinlan. This irreversibly unconscious patient was the subject of prolonged legal proceedings aimed at permitting her disconnection from a respirator. Prior to disconnection, she had not met the requirements for diagnosis of brain death, a fact which was amply confirmed by her resumption of spontaneous respiration after disconnection.[6] The Quinlan case, nevertheless, provided the stimulus for extensive discussion of cerebral death, during 1976 and beyond. It appears in retrospect that the philosophy underlying management of this case considered a diagnosis of death to be a mandatory pre-requisite for discontinuation of resuscitation.

The potential for confusion, at least in the minds of the general community, between the states of brain death and neocortical or cerebral death has been compounded by some semantic overlap. The two expressions "brain death" and "cerebral death" have, on occasion, been used with the intention of describing a state of total brain inactivity, as though synonymous:

"Strictly speaking, cerebral death is defined as irreversible destruction of both cerebral hemispheres exclusive of the brain stem and cerebellum. However, cerebral death has been and is often still [1978] used as a synonym for brain death."[7]

This confusion should lead to further concern about the value of informed consent in situations in which community understanding is likely to be most imperfect. Another, semantically based, argument in favour of the use of the expression "cerebral death" to encompass what was then understood as whole brain death was presented at the same meeting of the New York Academy of Sciences as the preceding observation:

"I balk at using a noun, brain, as an adjective, as in brain death. I have therefore fallen into the trap of using cerebral as the adjective derived from cerebrum."[8]

Whatever the origins of usage of "cerebral" as equivalent in value to "brain", the practice has recurred at intervals. A major multicentre study of the criteria for diagnosis of brain death reported by the US National Institute of Neurological and Communicative Disorders and Stroke in 1976 referred throughout the text, and in its title, to "cerebral death".[9] The term was clearly intended to represent "total destruction of the brain", as brain death was originally envisaged. The term "brain death" was substituted for "cerebral death" at several places in the text. The state in which "all functions attributed to the cerebrum are lost but certain vital functions...may be retained", which is commonly described as cerebral or neocortical death was referred to as "irreversible coma" in the study.

The arguments originally advanced for substitution of the less extensive cerebral death concept for that of brain death have evolved over two decades. In the aftermath of the Quinlan case, considerable emphasis was placed upon the retention of cognition as a benchmark in deciding upon provision of life support. Whilst the diagnosis of this patient as dead had not been the issue, one commentator on the New Jersey court decision in relation to Karen Ann Quinlan framed his discussion of its implications in terms of "cognitive death".[6] He noted that the court had decided that, provided cognition was irretrievably lost, "the patient's physicians and family could take steps that the court thought would lead to her death". Parenthetically, the commentary pointed out, the court arrived at its decision after making a number of assumptions that contradicted both medical and logical probability ("the court stated some conclusions that had limited evidentiary support"). Regardless of the underlying reasoning, the court effectively spelt out a precedent:

> "The state's interest in protecting life was not believed compelling in view of the evidence that she was a permanently noncognitive person...the noncognitive case like previable human fetuses whom the state cannot protect from abortion."[6]

Discussion of this commentary on the Quinlan case evoked the comment that "the next generation of problems" would involve cognitive death. If one recalls the sequence of events in the adoption of brain-death criteria, namely that they were used primarily as a guide for discontinuation of resuscitation and, to some extent, as an indemnity against legal action, but that subsequently they were used as the basis for the recruitment of organ donors, it is possible to speculate on the nature of "the next generation of problems". Recalling also, the manner in which the secondary objective of organ procurement from brain-dead patients has led to the continuation of resuscitative measures (from the imposition of which brain death criteria were originally intended to afford respite) the possibilities in relation to cerebral or cognitive death become much broader. One question about the extent of influence of the court decision, which was raised in discussion of the commentary, clearly anticipated some of the future problems:

> "If an individual with irreversible loss of cognition were declared dead, which could be possible, then one of the questions which could be asked is: why should the respirator be shut off? The irreversibly comatose person who has been labelled dead could be used for teaching, experiments or organ transplantation."[6]

The arguments that have been developed in order to establish cerebral death as an entity have centred more recently upon the proposition that cerebral death is tantamount to cessation of existence as a person. In the course of the presentation of these arguments, a number of similarities with the process of evolution of the original concept of brain death have become evident. It may be recalled that the term "brain death" arose originally as a device to accord recognition to a medical condition in which there was a certain and hopeless outlook for the patient who could no longer benefit from medical treatment. Having established that the patient no longer had any interests, a secondary influence, namely the possibility of organ harvesting, came into play and led to the development of strategies involving the continued provision of life support in the interest of potential transplant recipients. Some of the arguments that have been constructed more recently in relation to cerebral death may also have some implications for the current attitudes towards brain death itself. A good example of this is provided by a 1980 article "Brain death and personal identity" by Green and Wikler.[10] As implied in the title, the authors proposed that brain death has occurred when individual identity has been lost. According to this argument, a body stripped of identity is brain dead even if the body continues to live, as would be the case if brain-stem function continued. Whilst the authors equated the retention of capacity for cerebral function with the retention of personal identity, they did not nominate examples of clinical conditions to illustrate their point apart from indicating that an anencephalic infant would lack identity. To this end, they emphasized the distinction between the metaphysical question of what state of a body constitutes death and the biological one of how this is to be recognized. However, their article was concerned with individuals whose biological state is very different from that of the category of organ donor as it exists at present.

The alternative point of view, expressed by Lamb,[11] drew a sharp distinction between neocortical death and brain death. He described the concept of neocortical death in the following terms:

> "It has been argued that a diagnosis of death of the person could be linked to criteria for loss of certain characteristics (such as memory and behavioural patterns) associated with psychological aspects of human life. According to this view, if the cortex is totally destroyed, the patient has lost his or her personal identity."[11]

However, this basis for death is rejected because of its differences from brain death as recognized in 1985:

> "According to the concept of brainstem death so defined as the irreversible loss of function of the organism as a whole, the loss of psychological attributes is a necessary but not a sufficient condition of death. Psychological aspects may be absent but human life may continue as long as integrated functioning persists."[11]

A restatement of the position of the preceding article, but with more emphasis from a clinical perspective, was presented in the *American Journal of Law and Medicine* by Cranford and Smith.[1] Once again, the title conveys the major thrust of the article:

> "Consciousness: the most critical moral (constitutional) standard for human personhood."[1]

Apart from the incorporation of a more specifically medical perspective in its content, this article is notable for the forceful tones of its advocacy. Its starting point is the proposition that "consciousness is the most important characteristic that distinguishes humans from other forms of animal life". The argument runs that, with the onset of permanent unconsciousness, personhood is lost. It is contended that irreversible loss of consciousness can be diagnosed with certainty, after a certain period has elapsed, and also that this state results not only in a loss of all capacity to experience pain and suffering but also in the loss of all neocortical functions. The first contention may find validation in accumulated clinical observation, the others certainly can not do so as they lie outside the scope of objective proof. Nevertheless, their absolute accuracy has been trenchantly claimed in the most unequivocal terms by the authors:

> "These views on the medical reality of the persistent vegetative state patient are scientific medical positions—statements of facts, not values."[1]

Leaving aside the question of the extent to which "pain and suffering" may be experienced in subcortical structures such as the thalamus, Cranford and Smith quote the American Academy of Neurology to provide grounds for the conclusion that patients in a persistent vegetative state have no capacity to experience pain or suffering.[12] The first ground, namely that clinical experience fails to reveal any behavioural indication of awareness of pain or suffering, would seem to be of strictly limited value in a patient deprived of any of the motor functions required to make communication possible. The feasibility of a patient remaining sentient and conscious, but deprived of motor function, is demonstrated by the condition described as the "locked in" state. Such individuals, who should be distinguishable by a competent clinician from patients in the persistent vegetative state, appear to retain capacity for experience of some sensations accompanied by an extremely limited capacity to achieve any form of communication with others. The second point, namely that post-mortem examination of patients in a persistent vegetative state reveals damage to the cerebral hemispheres "incompatible with consciousness or the capacity to experience pain or suffering" begs the question of the extent and location of residual hemisphere function required to accomplish these functions. The third point is that the technique of positron emission tomography (PET) has indicated that the rate of metabolism of glucose in the cerebral cortex is greatly reduced in the persistent vegetative state "to a degree incompatible with consciousness". Once again, the question arises as to how the required level was ascertained. Reference is made to studies showing that metabolic rates in the neocortex of such patients are 50–60% lower than those in normal, conscious subjects.[12]

In interpreting the results of techniques for measuring residual cerebral activity, it is necessary to bear in mind that there will be a level of activity below which tests may fail to give a positive outcome. Tests of *any* biological activity will give a negative reading when the sensitivity of the technology becomes insufficient to detect a low level of that activity. As already indicated in discussing the use of studies of cerebral blood flow rate to understand the nature of brain death, it is possible to decide that blood flow is not detectable with the technique in use. It is not possible, using such a technique on its own, to certify that there is no flow. As the sensitivity of the technique increases, there is a reduction in the difference between the minimal function that is detectable and complete lack of function. The recently developed technique of position electron tomography (PET) allows activity within specific parts of the brain to be determined with a sensitivity unmatched by any other means. The demonstration that activity is reduced to approximately half of the normal level in vegetative patients (i.e. approximately to the level observed in deep anaesthesia) has been interpreted as consistent with the hypothesis that persistent activity is largely confined to ancillary cells in the brain, whilst function of neurons (the cells responsible for the observed activities of the nervous system) has been substantially lost. Whilst these ancillary cells are necessary for the survival and functioning of neurons, they are themselves unable to undertake any of the functions of neurons or nerve cells proper. The ancillary or neuroglial cells are believed to perform functions such as providing physical support to neurons and facilitating electrical conduction within and between neurons. However, neuroglial cells are unable to replace neurons in undertaking sensory or motor functions. Consequently, loss of neurons with retention of their ancillary cells would be expected to remove the possibility of brain function.

It seems highly likely that a major part of the loss of function detected by PET represents damage to neurons rather than to supporting cells, as microscopic examination of the brains of persistent vegetative state patients at autopsy has revealed damage to be selectively concentrated in the former cells. Nevertheless, correlations between levels of brain function measured by PET and the results of subsequent microscopic examination of brains from vegetative patients fall short of establishing that a diagnosis of a vegetative state, or "cerebral death" is uniformly indicative of complete loss of function in the cerebral hemispheres.

The original presumption that brain death itself represented total loss of function, as implied in framing the Harvard criteria, has been abandoned. Similarly, it is not possible to be certain from post-mortem examination of the brain of a patient who has been in a persistent vegetative state that all cerebral function had ceased. It is generally conceded that some parts, both of the cerebral hemispheres and the brain stem, may remain functioning, even when the US criteria are applied. The aspect of the clinicopathological correlation, which introduces the greatest difficulty, is the variability in pathological features that has been observed by the time of post-mortem examination. It is not feasible to infer on pathological grounds alone whether or not self-awareness was lost during life. As discussed in the preceding chapter, the question of the possible retention of subconscious activity in severely brain-damaged patients remains not only unanswered, but unposed.

Furthermore, as was the case with conventional brain death, it is not possible from post-mortem examination of the nervous system to determine the timing of the observed degenerative changes in relation to the clinical course, even if one is confident that those changes occurred before cessation of circulation. The best information that can be provided relates to the state of the brain at the time of circulatory arrest. Any conclusions about the extent of destruction that had occurred at earlier times remains inferential. Inferences about the extent of brain damage based upon reliable prognostic indicators are almost universally accepted to be adequate for purposes of discontinuing life support following brain death. Some neurologists argue that this should be so also in the case of cerebral death.

The arguments that have been presented in favour of treating patients with *cerebral death* in the manner generally thought to be appropriate for the *brain dead* will be examined in due course. The measures to be taken relate both to the cessation of life support and the removal of transplantable organs. It may be appropriate to consider briefly at this stage the extent to which the two states are separable or may overlap. The contention that I have already made with respect to brain death, namely that the nature of a structural entity has been inferred primarily on the basis of current clinical observation of the patient's functional state and of his or her prognosis, applies with equal force to cerebral death. In neither case have clear cut anatomical features, which can be objectively measured, been shown reproducibly to correspond with precise clinical deficits. This is not surprising, given that a comprehensive understanding of the role of the multiplicity of fine anatomical structures in the brain in mediating such complicated functions as normal consciousness has yet to be attained. However, because of the considerable uncertainty that remains in determining the extent of the pathological changes to which each clinical term corresponds, I believe it becomes increasingly difficult to sustain the proposition that brain death and cerebral death are completely discrete entities. (This is not to imply that the respective sets of diagnostic criteria developed to categorize these states are other than reliable. It is, rather, to question *just what is being categorized*.) Brain death, as understood in the USA, implies the coexistence of the demonstrable physical changes believed to be characteristic of cerebral death together with irreversible loss of brain-stem function. However, it has become clear that isolated functions may be retained in the cerebral hemispheres (in both brain death and cerebral death) and in the brain stem (in brain death).

ADVOCACY OF SUBSTITUTION OF "CEREBRAL DEATH" FOR "BRAIN DEATH"

As indicated in Chapter 2, brain death has been anything but a static concept since use of the term and intensive observation of patients meeting the relevant criteria began. Both concepts—brain death and cerebral death—were initially proposed as a means of sparing patients from intensive attempts at resuscitation. However, it is a matter of record that brain death has been used secondarily as a means of selecting patients from whom organs may be harvested. Similar proposals have been made with respect to cerebral death. As indicated previously, a diagnosis of brain death is often medically superfluous in determining whether life support should be maintained for any individual. The impact on medical practice of legal climates in which a diagnosis of death has become a necessary indemnity against litigation has likewise been noted. Proposals for novel uses of brain dead subjects, in particular for their incorporation in experimentation, have been advanced repeatedly and, as will be related on pp. 72–81, are now being acted upon. Meanwhile there has been an ongoing history of advocacy for the inclusion of patients diagnosed with cerebral death within the patterns of management, and useage, now accepted for the brain dead.

Within 7 years of the first attempts to define brain death by means of the "Harvard criteria", criticism of the outcome was forthcoming on the basis that the original approach was outdated. In an article entitled "The whole-brain-oriented concept of death: an outmoded philosophical formulation", Veatch argued that an anatomically based concept of death was inappropriate.[13] In its place, he advocated the substitution of a concept of death that was based primarily on retention or loss of specified capacities. He proposed that the loss of these capacities could coexist with retention of varying degrees of anatomical integrity. Adopting such an approach, evidence of continuing structural survival of various parts of the brain would sit comfortably with a diagnosis of brain-functional death, provided the surviving parts were not responsible for any of the functions the loss of which was specified. It could accommodate in its stride any discordant indications of retained brain activity, such as those already described in Chapter 2. In effect, the survival of these structures and the retention of any functions attributable to them and detectable by clinical or laboratory means simply would not matter. The question inevitably arises, what functions would be specified as the benchmark? What criteria would be defined? Who would define them?

Most commonly, those arguing in favour of radical changes in the conceptualization and diagnosis of brain death have required that increased emphasis be placed on irreversible loss of consciousness and cognition rather than on the loss of respiration. Taken to its conclusion, this approach would lead to the replacement of brain death as presently defined by a version of cerebral death. One of the arguments advanced by Veatch in support of this change was that others could be harmed if a "corpse" (his term for any patient in a persistent vegetative state) were to be treated as if it was still a living person. A complication that was envisaged in abandoning the whole-brain concept of death was that spontaneously breathing subjects would have to be treated as dead. In this context Youngner and Bartlett[14] recalled the comment of previous writers in favour of the whole-brain formulation:

"Disconnecting a ventilator from a recently declared dead patient fulfilling tests of permanent loss of whole brain functioning is one thing; suffocating a spontaneously breathing patient is another."[15]

However, this objection to changing the ground rules was countered on the grounds that it is irrational:

"The statement also equates an emotional reaction to the treatment of a breathing body with the rational determination of whether the patient is dead or alive. The repugnance associated with suffocating such a patient has no more relevance to establishing the life or death of a human than does the horror felt at the continuing growth of a dead person's hair."[14]

I am unable to agree with what I take to be the point of this statement, namely that (apparent) growth of hair and spontaneous respiration are of similar value as indicators of life. Additionally, I would question whether there is likely to be any of the comparability implied between the "repugnance" and the "horror" felt by observers of the two events described.

An inescapable consequence of redefining death as irreversible loss of cognition, as Youngner and Bartlett suggest, will be that the new criteria are concerned with loss of those functions that are confined to the human species, and ignore others that are shared with other living animals and which connote continued life in them. An objection that can be raised to any argument for higher brain function as the criterion of death is that it requires focussing on functions essential to one species. A more biological approach to death would require that its definition would encompass attributes, the loss of which connotes death in all animal species. Youngner and Bartlett's response to the proposition that being alive is something that is shared with other living things was that consciousness and cognition are essential features of *human* life. A similar approach was advocated by Veatch:

> "[O]ur concept of death must be further refined, and our technical criteria for death must be modified accordingly so that our concept and criteria most accurately reflect our understanding of what is essentially significant to the nature of man."[13]

Apart from the issue of whether it is reasonable to consider death in a "speciesist" manner, their position seems to me to make a substantial assumption about the capacities of some non-human species. The extent to which processes such as consciousness and cognition operate, for example, in the higher non-human primates, is unknowable. Younger and Bartlett's definition of death is influenced much more by social than biological considerations.

Discussion of having to suffocate a patient in whom spontaneous respiration is continuing raises one of the first of the new ethical problems that is likely to arise in any transition from whole-brain death to cerebral death: patients meeting criteria for diagnosis of cerebral death breath spontaneously without the requirement for a respirator. Recent commentaries on this issue have sometimes suggested that this need not present an insuperable problem to regarding them as dead. Puccetti summed up the situation as follows:

> "Many who have followed me so far [in advocating the adoption of a neocortical death standard] would nevertheless balk at the problem of disposing of human remains capable of breathing spontaneously. They would say that active intervention to stop the breathing prior to preparation for burial is not only presently illegal but morally murder."[16]

It is suggested that the "disposal problem in a more enlightened age" could run along the lines that "She's dead but her body is still breathing, so we're going to stop the breathing and prepare her body for burial".[16]

A similarly matter-of-fact approach to the subject of disposing of the neocortically dead was adopted by Gervais:

> "When the neocortically dead patient has been declared dead, we would simply stop the remaining bodily functions by an inexpensive, aesthetically tolerable procedure. Those who administer the means for stopping the remaining functions must understand that the person is already dead, and that their action is therefore not killing."[17]

Gervais finds no difficulty in managing

> "the sensibilities of those who cannot change their responses [in regarding a patient who is breathing spontaneously as still being alive], for the spontaneous functioning of the neocortically dead can be discontinued after death has been declared and before funeral services".[17]

The issue of withholding support from "neocortically dead" patients

inevitably becomes one of determining which other "treatment" is to be terminated. The answer to this question will depend upon whether one's primary
objective is to spare the patient from "treatment" or to procure an early death,
in the conventional sense. Simply "allowing" death will not ensure that it occurs
in these patients. There has been much discussion on the issue of whether basic
nursing care and the provision of hydration and nutrition should be designated
as the "treatment" to be terminated when a diagnosis of cerebral death is formulated. Perhaps the most explicit statement on this issue to have come from an
authoritative source is a position statement adopted by the Executive Board of
the American Academy of Neurology in April 1988.[12] This decreed that:

> "The artificial provision of nutrition and hydration is a form of medical treatment
> and may be discontinued in accordance with the principles and practices governing
> the withholding and withdrawal of other forms of medical treatment."[12]

In supporting this position the Academy drew an analogy between use of a respirator for a non-breathing patient and the feeding of patients unable to feed
themselves. The position paper contended that both procedures

> "serve to support or replace normal bodily functions which are compromised as
> a result of the patient's illness."[12]

The argument continued that provision of nutrition and hydration to an unconscious patient remains a medical rather than a nursing procedure because medical
judgement and monitoring are entailed in its management. I believe that it
would be difficult to frame any universally applicable solution to the question
of what constitutes "treatment". Circumstances can vary widely between
different cases. For instance, would intragastric and intravenous routes of
administration be regarded as equivalent procedures when deciding on
maintenance or withdrawal of nutrition?

The extent of the change in attitude that had occurred among American neurologists, as expressed in this 1988 position, can be gauged by a medico-legal
commentary published 11 years previously on the Quinlan case. In discussing
the implications of withdrawal of respirator support from patients in a persistent
vegetative state, two substantial difficulties were recognized. One of these concerned the reliability of a diagnosis of irretrievable loss of cognition. The other
concerned the question of *which* specific supportive measures were to be withdrawn.[18] The author commented upon the difficulty of determining irreversible
loss of cognition in patients who typically "move, make primitive sounds, and
grimace or withdraw when stimulated". Addressing the issue of withdrawal of
support, he speculated that

> "many physicians might be reluctant to discontinue treatment of a vegetative
> patient who retains enough vital functions to survive for a prolonged period

without respiratory support or drugs. As physicians well know, simply stopping major treatments does not ensure a prompt or tidy demise."[18]

An example of a demise which may not have been either prompt or tidy was provided by Nancy Cruzan, who died in December, 1990, some 12 days after cessation of "hydration and nutrition". Withdrawal of these medical measures followed the decision of a Missouri judge that Ms Cruzan had indicated that she would never have wanted to live "like a vegetable".[19] The case had entered the Missouri court after the US Supreme Court ruled against withdrawal of support on the grounds that the patient's wishes had not been clear. An issue likely to have a bearing on discontinuation of hydration and nutrition, but not on the interruption of spontaneous respiration, is the previously expressed wishes of the patient, to the extent that these are known. This became the crucial point in the management of Nancy Cruzan.

Projected legislative modifications that might eventuate if cerebral death were to replace whole-brain death as the standard have been discussed in anticipation of this change. The questions, "Should homicide laws refer only to persons rather than all live human beings?" has been raised.[1] A related suggestion was, "Not only should society consider increasing the criminal and civil sanctions for causing a person to become permanently unconscious, but society may also wish to reduce the criminal sanctions if a defendant causes the death of someone already in a persistent vegetative state". One stream of legal thinking has recognized even further opportunities for participation in the legal system by persistently vegetative patients. The potential for "keeping permanently unconscious patients alive for tax purposes and then timing the pulling of the plug to maximize insurance disability payments or pensions" has been pointed out by an American lawyer, David Smith.[20]

Smith's paper is of value in its presentation on one occasion, of a sequence of arguments which might have been expected to develop over an extended period. A summary of them provides a useful indication of the direction in which some speculation regarding cerebral death has proceeded. The point is made that:

"A more just and sensible position is to consider irreversibly unconscious noncognitive patients legally dead, but to recognize and account for the possibility of continuing biological existence."[20]

It is not considered essential that such "legally dead" patients must be buried or cremated. The patient, subject to family wishes (and funding), should be able "to obtain biological maintenance notwithstanding a legal certification of neocortical death". A possible resolution of the patient's predicament, similar to that advocated by Gervais, is suggested:

"if a neocortically dead patient biologically exists without the aid of artificial life-support machines, active termination by injection may be a more humane procedure to induce biological death than withdrawing fluids and nourishment."[20]

(As was subsequently done in the case of Nancy Cruzan.) Ten pages later, Smith advances a further stage of the argument:

"A neocortical death standard could significantly increase the availability of viable transplant organs. This raises the possibility that neocortically dead bodies, or part thereof, could be donated and maintained for long term research, for organ banks, or for other purposes such as drug testing or manufacturing biochemical compounds."[20]

The suggested range of uses was considerably in advance of what would then, or now, be generally regarded as acceptable for *brain dead* individuals. In recognition of this, a "concession" is introduced into the argument:

"If society is not yet ready to seek and accept donations of neocortically dead bodies for long term biological maintenance for transplantable or experimentation purposes, we may avoid the problem simply by treating neocortically dead bodies as we now treat whole brain donations ... Under this approach, biological existence would be maintained only for limited transplant purposes with the view toward terminating cardiopulmonary functions following the transplant procedure."[20]

It will be noted that this simple solution effectively assumes a favorable response to the highly contentious question of treating a spontaneously breathing patient as an object.

In a later paper, Smith repeated the proposal for "biological maintenance" of patients who had sustained cerebral death for prolonged periods and extended the catchment to include anencephalic infants.[21] It is notable that, whereas there does not appear to have been any published acknowledgement of the use of a patient meeting cerebral death criteria as a transplant donor, such use has been undertaken, with considerable publicity, in anencephalic infants. As will be discussed in Chapter 5, the numerical contribution that anencephalics could make to organ supply is miniscule. The number of patients in a persistent vegetative state is vast and it may be that the vigorous advocacy of anencephalic useage should be interpreted in that context. The changes to date in attitudes towards patients meeting cerebral death requirements recall the history of adoption of whole-brain death criteria. These were developed in the first instance for the purpose of deciding upon cessation of maintenance. Shortly afterwards they were used as an aid to the recruitment of organ donors. The newly sanctioned course of management for persistently vegetative patients, namely withdrawal of hydration and nutrition, would render them valueless as a source of organs. Gradual physical deterioration of the patient, consequent upon this step, would certainly *not* be compatible with the collection of organs in the optimal condition that is obligatory because of the duty of care owed to prospective recipients. As will be discussed on pp. 93–96, concern about deleterious effects on transplantable organs of circulatory cessation following disconnection of brain-dead patients from a respirator was responsible for initiation of the practice of prolonged resuscitation in order that they could be used as beating-heart donors. David Smith's discussion of use of the "neocortically dead" appears to have taken account of this difficulty and to have circumvented it by moving directly to their use (perhaps repeatedly) as beating heart donors. The most substantial limitation remaining to a concerted effort to classify cerebral death as a condition legitimizing use as an organ donor may be the degree of uncertainty remaining in diagnosing the condition and forecasting its course in the individual case.[22] As already indicated, this is a notable difference from the situation with brain death:

> "When and if certain diagnosis of persistent vegetative state becomes feasible for large classes of patients, a clearcut choice between stem-oriented and higher-brain-oriented definitions of death will be necessary."[23]

One prominent feature of the advocacy of programs for organ procurement from *whole-brain-dead* patients has been an invariable tendency to circumvent attitudinal obstacles to such programmes, not by adaptation of the programmes, but by well-planned strategies to manipulate community attitudes towards their less readily acceptable aspects. The manner in which this problem has been approached in relation to whole-brain death will be considered in detail on pp. 84–92. Similar solutions have been foreshadowed in the case of cerebral death. For instance, the article of Cranford and Smith which argued for the recognition of loss of cognition as the prime criterion of death did not call for scientific studies to attempt to validate the proposal. Rather it acknowledged that:

> "Society must be convinced that the diagnosis of the condition is certain, that these patients experience no pain and suffering and that the traditional goals of medicine cannot be served once a diagnosis of permanent unconsciousness has been made."[1]

If the general perception fails to accord with the opinion of the those who are responsible for regulating the certification of death, change of that perception is called for.

UTILIZATION OF BRAIN-DEAD SUBJECTS IN EXPERIMENTATION

Whilst there has been substantial community acceptance of the practice of using whole-brain-dead subjects as a source of organs for transplantation, the extension of use to include medical experimentation has been much slower. Nevertheless, such extension may be imminent. The subject has attracted limited attention in the past. It appears that this situation could be about to change. If this occurs, it seems highly likely that discussion of use of brain-dead subjects in experiments may have an impact on attitudes towards their principal use in transplantation programmes.

Incorporation of brain-dead patients into experimental procedures has been practised, albeit quite infrequently, since the 1970s. However, as the use of these patients as organ donors has burgeoned in recent years, so consideration of the possibilities that exist for using them for experimental or training purposes has attracted much more attention. The evident reticence of many clinicians to undertake experimentation, despite their commitment to transplantation programmes, raises the question of ethical similarities and differences between the two classes of procedure.

Speculation about possible use of brain-dead individuals in a range of procedures wider than transplantation began soon after acceptance of the concept of brain death. An editorial in the *Annals of Internal Medicine* reviewing the subject in 1988 recalled a 1974 article in *Harpers Magazine* by Willard Gaylin who suggested apprehensively that the use of "neomorts" for such purposes as experimentation, medical training, organ banking and immunologic manufacturing might come to be accepted practice.[24] These subjects, he speculated, might be maintained in "bioemporiums". The limited use, apart from transplantation, made of brain-dead subjects in the intervening years has not matched these suggestions. Nevertheless, experimentation has been undertaken and several types can be identified. However, before discussing them, it is appropriate to examine the question of the extent to which use of the brain dead in organ transplantation programs and in experimentation are separable entities.

In what ways does use of the brain dead for organ removal and for experimentation differ? Possible criteria that might be used to separate them include the aims of the procedure, its actual technical content, its perception by and impact upon participants and the immediacy of any benefits. The question that inevitably arises is whether every instance of use of a brain-dead subject can be confidently classified as clearly being either a case of organ removal for therapeutic transplantation or of experimentation. Alternatively, does the sharing of features result in a continuous spectrum extending from pure experimentation to clinical transplantation? Are there clearer lines of demarcation between some categories of experimentation than exist between organ collection and experimentation *per se*? Is it legitimate to consider the two subjects as discrete issues without substantial implications for each other?

The potential impact of experimentation on attitudes towards use of the brain dead in organ transplantation is probably its most important feature from the point of view of the medical community. If harvesting organs from, and experimentation upon, brain-dead subjects came to be regarded as closely related subjects, it is possible that any negative perceptions of the latter by the general community will attach to the former and so adversely affect donor recruitment. The most direct interaction between experimentation and transplantation relates to research aimed at improvement of techniques for organ preservation and harvesting.

When the two subjects are examined primarily from the aspect of procedural content, substantial affinities can be seen to exist between the use of brain-dead subjects as donors and as experimental preparations. The most prominent feature shared by transplantation and experimentation is the prolongation of life-support measures that would otherwise be discontinued because they were considered to be burdensome and useless to the patient. These measures are probably a more indispensable feature of the use of brain-dead subjects in experimentation than of their use as an organ source since, as will be discussed on pp. 93–100, there is reasonable experimental and clinical evidence to suggest that transplantation of organs from subjects who have already sustained cardiac arrest may be successful. In contrast, the usefulness of brain-dead subjects in experimentation depends upon the continuation of respiration and blood flow to the entire body that is as near normal as is achievable.

Many of the procedures that could be employed in an experiment may be already in use in the course of maintenance of brain-dead patients before organ harvesting. Possibly the most frequent aim of experimentation undertaken at present, or in the near future, is to improve the technical aspects of maintenance of patients so as to provide transplantable organs in optimal condition. Whereas in other types of experimentation on the brain dead, there may be procedures in common with organ procurement, although the aims differ, in this category of experiment both means and ends converge. Because of the existence of situations in which the demarcation between experimentation and organ harvesting practice becomes blurred, it is legitimate to ask *whether* there is a consistently identifiable "cut-off" between the two and, if so, where it is to be placed? What is considered to be experimentation at one location may be regarded as established practice at another. (Lack of a sharp distinction between established clinical practice and an experimental procedure is a feature that organ transplantation holds in common with many actively advancing fields of medicine.) Perhaps it would be more valid to classify some types of experimentation along with organ procurement, whilst others should be considered as "purely experimentation". Most of the arguments that have been raised in relation to classifying experiments on the brain dead may be more appropriately considered when possible regulation of the subject is discussed. However, one point that has been advanced as a consistent distinction between transplantation and experimentation is the immediacy of the impact of the former in clinical practice. This is expressed in the outcome that an "identifiable, critically ill recipient" may be benefitted within hours of the procedure.[24] In contrast, any beneficial outcomes of experimentation are likely to be more delayed and more impersonal in their application.

Why wasn't experimentation automatically approved once organ harvesting was accepted? Why distinguish between use of brain-dead individuals, whether it be in organ transplantation or in medical research, or for that matter in teaching, or whether it be in the ongoing production of renewable tissues or any of the other worthwhile purposes originally identified by Gaylin? Perhaps the major reason for the distinction has been that, whereas use for transplantation is regarded as laudable, use in experimentation is not necessarily perceived in a positive manner. A second, reinforcing motive might be that, if experimentation is currently perceived, rightly or wrongly, as an unacceptable practice by the community at large, then it is necessary that transplantation procedures be quarantined from it lest an adverse reaction is also directed towards them. As the majority of medical discussion of experimentation appears to have considered it to be either wholly or substantially unacceptable, the distinctions between it and transplantation, already mentioned, become of considerable importance.

A minority opinion has been that experimentation on brain-dead subjects is not only permissible but is a highly desirable activity. From this viewpoint, its proscription would be regarded as the unwarranted loss of an opportunity to achieve good. The outlook underlying this response has been that it is illogical to regard or treat a brain-dead individual any differently from a "conventional" cadaver, i.e. "brain dead" equals "dead". One of the most forceful advocates of this approach has been Joel Feinberg, professor of philosophy at the University of Arizona. His position on this subject will be considered later.

The extent to which experimentation has been undertaken on brain-dead subjects, as judged by published accounts, remains quite small. It is possible that some of the earliest instances of experimentation on brain-dead subjects were not recognized as such. Whilst discussion of its propriety has not usually considered the implications of variations in experimental detail, the responses that have occurred to specific examples of experimentation have often been strongly affected by the details of individual cases. The nature of these experiments may be conveniently classified, into three groups. One of these takes the form of a trial extension, after brain death, of procedures that may have been of benefit to the subject before that event. A second category, already mentioned, might include attempts to improve the preservation of potentially transplantable organs in brain-dead subjects. The third group of experiments could include protocols without any relationship to treatment of similar patients before brain death or to preparation of the subject to serve as an organ donor. These categories are best illustrated by specific examples.

An early example of the first category of experiment, intended to test the efficacy of a procedure, which could have been of benefit to the subject if brain death had not supervened, entailed the administration of lithium in an attempt to curtail excessive activity on the part of the pituitary gland in a child with tuberculous meningitis.[25] From the description of this case, it appears that preparations had already been made to initiate a trial of therapy when brain death was diagnosed. It was decided, nevertheless, to proceed, "the objective being to obtain information that could be useful in the future". After therapy for 3 days, it was clear that the desired effect of curtailing secretion of pituitary hormone had been achieved. The case report concluded with the enigmatic remark that "the study could not be continued because the child died from a mechanical ventilation problem". The discussion of the case did not give any indication of recognition that it represented experimentation on a brain-dead subject. However, an accompanying editorial in the *Journal of Pediatrics* drew attention to this feature. [26]

Experimentation on brain-dead subjects that was intended to increase their suitability for use as sources of organs for transplantation, or to perfect techniques to achieve this in others, is likely to have occurred, perhaps unwittingly, in the course of routine maintenance of patients during the interval between diagnosis of brain death and surgical intervention for organ removal. Some published accounts of such procedures exist. For instance, a 1979 report of trials of a perfluorochemical emulsion designed to substitute for blood as an oxygen carrier included its use for 24 h in several brain-dead accident victims. [27] The emulsion was found to be without harmful side-effects and the report appears not to have attracted comment at the time as an example of experimentation on the brain dead. The additional circumstance that the emulsion had also been tested in its inventor and several of his colleagues at the same time clearly indicated that the procedure was not expected to be harmful.

Another, somewhat related situation, which is uncommon but which raises a number of issues, concerns the maintenance of the brain-dead, pregnant woman. A 1982 editorial in the *Journal of the American Medical Association*, written in response to a report of such a case, identified a number of underlying attitudinal conflicts in the attending physicians. Noting the semantically contradictory objective of the obstetricians "to prolong maternal life in the face of brain death" the editorial observed:

> "The linguistic inconsistencies are, we believe, more than mere infelicities in usage. They reveal a deep—and in our view, justified—ambivalence about conventional wisdom on the definition of death, particularly the brain-death standard." [28]

There will inevitably be a substantial element of experimentation in prolonged maintenance of a brain-dead, pregnant patient. Loewy commented:

> "The farther from viability [of the foetus] maternal brain death occurs, the more does maintenance of the mother as an incubator come to resemble experimental therapy with its imperative for careful, informed consent." [29]

In considering this subject, Loewy felt that the differences between continued maintenance of a brain-dead patient in order to enable a foetus to attain viability and identical procedures embarked upon, either in order to preserve transplantable organs or for experimentation, justified different responses. He considered that the foetus "can be viewed as the biologic continuity of her life and the symbolic continuity of her being". [29] Whilst extended maintenance of a pregnant, brain-dead woman in order to improve the chances of foetal survival could be categorized as use of one individual for the benefit of another, it might be assumed that maternal consent to this procedure is likely to have been forthcoming.

It seems likely that the ethical acceptability of maintaining a brain-dead, pregnant subject will depend on the precise circumstances of the individual case. The unacceptable end of this spectrum could be represented, for example, by proposals for the use of female "neomorts" as incubators for IVF-produced embryos.

> "Even the many Australians unfazed by the idea [of surrogacy arrangements for IVF-produced embryos] were shocked last year when a Queensland bio-ethicist, Dr Paul Gerber. suggested using brain-dead women to gestate foetuses. It was a 'wonderful solution for the problem posed by surrogacy, and a magnificent use of a corpse' he reportedly said."[30]

The features of the latter type of proposal, in particular the initiation of gestation by medical attendants after the patient had sustained brain death and the very long period that would be required for any chance of foetal viability, appear to me to render this proposal not comparable with maintenance of the pregnant brain-dead subject. It is totally experimental.

The third form of experimentation on the brain dead, namely procedures undertaken without any relationship to possible benefit to that class of patients in which the subject would have been included before brain death, or to preservation of the subject's organs, has attracted more comment. The possible range of investigations has varied from ensuring the safety or efficacy of novel therapeutic procedures to observing the pattern of deleterious consequences of a potentially noxious intervention. In the former category, was a 1988 article describing the trial of an agent intended to lessen the chances of clot formation within the blood vessels.[31] In this case, consent for use of the brain-dead subject in the experiment was obtained from his next of kin. In discussing this experiment, the researchers nominated the outcome that they were able as a consequence of it, "to provide prospective volunteers (in further trials) with the data obtained in this study so that they can make.their decision on a more informed basis". In its combined application to brain-dead and normal subjects, this experiment resembled that described above in relation to use of a blood substitute. The authors included a discussion of the principles which, they believed, should apply to research on the brain dead. Their report did not attract criticism.

Finally, at the other end of the range, a recent experiment specifically intended to study the damage produced in a brain-dead subject by a noxious stimulus, attracted widespread condemnation. The experiment, undertaken in an Amiens hospital, entailed the administration of potentially lethal doses of the anaesthetic nitrous oxide to a brain-dead subject. Its stated purpose was to obtain data, which could be introduced in defence of several doctors accused of negligence in relation to death of a patient under anaesthesia.

"It was apparently carried out with the sole purpose of discovering whether the inhalation of pure nitrous oxide led to a cyanosis [blue discoloration] of the skin, which had not been observed in the dead patient's case."[32]

(My understanding is that cyanosis would be invariable under these circumstances and experimentation to establish this would be unnecessary.) The experimenter was Professor Milhaud, a professor of anaesthesiology, described as "a pioneer in techniques aimed at prolonging the biological functioning of the bodies of individuals declared clinically dead".

Responses within France to the experiment varied across the full range of possibilities. The National Association of Medical School Teachers appeared to close ranks in deciding that Milhaud "was only carrying out his duty". However, President Mitterand was considered to be referring to the case when he stated:

"We must never forget that the human being is not an instrument...neither the search for the truth, nor scientific progress should be allowed to challenge this basic value of civilisation."[32]

Defenders of the experimenter, in their turn, asserted that to preclude experimentation on the brain dead was comparable to the ecclesiastical prohibition that once applied to the dissection of corpses as a means to study anatomy. If death is a single state, albeit with a number of different manifestations one of which is brain death, then there would appear to be little rationale for discriminating between organ harvesting and experimentation.

Whilst most of the examples cited above have been characterized by a perceived need to defend from condemnation the use of the brain dead in experimentation, a considerably more assertive approach to the question of experimentation has been to equate conventional death and brain death without any questioning of the legitimacy of this assumption. A 1985 article by Feinberg in the *Hastings Center Report* provides the best possible example of such an approach to the issue. The question of the equivalence of the "dead" and the "brain dead" is effectively begged as early as the article's title, "The mistreatment of dead bodies".[33] Whilst the context of the article clearly relates to the experimental use of the brain dead, the opening discussion is effectively confined to the legitimacy and morality of employing conventional cadavers in the design of safer passenger restraints in motor vehicles.

Feinberg illustrated his argument by reference to a 1978 report entitled, "The quick, the dead and the cadaver population".[34] This described an incident in which the use of cadavers to facilitate the design of realistic dummies for testing the effect of motor vehicle collisions on passengers was aborted because of opposition to use of the human body in this way. As a result, it was likely that vehicle testing in order to design safer automobiles was significantly retarded and, ultimately, some deaths, which otherwise may have been preventable, could have occurred. Opposition to use of cadavers in testing in this instance was based on the belief that it entailed disrespect for the body and was a violation of human dignity.

I do not find it difficult to agree with Feinerg that the withholding of cadavers from vehicle tests, if these offered a real prospect of improving automobile safety and saving lives was a mistaken ordering of priorities. However, I disagree with both of the arguments that he employs to equate this incident with the subject of experimentation on the brain dead. The first argument is that objections to experimentation represent no more than apprehension about disrespect for a dead body. Its thrust was foreshadowed in the article's subtitle "The moral trap of sentimentality". Feinberg attributes the existence of distaste for experimentation to sentimentality:

"But the problems to which I call attention here involve possible conflicts not between interest and interest, or life and life, but between interest or life on one side and symbolism and sentiment on the other."[33]

He regards a newly dead body as "a sacred symbol of a real person" and suggests that to deny the possibility of using it for potentially beneficent experimentation is effectively attaching such a value to the symbol that it is favoured at the expense of the real interests of those who might benefit from the experiment. I believe that his suggestion is incorrect on at least two grounds. In the first place, "symbolism and sentiment" constitute an integral part of human life that cannot be dismissed in an offhand fashion. Secondly, I suggest that concern about use of brain-dead subjects runs much deeper than worry about disrespect to a cadaver.

Feinberg's second ground for supporting the use of the brain dead in experimentation is that such subjects, maintained on a ventilator and with continuing cardiac action, are equivalent to cadavers delivered from the mortuary to a vehicle testing laboratory. I consider that this proposition fails completely to address the question of *whether* the brain-dead subject is identical with, or is commonly regarded as identical with, a dead subject. The retention of the term "brain death" adequately testifies to me that a difference is *still* recognized between this state and conventional death.

Use in experimentation clearly can not benefit a brain-dead subject: can it be a burdensome imposition? If the brain-dead subject is considered to be equivalent to the "conventional" cadaver, inhibitions about his or her use in experimentation carry little weight on these grounds. Earlier discussion of attitudes towards the use of brain-dead subjects as organ donors has noted that such patients are commonly regarded as the equivalent of conventionally dead *for purposes of organ removal*. As described in Chapter 2, criteria originally developed as a guide to discontinuation of treatment were subsequently adopted as a basis for designating patients as a source of organs for transplantation. With a large measure of acceptance having been gained for this change of purpose, a second proposition has now become that of whether suitability for organ donation should automatically qualify a subject to be used in experimentation. The issue of the use to which a subject may be put following diagnosis of brain death has not yet generated extensive discussion. Nevertheless, two divergent approaches to the problem have been adopted.

One approach has been to query whether the subsequent use that one has in mind for a subject has to be taken into account in categorizing him or her as brain dead. An editorial comment of 1980 in the *Journal of Pediatrics*[26] in response to use of lithium therapy in a brain-dead child observed that:

> "Although there is increasing statutory and judicial approval of treating brain-dead patients as dead in the total sense, there is no law commenting explicitly on the use of brain-dead subjects for research, What rules, if any, should apply to research on a brain-dead subject? Should they be the same as those pertaining to research on the clearly living? Should they be the rules covering those who are dead in the total sense? Or should there be special consideration for patients whose brains have ceased to function but who are alive in most other respects."[26]

The editorial writer has effectively presented the question of whether thinking should be adjusted to accommodate not two, but three categories of individual: the live, the dead and the brain dead.

Having explicitly taken the point that brain death is a valid reason for ceasing treatment, not necessarily because a patient is dead but because he or she no longer has any interest in being maintained, the editorial noted that brain death was not a necessary prerequisite for this. It then proceeded to grasp the nettle almost invariably passed over in other commentaries:

> "We do not know whether patients who meet the Harvard criteria of brain death experience discomfort. It is extremely unlikely and probably unknowable, but the risk-averse individual might prefer that painful procedures not be done on him, or that his life not be prolonged to allow even painless procedures."[26]

Having raised the question of whether a set of criteria intended to serve as a basis for cessation of treatment can legitimately be applied to recruitment as an experimental preparation, the article queries the extent to which prior consent to this by a brain-dead subject can provide justification. The author arrives at the position that use of brain-dead subjects without previous consent may be permissible "provided the purpose of the research is important". An inconsistency that is introduced if consent is considered to authorize experimental use derives from the impossibility of such consent being genuinely "informed" given the "unknowability" of the ability of the brain dead to experience discomfort. It would be necessary to reconstruct the patient's likely wishes on the basis of his or her known views. There would appear to be an absolute proscription on making such a reconstruction in the case of children not competent to provide informed consent.

It can become a short step from arguing that a practice is permissible to proposing that it is a requirement to adopt without further question. This step has been taken in the course of some arguments for experimentation with the brain dead. For instance, the response of some of the supporters of Professor Milhaud after the experiment described above, as reported in *Science*, was that "experiments on the human body had always been a necessary element of medical progress".[32]

Irrespective of the attitude that one adopts towards experimentation on the brain dead, the subject draws attention to an issue that has previously been almost totally ignored. This is the question of whether different courses of management of a patient may all be automatically validated once brain death is diagnosed. As discussed in Chapter 2, the original reason for creating the concept of brain death was to provide reliable guidelines for discontinuing treatment, which was no longer of advantage to the patient. The extension of the possible courses of management that would be permissible following brain death to the use of the patient as a source of organs soon followed without serious discussion of the issue of whether both courses were equally validated by the diagnosis. General reticence to undertake experimentation clearly indicates that end use of the brain dead may be regarded as an issue to be debated. Is brain dead, indeed dead enough to be submitted to organ harvesting but not dead enough to become an experimental subject?

THE IMPACT OF MANAGEMENT OF BRAIN-DEAD SUBJECTS ON OTHERS

> "There still remains an uneasiness about the provision of meticulous care to a human being who may be physiologically stable but legally dead, and this is enhanced by the fact that sophisticated medical care is suddenly and irrevocably withdrawn once organs are harvested from such patients."[35]

Reticence on the part of many medical personnel to become involved in soliciting permission from the families of brain-dead subjects for their use in transplantation has been identified as a major factor in retarding the development of transplantation programmes.

> "Denny [a transplant coordinator] described physicians and nurses as 'the weak link' between the organ-procurement programs and the public, because they often 'shirk' the task of explaining to families the meaning of brain death."[36]

A number of commentators have referred to the potential that exists for unfavorable impact on the attendant medical personnel of involvement in organ harvesting from brain-dead patients. In a discussion in the *New England Journal of Medicine*, of the psychosocial implications of organ retrieval, a group from Cleveland made the point that, even though health professionals may be familiar with the definition of brain death, they may be swayed by the evidence of their senses into regarding brain-dead individuals as still alive.[37] Furthermore, it is suggested that deliberate choice of an operating theatre workplace by medical and paramedical staff may reflect a wish to avoid the exposure to patient death, which is a feature of work in the wards. Death rarely occurs in theatre. If this wish to avoid contact with death influenced choice of workplace, then participation in organ harvesting from brain-dead patients brought into theatre could prove especially disturbing.

Another group who were reported to experience resentment as a result of involvement in organ harvesting were neurosurgeons:

> "We do it for somebody else. It is an inconvenience. I'm busy enough. It is not a role I choose and I wish I didn't have it."[35]

It was concluded from interviews with neurosurgeons that this resentment springs from a number of factors. These include displeasure with the frequent calls at irregular hours and apprehension (at least in the USA) about the possibility that litigation could be directed against them in the future. Perhaps the necessity for extended involvement with brain-dead subjects manifesting many of the normal signs of life was also a contributing factor. An additional group of medical personnel likely to experience a severe impact as a result of their rare exposure to brain-dead subjects are obstetricians. As already mentioned, there have been a small number of reports of prolonged maintenance of brain-dead pregnant women in an endeavour to secure the birth of a live infant.

Whilst some consideration has been given to the psychological impact on medical personnel of involvement in maintenance of the brain dead for purposes of organ harvesting, this has usually been motivated by concern about the possible retarding effects of this impact on their effectiveness in donor recruitment rather than by primary concern about the basis for the impact or its significance for the welfare of affected personnel. Even less attention has been given to the subject of possible longer term impact of organ donation on the donor's family. This contrasts with the considerable effort that is currently being expended in order to counteract any attitudes, held by the relatives of *potential* donors, which might inhibit their participation in donation. For example, factors which have yet to attract serious attention include any subsequent impact on the donor family of death of the transplant recipient or of an increased awareness, after the event, of the technical procedures that organ collection from beating-heart donors entails. As regards the former, the very limited evidence available does not suggest that donor families experience a "second grief response" or a feeling that the donor had "finally died completely". A 1971 article on this subject from Stanford University Hospital suggested that:

> "Donor families appeared to view donorship as a positive experience even when the heart transplant patient died."[38]

Nevertheless, as this review was based on the experience of some 20 donor families assessed 1–2 years after heart transplantation, its results may have little bearing on the longer term impact of the event on the surviving family. Reliable information about the possibility of residual impact at a later stage is virtually non-existent. As regards the second influence identified above, namely the possible impact on donor families of a subsequent realization that the semantics used in relation to organ harvesting from beating-heart donors convey an inaccurate impression of the procedure, no research appears to have been undertaken. Any investigation of this type would become feasible only when the community gains a more accurate understanding of both brain death and organ transplantation procedures.

The assessment of one experienced neurologist that "A currently uninformed public will sooner or later discover how misleading this simple formulation [of brain death] really is"[39] implies that this impact may have unfavourable consequences for future donor recruitment. Conceivably, subsequent realization by the family that the circumstances surrounding removal of organs from beating-heart donors differed considerably from the impressions held by the donor's family at the time of decision may lead to a later reappraisal. As indicated above, virtually all medical study to ascertain attitudes of the families of donors seems to have been motivated primarily by a wish to influence relatives to consent to organ transplantation.

Two remedies might be envisaged for the reticence frequently expressed by medical personnel in relation to participation in organ-donor recruitment. Perhaps reticence about participation on the part of medical staff suggests that it is premature to assume that recruitment of patients to provide organs is acceptable to the community. Alternatively, if it is believed that the community both understands and supports the practice, it will be necessary to devise means to circumvent any hindrance produced by medical personnel.

Certainly, by far the most frequent response to the possibility that use of brain-dead subjects as organ sources may have a negative impact on associated medical personnel has been to seek to neutralize that impact even if this requires measures that verge on coercion. The alternative strategy of identifying the basis of any negative impact, so that donor-management practices may be modified to remove or lessen it seems to have been overlooked. This choice of response recalls the typical responses to observations that tend to undermine the validity of the brain-dead state, as exemplified in Chapter 2. These responses have taken the form of reasserting the concept while discounting the reliability of the discordant observation as an indicator of brain death. In similar fashion, the usual response to concern about psychological effects of organ donation, has been to encourage and assist affected medical personnel to accept donation procedures *as currently practised*, not to question them. An example of this solution was provided in an article that reported retention of the capacity of brain-dead subjects to respond to surgical incisions in the course of organ removal by changes in blood pressure. It was suggested that:

> "Although these responses may suggest partial lower medullary functions, the
> medical personnel caring for the donor should be reassured that such a response
> does not invalidate the diagnosis of brain death."[40]

The question of the identity of the individual providing reassurance was not
taken further.

Examples of the institutional response to any expression of reservations about
organ collection on the part of medical personnel, are contained in the
proceedings of a US Congressional inquiry into organ transplantation. The sub-
mission from a "director of organ procurement" quoted at the commencement
of this section is typical of the responses presented. The most common response
to this perceived failing on the part of medical personnel has been to undertake
conditioning regimes designed to minimize their ambivalence. However, such
preparation has not been restricted to medical personnel likely to be responsible
for donor recruitment. The introduction into high school courses of conditioning processes designed to inculcate positive attitudes towards organ
harvesting from brain-dead subjects has been advocated:

> "Classroom discussion will generate discussion within the family with the result
> that organ donation will be an expected, normal form of activity, rather than some-
> thing unusual and tumultuous."[41]

To advocate the facilitation of a situation in which the death of a loved one
would be accepted as a normal activity suggests to me that the author was not
in touch with reality. The circumstances associated with death and decisions on
organ removal will always be catastrophic and tumultuous for any psychologically normal individual. Consequently, the extent to which use of brain-dead
family members can be successfully promoted as an unquestioned "normal form
of activity" within the community remains to be seen.

PROBLEMS OF DONOR RECRUITMENT

> "Things are not going well for the organ transplantation enterprise. Despite
> universal legal recognition of brain death and sanction of organ procurement in the
> United States, the ratio of actual to potential donors remains woefully inadequate.
> In fact, the situation seems to be growing more critical as organ transplantation
> becomes the treatment of choice for more and more Americans whose own
> kidneys, livers and hearts can no longer sustain them. Efforts to correct this situa-
> tion with donor cards, public education programs, and, more recently, required
> request laws have met with limited success."[42]

This assessment of the current situation was presented in 1990 to the Transplantation Society.

"Cyclosporine, introduced as a new immunosuppressive drug in the early 1980s, is credited with remarkable improvements in kidney transplantation and with the transition of heart and liver transplantation from experimental to effective therapy."[43]

There is little doubt that most, if not all, communities are currently experiencing a sharp donor/recipient imbalance in respect of all transplantable organs. This is probably a reflection of improvements in success of transplantation during the last decade with a consequent burgeoning of waiting lists. A 1988 editorial in the *New England Journal of Medicine* noted that the annual number of kidney transplants performed in the USA had increased from 6000 to 9000 between 1983 and 1986, whilst heart transplants had increased from 172 to 1368 in the same period. Nevertheless, the numbers of potential recipients for kidneys, hearts and livers had continued to increase rapidly, despite the large numbers treated over this period.[43] Whilst it would be hazardous to attempt to identify future trends based on recent data from a limited number of years, it appears highly likely that waiting lists for organ transplants will continue to lengthen. An earlier editorial review of heart transplantation, published in 1984,[44] concluded that the number of heart donors potentially available at that time appeared to be "about appropriate". However, it cautioned that, "if indications for heart transplantation are considerably expanded in the future, a major donor shortage can be anticipated".[44]

The pressure that the waiting list for heart transplants generates is accentuated by the probability that many, assessed as suitable recipients, will die before they reach the head of the waiting list. The number of potential USA recipients likely to die before an organ becomes available was estimated at one-third in 1986.[45] At the same time, it was also estimated that only 14% of potential donors (i.e. patients in the appropriate age range, free of contraindicating disease but diagnosed as brain dead) were actually used as donors in 1984. This was considerably less than the frequency with which the community at large expressed a willingness in opinion polls to serve as organ donors. Before outlining the measures that have been advocated to bring the frequency of actual donors closer to its potential, it should be noted that the reticence of doctors to take part in organ retrieval procedures discussed in the preceding section has been accorded considerable importance in failure of donations to approach the potential level. Reasons adduced for this attitude range from "fear of legal repercussions to simple ignorance of who is a suitable donor and whom to call."[46]

"Early donor recognition, rapid and accurate declaration of 'brain death', physiological maintenance, and coordination with the local organ procurement agency are all important aspects of organ donor management."[47]

Efforts to increase the frequency with which suitable patients, diagnosed as brain dead, are used as a source of organs for transplantation have been directed both towards potential donors, before the occasion, to their families at the time of it, and to medical personnel. The use of "donor cards", either as a separate entity or as part of a driver's licence, by means of which an individual can indicate a willingness to be used as a source of transplants, in the event of their being diagnosed as brain dead, appears to have made little impact. It is likely that most doctors would wish to obtain family consent before referring patients as organ donors. In the light of the existing community misconceptions about brain-dead patients, discussed above, it is not clear that "consent" would necessarily equate with "informed consent".

Concerted efforts to increase community knowledge about organ transplantation have been suggested frequently. An article entitled "Getting organ...ized", from a member of a Californian Regional Organ Procurement Agency called on the medical profession to find "ways to differentiate between the layperson's understanding of death, and more clinical criteria". She continued:

> "How can the public or even media reporters understand 'brain death' when hospital spokespersons announce that someone has been declared brain dead but is being kept 'alive' on 'life-support' systems?"[48]

Her conclusion in relation to presentation of information was:

> "'Death' must mean death and there must be clarity and confidence in the public's mind that organs are removed only after death has been declared."[48]

Related reservations about the impression in the community concerning brain death in relation to organ retrieval came from another individual involved in transplantation:

> "The notion that we can quickly resolve our society's ambivalence with laws and regulations is misguided."[42]

Presentation of organ transplantation in a positive light to the families of brain-dead patients, who are potentially available as donors, has been suggested as a worthwhile strategy. The director of organ procurement at the University of Pittsburgh reported that he always wrote to donor families to tell them what happened to donated organs:

> "Frequently the families write back saying that it was a source of comfort to them to know that someone else benefited from the death."[46]

In a more pragmatic vein, an Australian Health Department paper on "Co-ordination of donor organ acquisition" identified as a priority:

> "... support of the donor families, lest any adverse experiences jeopardise the reputation of organ donation."[49]

One aspect of management of the donor family, in the period after transplantation, to have received attention relates to the provision of information about the
recipient and to communication between the recipient and the donor family. A
survey undertaken by the Transplant Service, Cleveland, USA reported positively on the outcome of transmission of letters of thanks from organ recipients
to donor families:

> "Some of the families expressed relief knowing their gift was a success, and happi-
> ness that a part of their loved one lived on in the recipient." [50]

The concept of "living on" of the donor in the transplant recipient was commonly expressed by donor families, as also was the proposition that, as a result
of transplantation, the death of the donor had not been in vain. As such studies
of the impact of the use of a family member as an organ donor on the bereave-
ment process have been infrequent, it is difficult to draw any long term conclusions about its effect on further donor recruitment. The possibility of tapping
in to patients who have already received transplants has been raised:

> "[T]hey, and their ever-increasing corps of new beneficiaries (10,000 per year of
> kidney, liver and heart) could form a self-perpetuating advocacy group." [51]

A significant factor that would require consideration in any substantial study
of these subjects is the nature of the circumstances surrounding the occurrence
of brain death of the donor. For instance, it has been reported that over one-
third of the donors in 40 cases of heart transplantation undertaken at Louisville,
Kentucky had become available as a result of suicide. [52] It has been recognized
that families of suicide victims are more likely to consent to multiple organ donation than are those of other categories of brain-dead patient. It is highly likely
that an underlying wish to ensure that the death of the family member has not
been entirely in vain provides adequate motivation for this response.

Whether the longer term outcome for the families of organ donors remains in
accord with the short-term reaction is undetermined. A bizarre variant of the
involvement of suicide victims in transplantation, but one which provides an
insight into one aspect of the impact of organ procurement on the community,
concerns "living would-be donors" of organs indispensable to life:

> "One man who telephoned claimed to be holding a pistol to his head and clicked
> the safety catch throughout the conversation. He stated that he intended to shoot
> himself but wished to donate his heart for transplantation. He offered to shoot
> himself at the time and place of our choosing." [38]

Apart from the need to undertake later surveys to determine the ultimate impact
of organ donation on donor families, the possible effect on them of knowledge
of the longer term course of the transplant recipient requires investigation. If the
notion that part of the loved one "lives on" in the recipient is to be fostered,

or not actively discouraged, are unfavorable outcomes, perhaps after initial success, also to be transmitted to the donor family? If, as the limited available surveys suggest, this notion of "living on" acts as an incentive to some families to participate, is it fair to release only information which reinforces the family decision? There do not appear to be specific answers available to this type of question.

The subject of direct identification of recipient and donor's family to each other is a different issue. There have been some florid examples in the USA of publication of donor identity:

> "A Nashville newspaper headline read, 'Heart–Lung Transplant Underway'. Beneath this were the name and address of a donor who 'shot herself in the head with a rifle about 3 pm Friday while at a friend's house."[52]

Similarly there have been some highly questionable media attempts to uncover the identity of organ donors for celebrity recipients:

> "In the case of Linda Machiano ("Linda Lovelace") of 'Deep Throat' notoriety, a tabloid offered $5000 for the identity of her liver donor."[52]

The use of an anencephalic infant as a heart donor has been accompanied by the introduction of donor and recipient families on television. Fortunately, such episodes are rare. However, the issue of the appropriate response to later requests by donor family or recipient to meet the other, may have to be met. The reversal of attitude that has recently occurred, with release of information about the identity of biological parents to children after adoption and artificial insemination by donor may affect practice in transplantation. If so, contact between transplant recipients and donor families may become more frequent with the objective of strengthening community inclinations towards organ harvesting from brain-dead relatives.

Whilst strategies to increase the availability of donors have been directed to the community as a whole, major effort has been directed to medical personnel likely to have the responsibility of caring for potential donors. As indicated above, the unwillingness of doctors to be involved in referral of brain-dead patients to transplant programmes is thought to be an important reason for the low frequency of use of such patients. The tactics advocated to modify doctors' behaviour frequently verge on the coercive. This approach is also apparent in the coercive response to donor management of "contracting out". In the "contracting out" system, which has been in place for some years in a number of European countries, it is legally permissible to remove organs from any brain-dead patient, unless he or she has explicitly indicated unwillingness at some earlier date. However, in these countries:

> ". . . little improvement has been seen, underlining the necessity for the cooperation

of the medical profession in the referral of a brain stem-dead patient as a potential organ donor."[53]

Another form of coercion of medical personnel is embodied in the concept of "required request", which has been adopted in the USA for some years. This requires that inquiry of the family of brain-dead patients about the possibility of organ harvesting be made, as a routine, at the time that discontinuation of life-support measures is discussed. In advocating the introduction of this legislation, an ethicist identified its objective as being that of mandating that:

"No-one on a respirator who might serve as an organ donor could be declared legally dead (assuming that the medical requirements for such a declaration had been met) until a request for donation had been made of any available next of kin or legal proxy."[54]

Use of the verb "to serve" together with the idea of being a donor might strike some as incongruous.

A variant of the "required request" policy has been advocated in an Australian report on donor organ acquisition:

"It could be made mandatory that doctors in Intensive Care Units consider all patients for organ donation before withdrawing support...Hospitals should be compelled by law to institute mechanisms whereby all brain dead victims are assessed as possible donors of organs. Permission for multiple organ donation should be sought, but such an approach should be sympathetic to donation of specific organs. A voluntary system which allows for potential donors to opt out may not be able to keep up with the demand for organs."[49]

These are strongly expressed points of view. Undoubtedly, organ transplantation can offer great benefit to recipients. Equally clearly, the present availability of suitable organs is insufficient for the treatment of those who are on waiting lists or likely soon to become so. Many medical personnel, I suspect, would regard these administrative stratagems as unreasonable. Irrespective of the issue of their propriety, their likely efficacy remains an open question.

The institution of policies such as "contracting out", and of other measures that are expected to increase the frequency of organ retrieval, in some countries, but not in others, can result in significant changes in the exchange of organs between transplantation clinics. For example, a 1990 report from Belgium documented the occurrence of an increased export of organs harvested in that country, following the introduction of a "presumed consent" law. It warned that:

"The existence of different organ procurement policies among countries collaborating within the same organ exchange organization leads to a permanent imbalance in organ availability which could ultimately jeopardize the survival of these institutions."[55]

Differences in transplantation practice between countries may result in a traffic not only in organs, as in the European exchange system, but in prospective recipients. The most evident of such migratory tendencies at present is the movement of patients from Japan, where unwillingness to utilize beating-heart donors has retarded the extension of transplantation practice, to other countries in which beating-heart donors are available:

"To Tokyo's embarrassment, Japanese are starting to travel abroad for transplant operations they cannot get at home...With transplant organs in short supply everywhere in the world, Japanese patients in the hospitals of developing nations would seem incongruous. The Phillipines is already considering legislative action to control visits by foreign patients."[56]

A common approach in advancing an argument is to identify any alternative positions that an audience is likely to find less attractive. Coercion of subjects or of their medical attendants, in order to procure transplantable organs, may be unappealing to many. However, proposals to allow unrelated persons to donate a kidney, for a price determined by the "free market", are likely to be even less acceptable. A letter from several American transplant physicians identified the prospect of a "free-market" approach to organ donation as likely to evolve because of the scarcity of cadaveric organs:

"It is ethically impossible for physicians to justify removal of kidneys from living unrelated persons when we are using only a small fraction of the available cadaveric organs. Efforts must be directed toward development of procedures that will bring home to each person the need and mechanism for allowing himself or his loved ones to become organ donors."[57]

Apart from the movement of Japanese patients to hospitals in neighbouring countries that was referred to above, a substantial trade in transplantable organs appears to have developed. Fuelled by entrepreneurial "organ brokers", this takes the form either of importing healthy individuals from underdeveloped countries to Western hospitals in order to serve as paid "donors" of a paired organ, or of arranging the supply of organs from a similar source for prospective recipients from the West who have travelled to the home country of the "donor". The first pattern was brought to attention by an article entitled "Kidney for sale by live donor" published in 1989 in the *Lancet*.[58] It claimed that four healthy but impoverished Turks had been flown into Britain and paid to have a kidney removed for transplantation to wealthy patients at the Humana Hospital Wellington. The second pattern, according to a 1991 Australian report, operates openly in Bombay:

"Entrepreneurs will round up young peasants, and, for a fee allow surgeons to take life-saving kidneys and transplant them into wealthy Arab patients."[59]

Apart from the active inducement of organ "donation" by the provision of financial incentives to the impoverished, an increasing tendency to use the power which the state has over prisoners to tap this source of material has become apparent. In cases in which one of a pair or organs is to be removed from a living prisoner, an incentive may be provided. For instance, in the Phillipines, "it is quite common for prisoners to have their sentences shortened in return for donations of kidneys." [59] The other situation, which has been adequately documented in recent years, has entailed the use of executed prisoners. In the case of the People's Republic of China, this practice has given rise to a profitable industry for earning hard currency.

A report carried in *The Australian* in June, 1990 and sourced to The *Sunday Times* carried the headline "Executed Chinese prisoners source of kidneys for sale." [60] The article continued:

> "The practice has been carried on without the permission of the prisoners or their families contravening an international convention against torture and other cruel, inhuman or degrading acts which China signed in 1986...The normal practice is for the Chinese police to notify hospitals before any executions. Patients are alerted by telephone, telex or fax that a kidney will soon be available so that they can reach the transplant centre in time." [60]

Judging from the report, the organ procurement and transplantation procedures are closely co-ordinated:

> "The usual Chinese form of execution is a rifle shot in the base of the skull, a method which gives doctors a good chance of retrieving such useful organs as kidneys...But human rights observers say executions are so carefully planned that if eyes [presumably corneas] are needed, prisoners are shot in the heart." [60]

Several months after the preceding article, Melbourne's *The Age* carried a report [61] from a Hong Kong correspondent, which provided some recipient insights into the process of organ procurement from prisoners. An interview with Mrs Yeung, a 40-year-old Hong Kong woman who had received a kidney transplant, elicited the response that:

> "In China, the prisoners have to die. And if I don't take the kidney someone else will take it." [61]

The chairman of the Hong Kong Society of Kidney Specialists, Dr Man Kam Chan explained his position:

> "Provided the sentence is justified and the chap did commit a crime which is dealt with by capital punishment in that country, whatever happens after death is very immaterial." [61]

The open and shut nature of the case, as interpreted by Dr Man, has been complicated to some extent by the concern that some of the executed "donors" had met their fate for political dissent.

The inevitability of considerable interaction between suppliers and clients in the situation of organ collection from executed individuals will become, I suggest, increasingly evident to all except the clients and their medical attendants. Dr Man's allusion to the nature of the crime for which a prisoner had been executed is tantamount to introducing a requirement that the medical personnel intending to use each organ have to satisfy themselves that the circumstances under which it was obtained are acceptable to them. Similarly, the refinement of tailoring the technique of the execution to suit the requirements for organs to be removed from the individual patient brings supplier and user into close liaison.

An illuminating, albeit grotesque, insight into the manner in which the processes of organ procurement and use may become intertwined was afforded by an incident in Taiwan:

> "Huang Ching-chia, 25, sentenced to death for robbing and stabbing to death a fellow taxi driver was shot once in the back of the head instead of the heart on Monday because he had agreed to donate his organs...His remains were rushed to the Veteran's General Hospital so that his organs could be preserved, but he survived and his condition was 'getting better and better', the hospital administrator, Dr Lei Yung-yao said." [62]

The newspaper report which provided this information did not clarify the nature of the improved status of Huang. Following a recent gunshot wound to the head, it would be surprising if he were other than comatose, in which case some of the considerations applying to his treatment and/or use as an organ source that have been discussed on pp. 57–66 may be relevant. His case would certainly seem likely to bring the question of separation of these two aspects of management (i.e patient versus donor) into focus. The difficulties of the medical personnel at the Veteran's General Hospital may have been resolved in this case by Mr Lin Shyi-hwu, the Taiwanese Vice-Minister for Justice. He was reported as saying that Huang should be executed again. In accord with his directive, Huang was shot in the back of the head on a second occasion, this time with a fatal outcome.

I do not believe that many would find the patterns of organ procurement outlined in the preceding half-dozen paragraphs appealing. Coercion of medical personnel, exploitation of the impoverished and blatant conversion of individuals, irrespective of their guilt, into objects to be exchanged for hard currency are likely to be regarded as generally repugnant to a majority in most, if not all, communities. The context in which these topics were introduced and, I suggest, that in which their greatest influence is likely to be exerted, is that of alternatives to organ procurement procedures, currently practised in most Western countries. In this context, it is highly likely that they will be seen as socially unacceptable and, consequently, reasons for entrenching existing practices and extending the scope of their operation. An outcome of this response may be that another alternative to existing practice, namely the use of non-heart-beating donors, is overlooked. The following section will be concerned with this subject.

THE USE OF ORGAN DONORS FOLLOWING CARDIAC ARREST

"The regrettable trade in organs can only be stopped by procurement efforts that are directed in such new directions as non-heart-beating donor programs and research into the usability of animal organs."[63]

Replacement of "conventionally dead" donors who had already sustained cardiac arrest by patients with a beating heart, but satisfying the criteria for brain death, occurred when heart transplantation became a reality. Norman Shumway, one of the pioneers of heart transplantation, wrote in 1971 that:

"Prior to the advent of human cardiac transplantation, it was anticipated that the development of techniques for organ resuscitation and preservation would allow the removal of a donor heart after asystole [cardiac arrest] had occurred."[64]

Shumway's revised judgement that cardiac transplantation should only be undertaken using beating-heart donors was cited several years later in a British review of the subject:

"The surgeon most experienced in heart transplantation considers it unethical to use a heart for transplantation unless it has come from a donor whose heart was still beating, for to transplant a heart that has stopped as a result of anoxia will give the recipient a severe initial handicap which he may not overcome."[4]

This represents one of an increasing number of situations in which a duty of care to a prospective recipient has mandated changes to donor management.

By the late 1960s when heart transplantation was introduced, kidney transplantation had become a well-established procedure. Donors were either appropriately matched relations or unrelated individuals who had sustained cardiac arrest. However, the impression that collection of kidneys from beating-heart but brain-dead donors would permit a better outcome was prevalent. This belief was expressed by one author as follows:

"It is suspected...that the better results obtain with living related donors compared with cadaveric donors are, in part, a reflection of the physiologic condition of the kidney at the time of removal rather than the closeness of tissue match."[64]

Failure to obtain kidneys in optimal condition for transplantation had become a cause for concern in the UK by 1975. A report of a subcommittee of the British Transplantation Society remarked upon the poor quality of kidneys transplanted in the UK, "the poor quality being caused in large measure by the shortage of available kidneys and the legal uncertainties concerning their removal". They observed that:

"... many continental transplantation centres refused to accept kidneys from the UK because of the relatively high proportion of organs that were damaged by ischaemia [reduction of blood and oxygen supply]. The solution proposed by the subcommittee centred on the use of brain dead subjects with beating hearts."[4]

The question of whether intervention to remove organs should be undertaken before cardiac arrest has occurred was canvassed by the subcommittee:

"To remove the organ with the circulation intact has obvious advantages to the recipients, as there will be no anoxic damage."[4]

The report indicated that this was already accepted practice in a number of other European countries. An argument advanced in favour of this was:

"When a ventilator is stopped the heart may continue beating for more than an hour, but the organs may suffer greatly from anoxia and acidosis. Many surgeons with experience of this type of organ donation feel that the procedure of waiting for the heart to stop is unsatisfactory from every point of view."[4]

(It could be noted that these comments relate to the state of the technology in the mid 1970s. Experience obtained 15 years later using non-beating-heart donors is not in accord with them as will be described below.)

Recognizing a need to gain acceptance of the removal of organs from beating-heart donors, the British Transplantation Society report suggested that:

"Though the concept of brain death is not easy to explain to the layman, the extreme example of the victim of the guillotine is perhaps helpful. Nobody would consider the body, after the head has been severed, to represent an individual living being."[4]

As has been discussed previously, nobody who was accurately informed would consider the brain dead and decapitated individuals to be synonymous. The analogy is spurious. There do not appear to have been substantial attempts to modify this image of brain death in the public perception during the past two decades, despite increasing indications that the condition of many brain-dead subjects does not correspond to the original, simplistic concept.

An alternative opinion to those cited above on the necessity for substitution of beating-heart donors for the non-beating-heart or cardiac-arrest donors, who had been used during the 1960s, is available from a most authoritative source. Professor Roy Calne of Cambridge was more responsible than any other surgeon for the development of successful liver transplantation, a procedure that exceeds the more widely publicized heart transplantation in regard to its requirements both for surgical dexterity and control of organ preservation. Writing on the state of clinical transplantation in 1971, Calne reviewed events to that time:

"Initial unwarranted optimism and adulation were followed by bitter criticism. In particular, since the operation [heart transplantation] can be performed by any competent cardiac surgeon, the prestige of the individual and institution appeared to influence some centres in deciding to pursue heart grafting even in the absence of any previous interest or research background in the subject."[65]

He proceeded to examine the question of conversion to the use of beating-heart donors, which was then at issue:

"A powerful argument has been advanced and is gaining increasing acceptance in America and the continent of Europe to permit organ removal from patients with established brain death—coma depassé—whilst ventilation of the lungs is continued and the circulation is intact. This allows the surgeon to remove the organs unhurriedly whilst they are perfused with oxygenated blood and undoubtedly improves the transplantation results."[65]

Despite the potential advantages of removing organs whilst the circulation was intact, Calne noted that:

"If however resuscitation is abandoned and the organs are not removed until the circulation has ceased, then the brain must be dead from ischaemia and the irreversibility of the process will have been demonstrated. Following this conventional diagnosis of death, livers have been transplanted successfully. Since the liver is the most sensitive organ to ischaemic damage [deterioration resulting from lack of blood supply and oxygenation] with the exception of the brain itself, conventional diagnosis of death is compatible with all types of organ transplantation and has the immensely reassuring feature of *revealed* irreversibility of death that provides the public and the profession with adequate safeguards."[65]

Calne's arguments appear to have attracted little support as the transition from non-beating-heart to beating-heart donors occurred in most countries during the 1970s. The sequence of events was subsequently summarized by a British neurosurgeon:

"Renal transplantation became a routine procedure some time after brain death had become well recognized, and for some years only a proportion of cadaveric kidneys came from brain-dead patients, [that is, they were obtained *after* cardiac arrest]. In the West Midlands, for example, only 25% of donors offered in 1969 were receiving ventilation [that is, had a continuing beating heart]; by 1977 the proportion had risen to 65% and since 1978 all donors have been brain dead."[66]

As the use of beating-heart donors had replaced collection of organs after cardiac arrest in most countries by the late 1970s, it is not possible to apportion relative responsibility between this measure and other factors, such as better cross-matching, better preserved grafts and better immune suppression, in accounting for improvements in the results of transplantation during the past 20 years. Furthermore, with the widespread adoption of the use of beating-heart donors, development of technology to improve the quality of organs recoverable from cardiac-arrest donors has been relatively neglected. Another factor that seems to have assisted in the substitution of beating-heart for cardiac-arrest donors may have been an increasing tendency towards use of multiple-organ donors.

As regards the use of a single subject as a source of a number of organs, it should be observed that, whereas there was a well-established pattern of use of cardiac-arrest subjects as renal donors in some clinics during the 1960s, no such precedent existed in the case of heart donors. It is likely that any hospital with a commitment to recruiting organ donors in general would apply a regime of selection and management of prospective donors that was compatible with the most demanding procedures, namely heart and liver transplantation.

One argument that was identified by Jennett and Hessett as having made the removal of organs from beating-heart donors a more useful option than waiting for cardiac arrest, was the likelihood of an increased degree of agreement from donor families:

"Relatives are more likely to consent to donation when their family member is receiving ventilation perhaps because the process of seeking permission and arranging nephrectomy can then be conducted in an unhurried and seemly way."[66]

This proposition appears to me to be quite irrelevant to any comparison between beating-heart donors and donors who are disconnected from ventilator support, so that cardiac arrest is permitted, *after* consent for organ removal has been obtained. The latter class of patients will be receiving ventilation whilst decisions as to organ removal are being made and so it is quite feasible to proceed in an unhurried and seemly way. One consequence of changing to beating-heat, brain-dead donors has been the introduction of additional considerations into the management of prospective donors. For example:

"Aggressive hydration to preserve organs for transplant in patients not yet fully brain dead is standard donor maintenance procedure once a case is hopeless, even though this management increases brain swelling and hastens total brain death."[67]

As mentioned above, a frequent outcome of the general acceptance of any form of therapeutic procedure is that an extended period of neglect of alternative procedures is likely to occur. An obvious example of this negative effect during the 1980s was the waning of support for research on microsurgical reconstruction of the uterine tube following the introduction of *in vitro* fertilization. In the case of transplantation, the outcome of adoption of the use of beating-heart donors has been that techniques for retrieval of organs for transplantation from cardiac-arrest patients have received little attention in many clinics since the late 1960s . Two factors have operated to prevent the complete abandonment of research on this subject. The first of these has been the unwillingness of some communities to accept the use of beating-heart donors; the second has been the increasing shortfall between demand for organ transplants and the supply that has been available from beating-heart donors. It is abundantly clear that the demand for transplantable organs can not be met from the foreseeable supply of beating-heart donors. One possible response to this situation, as discussed on pp. 66–72, is the extension of the criteria for donor selection to include patients in the persistent vegetative state. An alternative, which I believe, is much more likely to obtain approval in most communities is that spelt out by Kootstra:

> "If only 10% of all traffic accident victims who die on the spot could be brought into a hospital within 45 minutes of death and if *in situ* cooling and nephrectomy could then be performed, the whole problem of supply in the Western world would be solved."[63]

Whilst there have been restrictions upon the removal of organs before cardiac arrest in a few European countries, the major opposition to the use of beating-heart subjects has occurred in Japan. This opposition reflects the attitudes of communities which apparently have not accepted a diagnosis of brain death as adequate grounds for organ removal. Two consequences of the unavailability of beating-heart donors have become apparent. The first, which was mentioned on p. 90, is an increasing tendency of Japanese patients to travel to other countries to receive transplants (from local beating-heart donors). The second has been the generation of a considerable impetus to improve procedures for the use of cardiac-arrest donors in Japan. This, in its turn, has lead to some major improvements in technology for organ preservation in the late 1980s. Concurrently, inadequacy in the supply of beating-heart donors has been responsible for similar research into use of non-beating-heart donors in other locations.

Studies reported from the Netherlands and Spain in 1988 provided qualified support for the use of cardiac-arrest kidney donors. The Dutch report, summarized the results from 1981 to 1988 of a new procurement programme.[68] It was directed to donors who had already sustained cardiac arrest, including some patients who were already brain dead and awaiting kidney removal when cardiac arrest intervened. The authors concluded that, even though the recipients of kidneys from cardiac-arrest donors had experienced a higher incidence of acute renal malfunction, survival of both recipients and grafts was similar to that of matched patients who had received grafts from beating-heart donors. Survival of both patients and grafts 1, 2 and 3 years after transfer from non-beating-heart and beating-heart donors was not different. The Spanish study found that the success rate of kidney transplants was lower in cardiac-arrest than in beating-heart donors but nevertheless concluded that use of the former "may be a significant alternative to prevent kidney wastage".[69] A similar outcome, implying that kidneys collected under relatively unfavorable conditions from non-beating-heart donors were suitable for transplantation, was reported in 1990 by a Polish group.[70] The brain-death criteria in force in Poland are considerably more demanding than those prevailing in Europe in general. There is a requirement for performance of angiography (visualization of a radio-opaque infusion in the blood vessels of the brain) and EEG before the diagnosis can be made. As a result of the prolongation of time before diagnosis occasioned by these requirements, prospective donors have often experienced prolonged periods in which their blood pressure has remained abnormally depressed. In a substantial number, cardiac arrest occurs before the brain-death criteria are met. Nevertheless, despite markedly suboptimal conditions, only 8% of transplanted kidneys failed to regain function.

The use of newer techniques to perfuse the kidneys of cardiac arrest donors either before and/or after their removal has been reported from a number of clinics to produce results after transplantation that are comparable with those observed after organ retrieval from beating-heart donors. For instance, a 1989 issue of the journal *Transplantation Proceedings*[71] contained four such reports. A transplant team from the University of Wisconsin reported that they had obtained excellent results using machine perfusion, "even with kidneys harvested from 'non-ideal cadavers'" (non-heart-beating).[71] Two Japanese reports, published at the same time, described the results of successful transplantation of kidneys from non-heart-beating subjects using organ perfusion. In both hospitals, tubes were placed in arteries and veins of prospective donors so that cooled, oxygenated fluid could be perfused through the circulation from the time of cardiac arrest until kidney removal had been completed.[72, 73] A similar approach, namely perfusing prospective donors with cooled fluid, was undertaken by a group from Baltimore in order to improve the outcome when multiple organs were to be collected from a single individual.[74] In this instance, perfusion was initiated in a brain-dead patient before cardiac arrest, which was actually precipitated by lowering of body temperature as a result of the perfusion. Nevertheless, in discussing the technique of "cardiopulmonary bypass with profound hypothermia", the authors made the point that, "The potential for application in non-heart-beating donors is also evident and has already found application".

It is probably too early to assess the potential for application of techniques in which brain-dead patients in whom cardiac arrest has occurred following disconnection from a ventilator, are perfused with cooled fluid before organ removal as a strategy for recovering organs suitable for transplantation. Japanese studies with experimental animals suggest that further development of this technology may lead to the use of cardiac-arrest subjects as sources of other organs in addition to kidneys. A report of a study undertaken in pigs noted that the liver could be successfully removed in a viable state from non-beating-heart donor animals submitted to perfusion and cooling, provided the warm ischaemia time (i.e. the interval during which the animal's tissues remained deprived of oxygen at body temperature) elapsing between cessation of circulation and the beginning of perfusion did not exceed 20 min.[75]

Another study from the State University of New York examined the effects of *in situ* cooling of organs in dogs. Cardiac arrest was produced by means of haemorrhagic shock (a state which would itself be expected to accentuate anoxia in the donor) and, after an interval, perfusion and cooling was initiated to improve organ preservation. Following their removal, after adequate cooling, kidneys were successfully transplanted.[76] The rationale behind this experiment was to attempt to utilize the "large as yet untapped source of transplantable organs" from accident patients "who succumb to their injuries before or on arrival in emergency rooms". Having shown that retention of organs in condition suitable for transplantation might be feasible if cooling and perfusion are instituted sufficiently early after cardiac arrest, the authors speculated on the possible implications of the experiment for donor-recruitment practice. They suggested that, provided adequate cooling of organs that are potentially transplantable could be maintained for some hours, adequate time would be available for preparing an operating theatre and securing the consent of the patient's family.

Arguing from the analogy of corneal harvesting from conventionally dead subjects, Anaise et al. suggested that the frequency of family consent to removal of other organs from cooled, perfused, cardiac-arrest patients might approximate that experienced with corneas rather than the much lower rate applying to beating-heart subjects.[76] They pointed out that the acquisition rate for corneas was almost seven-fold that for kidneys in New York:

> "These data suggest that when donor families are not faced with decisions on brain-death and termination of life support, but are faced only with the issue of organ donation, such families may be more likely to decide to donate these desperately needed organs, even if the donation were to result in deformation of the deceased's body (as occurs with removal of the eyes). The insertion of a femoral vascular line *after death* is clearly not a deforming procedure, and is already in common usage by morticians to embalm the body."[76]

Conceivably, if the technique were to be sufficiently refined, such an approach might eventually obviate the need for removal of organs from beating-heart subjects and might also resolve the shortage in supply of organs for transplantation.

As indicated earlier, when outlining the historical background to the replacement of beating-heart by cardiac-arrest patients as organ sources, the change occurred in a gradual manner. Consequently any extensive source of information on the results of use of cardiac-arrest subjects that was adequate for comparison with results currently obtained with organs from beating-heart donors would probably be 20 years old. There is little doubt that more recently developed techniques for preservation of organs from cardiac-arrest donors would be expected to lead to superior results. One assumption, that appears to have been made frequently, was that most deterioration in organs obtained after cardiac arrest is attributable to deprivation of oxygen during the period *before* organ removal. A second common assumption has been that delay in removal of organs after cardiac arrest would be produced primarily as a result of the time taken up during the surgical intervention itself. It now appears that both assumptions should be heavily qualified. As regards the first, experimental examination of perfused livers[77] has suggested that damage is produced by both warm ischaemia and the subsequent reperfusion after removal of the organ.[78]

Furthermore, there are some indications that much of the damage is attributable to the production of oxygen-derived free radicals. It is possible that the use of free radical scavengers before and during hepatic reperfusion may reduce damage.

On the subject of the contribution of delay between circulatory arrest and organ removal to deterioration, recent evidence suggests that the use of inefficient preservation techniques on organs *following* their removal may play a larger part in organ damage than changes produced by warm ischaemia *before* removal.[71] Furthermore, the indications are that the duration of warm ischaemia before an organ is removed from a cardiac arrest subject is more dependent (at least in the USA) upon completion of the necessary legal requirements than it is on the time required to prepare for surgical removal. Introduction of a reliable procedure for maintenance of a cooled, perfused subject *after* cardiac arrest, as discussed above, could radically alter this situation.

REFERENCES

1. Cranford, R. E. and Smith, D. R. (1988) Consciousness: the most critical moral (constitutional) standard for human personhood. *American Journal of Law and Medicine*, **13**, 233–248.
2. Levy, D. E., Sidtis, J. J., Rottenberg, D. A., Jarden, J. O., Strother, S. C., Dhawan, V., Ginos, J. Z., Tramo, M. J., Evans, A. C. and Plum, F. (1987) Differences in cerebral blood flow and glucose utilization in vegetative versus locked-in patients. *Annals of Neurology*, **22**, 673–682.
3. Gervais, K. G. (1986) *Redefining Death*, p. 25, Yale University Press, New Haven.
4. Brent, L. (1975) The shortage of organs for clinical transplantation: document for discussion. *British Medical Journal*, **1**, 251–256.
5. Shannon, T. A. (1978) Death and 'brain death'. *New England Journal of Medicine*, **299**, 1314.
6. Beresford, H. R. (1978) Cognitive death: differential problems Quinlan Commentary and legal overtones. *Annals of the New York Academy of Sciences*, **315**, 339–345.
7. Korein, J. L. (1978) Brain death: terminology, definitions and usage. *Annals of the New York Academy of Sciences*, **315**, 6–10.
8. Molinari, P. Page 96 in: discussion of Allen, N. (1978) Clinical criteria of brain death. *Annals of the New York Academy of Sciences*, **315**, 70–95.
9. Walker, A. E. (1977) An appraisal of the criteria of cerebral death. *Journal of the American Medical Association*, **237**, 982–986.
10. Green, M. and Wikler, D. (1980) Brain death and personal identity. *Philosophy and Public Affairs*, **9**, (no 2, Winter), 105–133.
11. Lamb, D. (1985) *Death, Brain Death and Ethics*, p. 84. Croom Helm, London.
12. Executive Board, American Academy of Neurology. Position of the American Academy of Neurology on certain aspects of the case and management of the persistent vegetative state patient (1989) *Neurology*, **39**, 125–126.
13. Veatch (1975) The whole-brain-oriented concept of death: an outmoded philosophical foundation. *Journal of Thanatology*, **3**, 13–30.
14. Youngner, S. J. and Bartlett, E. J. (1983) Human death and high technology: the failure of the whole-brain formulations. *Annals of Internal Medicine*, **99**, 252–258.

15. Bernat, J. L., Culver, C. M. and Gert, B. (1981) On the definition and criteria of death. *Annals of Internal Medicine*, **94**, 389–394.
16. Puccetti, R. (1988) Does anyone survive neocortical death. In R. M. Zaner (Ed.) *Death: Beyond Whole-Brain Criteria*, pp. 75–95. Kluwer Academic Publishers, Dordrecht.
17. Gervais, K. G. (1986) *Redefining Death*, p. 89. Yale University Press, New Haven.
18. Beresford, H. R. (1977) The Quinlan decision: problems and legislative alternatives. *Annals of Neurology*, **2**, 74–80.
19. *Canberra Times*, December 28, 1990.
20. Smith, D. R. (1986) Legal recognition of neocortical death. *Cornell Law Review*, **71**, 850–888.
21. Smith, D. R. 1988 Legal issues leading to the notion of neocortical death. In R. M. Zaner (Ed.) *Death: Beyond Whole-Brain Criteria*, pp. 111–114.Kluwer Academic Publishers, Dordrecht.
22. Cranford, R. E. and Smith, H. L. (1979) Some critical distinctions between brain death and the persistent vegetative state. *Ethics in Science and Medicine*, **6**, 199–209.
23. Wikler, D. (1990) Brain-related criteria for the beginning and end of life. *Transplantation Proceedings*, **22**, 989–990.
24. La Puma, J. (1988) Discovery and disquiet: research on the brain-dead. *Annals of Internal Medicine*, **109**, 606–608.
25. Casado de Frias, E., Balboa de Paz, F., Perez Martinez, A. and Palacio Mestres, C. (1980) Inappropriate secretion of antidiuretic hormone and the effect of lithium in its treatment. *Journal of Pediatrics*, **96**, 153–155.
26. Fost, N. (1980) Research on the brain dead. *Journal of Pediatrics*, **96**, 54–56.
27. Maugh, T. H. (1979) Blood substitute passes its first test. *Science*, **206**, 205.
28. Dillon, W. P. (1982) Life support and maternal brain death during pregnancy. *Journal of the American Medical Association*, **248**, 1089–1091.
29. Loewy, E. H. (1987) The pregnant brain dead and the fetus: must we always try to wrest life from death? *American Journal of Obstetrics and Gynecology*, **157**, 1097–111.
30. Editorial. Surrogate Mothers: a legal dilemma. *The Australian Financial Review*, March 13, 1989, p. 14.
31. Coller, B. S., Scudda, L. E., Berges, H. J. and Iuliucci, J. D. (1988) Inhibition of human platelet function *in vivo* with a monoclonal antibody. *Annals of Internal Medicine*, **109**, 635–638.
32. Dickson, D. (1988) Human experiment roils French medicine. *Science*, **239**, 1370.
33. Feinberg, J. (1985) The mistreatment of dead bodies. *Hastings Center Report*, **15**, 31–37.
34. Wade, N. (1978) The quick, the dead and the cadaver population. *Science*, **199**, 1420.
35. Corlett, S. (1985) Professional and system barriers to organ donation. *Transplantation Proceedings*, **17** (Suppl. 3), 111–119.
36. Iglehart, J. K. (1983) Transplantation: the problem of limited resources. *New England Journal of Medicine*, **309**, 123–128.
37. Youngner, S. J., Allen, M., Bartlett, E. T., Cascorbi, H. F., Hau, T., Jackson, D. L., Mahowald, M. B. and Martin, B. J. (1985) Psychosocial and ethical implications of organ retrieval. *New England Journal of Medicine*, **313**, 321–324.
38. Christopherson, L. K. and Lunde, D. T. (1971) Heart transplant donors and their families. *Seminars in Psychiatry*, **3**, 26–35.
39. Pallis, C. (1985) Defining death. *British Medical Journal*, **291**, 666–667.
40. Wetzel, R. C., Setzer, N., Stiff, N. L. and Rogers, M. C. (1985) Hemodynamic responses in brain dead organ donor patients. *Anesthesia and Analgesia*, **64**, 125–128.

41. Stiller, C. R. (1985) Transplantation in the 80s: a blueprint for success. *Transplantation Proceedings*, **17** (Suppl. 13), 19–31.
42. Youngner, S. J. (1990) Organ retrieval: can we ignore the dark side? *Transplantation Proceedings*, **22**, 1014–1015.
43. Salvatierra, O. (1988) Optimal use of organs for transplantation. *New England Journal of Medicine*, **318**, 1329–1331.
44. Austen, W. G. and Cosimi, A. B. (1984) Heart transplantation after 16 years. *New England Journal of Medicine*, **311**, 1436–1438.
45. Casscells, W. (1986) Heart transplantation. Recent policy developments. *New England Journal of Medicine*, **315**, 1365–1368.
46. Kolata, G. (1983) Organ shortage clouds new transplant era. *Science*, **221**, 32–33.
47. Darby, J. M., Stein, K., Grenvik, A. and Stuart, S. A. (1989) Approach to management of the heartbeating 'brain dead' organ donor. *Journal of the American Medical Association*, **261**, 2222–2228.
48. Schulman, B. (1988) Getting organ...ized. *Transplantation Proceedings*, **20**, (Suppl. 1), 1025–1027.
49. Published by Dept. as noted, without mention of any individual author. Co-ordination of donor organ acquisition (1988) Australian Commonwealth Department of Community Services and Health, Canberra.
50. Bartucci, M. R. and Seller, M. C. (1988) A study of donor families' reactions to letters from organ recipients. *Transplanation Proceedings*, **20** (Suppl. 1), 786–790.
51. Terasaki, P. I. (1989) A proposal to increase donations of cadaveric organs. *New England Journal of Medicine*, **321**, 618–619.
52. Pennington, J. C. (1988) Public information and transplantation from a recipient's point of view: the case for donor confidentiality. *Transplantation Proceedings*, **20**, 1036–1037.
53. Wight, C. (1988) Organ procurement in Western Europe. *Transplantation Proceedings*, **20**, 1003–1006.
54. Caplan, A. L. (1984) Ethical and policy issues in the procurement of cadaver organs for transplantation. *New England Journal of Medicine*, **311**, 981–983.
55. Roels, L., Vanrenterghem, G., Waer, M., Gruwez, J. and Michielsen, P. (1990) Effect of a presumed consent law on organ retrieval in Belgium. *Transplantation Proceedings*, **22**, 2078–2079.
56. Anderson, A. (1989) Japan grapples with definition of death by brain death. *Nature*, **337**, 592.
57. Carpenter, C. B., Ettenger, R. B. and Strom, T. B. (1984) "Free-market" approach to organ donation. *New England Journal of Medicine*, **310**, 395–396.
58. Brahams, D. (1989) Kidney for sale by live donor. *Lancet*, **1**, 285–286.
59. Wilson, P. (1991) Body-snatching is alive and well. *Australian Dr Weekly*, July 19, 1991.
60. Swain, J. Executed Chinese prisoners source of kidneys for sale. *The Australian*, June 25, 1990.
61. Hawksley, H. Transplant organs being taken from executed Chinese prisoners. *The Age* (Melbourne), August 22, 1990.
62. Saved, then re-executed. *The Australian*, April 17, 1991.
63. Kootstra, G. (1988) Will there still be an organ shortage in the year 2000? *Transplantation Proceedings*, **20**, 809–811.
64. Griepp, R. B., Stinson, E. B., Clark, D. A., Dong, E. and Shumway, N. E. (1971) The cardiac donor. *Surgery, Gynecology and Obstetrics*, **133**, 792–798.
65. Calne, R. Y. (1971) Ethics, the law and the future. In R. Y. Calne, (Ed.) *Clinical Organ Transplantation*, pp. 517–524. Blackwell, Oxford.

66. Jennett, B. and Hessett, C. (1981) Brain death in Britain as reflected in renal donors. *British Medical Journal*, **283**, 359–362.
67. Robertson, J. A. (1987) Supply and distribution of hearts for transplantation: legal, ethical and policy issues. *Circulation*, **75**, 77–87.
68. Vromen, M. A. M., Leunissen, M. A. M., Persijn, G. G. and Kootstra, G. (1988) Short- and long-term results with adult non-heart-beating donor kidneys. *Transplantation Proceedings*, **20**, 743–745.
69. Castelao, A. M., Sabater, A. M., Grino, J. M., Gil-Vernet, S., Andrés, E., Franco, E., Serrallach, N. and Alsina, J. (1988) Renal function of transplanted kidneys from non-heart-beating cadaver donors. *Transplanation Proceedings*, **20**, 841–843.
70. Walaszewski, J., Rowinski, W., Zawadzki, A., Chmura, A. and Kowalczyk, J. (1990) The influence of preagonal hemodynamic disturbances in the donor on the incidence of acute tubular necrosis after cadaveric kidney transplantation. *Transplantation Proceedings*, **22**, 1381.
71. Southard, J. H. (1989) Advances in organ preservation. *Transplantation Proceedings*, **21**, 1195–1196.
72. Koyama, I., Hoshino, T., Nagashima, N., Adachi, H., Veda, K. and Omoto, R. (1989) A new approach to kidney procurement from non-heart-beating donors: core cooling on cardiopulmonary bypass. *Transplantation Proceedings*, **21**, 1203–1205.
73. Fujita, T., Matsui, M., Yanaoka, M., Shinoda, M. and Naide, Y. (1989) Clinical application of *in situ* renal cooling: experience with 61 cardiac-arrest donors. *Transplantation Proceedings*, **21**, 1215–1217.
74. Williams, G. M., Cameron, D. E., Fraser, C. D., Reitz, B. A., Gardner, T. J., Burdick, J. F., Augustine, S., Gaul, P. D. and Baumgartner, W. A. (1989) Cardiopulmonary bypass with profound hypothermia: an optimal preservation method for multi-organ procurement. *Transplantation Proceedings*, **21**, 1199.
75. Hoshino, T., Koyama, I., Nagashima, N., Kadokura, M., Kazui, M. and Omoto, R. (1989) Liver transplantation from non-heart-beating donors by core cooling technique. *Transplantation Proceedings*, **21**, 1206–1208.
76. Anaise, D., Yland, M. J., Ishimaru, M., Shabtai, M., Hurley, S., Waltzer, W. C. and Rapaport, F. T. (1989) Organ procurement from non heart-beating cadaver donors. *Transplantation Proceedings*, **21**, 1211–1214.
77. Marubayashi, S., Dohi, K., Ochi, K. and Kawasaki, T. (1986) Protective effect of α-tocopherol administration on ischemic rat liver cell injury. *Transplantation Proceedings*, **18**, 596–597.
78. Toledo-Pereyra, L. H. (1988) Liver preservation: experimental and clinical observations. *Transplantation Proceedings*, **20**, 965–968.

4 Brain Absence: the Case of the Anencephalic Infant

"Any day now, Brenda Winner is going to have a baby—and it is going to die,"

began the report in the Melbourne *Sun* in late 1987. The story continued:

> "Brenda's child is set to become a source of rare and precious parts—a heart, a lung, a kidney, an eye perhaps. The 30-year-old Californian has won possible life for others' babies, but at the same time there is no hope for her own. The strange case of Baby Winner has focused attention on one of the most wrenching of medical issues—the use of babies born without brains as organ donors."[1]

Leaving aside, for the moment, the categorization as "babies born without brains", this or a similar article may well have been the first contact of many in the community with the condition of anencephaly. It is unlikely that any other circumstances, with the possible exception of reports of clusters of cases of anencephaly and spina bifida in particular districts would have focussed the attention of the media on infants with this malformation.

Baby Winner suffered from a congenital malformation termed "anencephaly". As events transpired, this baby was stillborn, a frequent outcome of the condition and, as a result, its use as a source of organs for transplantation (with the possible exception of the cornea) was not feasible. Whilst anencephalics have been used as organ sources at least since 1962, it is only since the mid 1980s, that prominence has been accorded these infants in either the medical or in general literature, as a source of transplantable organs for other infants and young children. As will be discussed in Chapter 5, it is likely that this prominence has been far in excess of that to be reasonably expected from their likely numerical impact on transplantation programmes.

After two decades of relative neglect, an explanation is not immediately apparent for the recent direction of attention to the issue of organ harvesting from anencephalics. The condition is not new. As will be indicated on p. 148 it is decreasing in frequency. As remarked above, anencephalics have been used as a source of organs for more than a quarter of a century. Why, then, has the subject only attracted substantial media attention in the last 5 years? As a preliminary to considering the question of the use of anencephalics, this chapter will examine some of the features of anencephalic infants. These include the structural (morphological) nature of the abnormality, the functional (physiological) capacity of anencephalic infants, their future and their status as human organisms. It will also be necessary to consider the problem of diagnosis of brain death as this relates to infants.

When transplantation of an organ, such as the heart or liver, to an infant or a young child is to be attempted, the physical constraints of accommodating that organ within the recipient's body necessitates the selection of a donor of appropriately small size. This requirement immediately introduces two major difficulties. In the first place, donors of the appropriate size are scarce. One reason for this relative scarcity of very young donors in comparison with their adult equivalent soon becomes apparent when it is realized that a substantial proportion of adult donors are recruited from among previously healthy, young adults involved in motor vehicle accidents. The number of infants or very young children who become available as donors in these circumstances is very limited. Secondly, early diagnosis of brain death, a prerequisite for organ removal, may be technically impossible in infants. This difficulty in making a confident diagnosis effectively compounds the obstacle already imposed by numerical shortage.

DIAGNOSIS OF BRAIN DEATH IN NEONATES

Diagnosis of brain death in adult patients provides a highly reliable forecast of the patient's future course. What that diagnosis *actually implies* in relation to the current state of structure and function of all parts of the patient's brain remains a more debatable subject, as discussed in Chapter 2. The first difference to become apparent between diagnosis of brain death in infants and in adults is the much greater difficulty encountered if one is dealing with neonates. This difficulty in diagnosing brain death in very young subjects does not reflect any difference, between adult and neonate, in the concept of the state that one is seeking to detect. This point was emphasized by the Secretary of the British Medical Association when the subject of diagnosis of death in neonatal organ donors was brought to public attention in 1986 following the well-publicized use of an anencephalic infant as the source of a heart for transplantation:

"The legal definition of brain death in Britain is the irreversible cessation of function in the brain stem and that is the same at 70 years or two hours."[2]

Nevertheless, whilst the concept underlying the term brain death is considered to be equally applicable, the historical background to the adoption of brain-death criteria in relation to the adult and the neonate followed quite different courses.

The original procedures for formal diagnosis of brain death in subjects other than young children were developed primarily, if not exclusively, as a guide to patient management. In essence, they were devised so as to afford benefit to the patient and his or her family. This occurred independently of, and historically some time in advance of, any requirement for organ donors for transplantation.

That is, the *primary* objective of the brain-death concept had nothing to do with its use in transplantation, but everything to do with management for the welfare of the patient. However, the course of events was significantly different from this in the case of formal diagnosis of brain death in young children. Addressing this subject, two experienced American paediatricians made the point, quite succinctly, that the only reason that could be advanced in support of defining criteria of brain death applicable to young children was to facilitate their subsequent use as organ donors:

> "We do not need to diagnose brain death to terminate care, to discontinue ventilator support, or to withhold further medical intervention. For these decisions we have the long tradition of doing what is best for the child (and family). These decisions can be made with some degree of leisure unless the child is a potential donor."[3]

As has been stressed in Chapter 3 when considering the procurement of organs in ideal condition for transplantation, there is no opportunity for leisure if harvesting of organs is contemplated. This is because of the risk of tissue deterioration with lengthening of the period during which blood supply is potentially inadequate. The possibility of subsequent use in organ transplantation has introduced considerable urgency into efforts to diagnose brain death in neonates in order that tissues are procured in optimal condition. Despite considerable pressure to respond to this need, the diagnosis of brain death in the infant is still regarded by most paediatricians as a difficult process that requires adequate time.

A combination of a steadily increasing demand for the provision of neonatal organs together with the innate difficulty in diagnosing brain death in infants led, in 1987, to the framing of no less than three sets of guidelines by American paediatricians and neurologists. These guidelines differed from each other in the specified duration of observation of the infant required before death could be confidently diagnosed. However, in other respects, they nominated quite similar clinical features as a basis for that diagnosis.

When comparing the various sets of guidelines and commenting upon them, an American paediatrician, Joseph Volpe, cited several reasons for the difficulties experienced in diagnosing brain death in the neonate.[4] The first of these was the frequent absence of an accurate history of the preceding events *in utero*. The most common cause of death in the neonate is brain damage following asphyxia of unknown duration before or during birth. When diagnosing brain death in adult subjects, a knowledge of the preceding medical history is essential because confident diagnosis of a specific condition producing brain damage is a prerequisite to diagnosing brain death. However, such history is usually unobtainable in the case of the neonate because of the difficulty of accurately observing the foetus during a prolonged delivery. Consequently, it may not be possible to decide from the infant's history whether brain damage is likely to be irreversible.

A second difficulty that may complicate diagnosis of brain death in the neonate is the occurrence of hypotension (abnormally low blood pressure), which is a common sequel of perinatal asphyxia (deprivation of oxygen during the process of birth). Lowering of blood pressure may severely depress brain function in the neonate. At least in its early stages, this depression is reversible. A third factor impeding the diagnosis of neonatal brain death is the relative inefficiency of the brain-imaging techniques that could be used during the first week of life to measure the extent of brain injury. A final impediment to which Volpe drew attention was the requirement for employing much longer observation periods to diagnose brain death in the infant, compared with the adult, because of the frequency with which errors could be introduced by isolated observations. This could be a major obstacle in possible organ transplantation situations in which the available time is limited. This is especially the case if the infant to be used as an organ source is to be transported over a long distance as has been the practice with some anencephalics. This form of management is not conducive to extended observation under stable conditions.

Other factors, apart from the requirement for additional time, are likely to compound the difficulties of neonatal brain death diagnosis. Regardless of the means employed, diagnosis of brain death in the neonate is much more prone to error because many of the neurological functions which are to be assessed have only been partially acquired by the *normal* neonate. As a result, these brain functions may be especially susceptible to temporary interruption, with a possibility for recovery that is lacking in an adult, following brain injury. Examples of this possibility are provided by cases in which comatose infants, lacking any detectable brain-stem function, are reported to have recovered. In one case of this type, a neonate was not breathing, had fixed, dilated pupils and lacked spontaneous or reflex movements.[5] This group of symptoms, which the attending paediatricians considered to be characteristic of haemorrhage into the brain, is usually followed by death. However, in the reported case, the infant not only survived but had attained near normal development of the nervous system by 8 months of age. The significant feature of cases such as this is not the eventual recovery of normal function. This is likely to be an uncommon occurrence even in neonates. Rather, their significance lies in the potential unreliability which they expose in diagnosis of *neonatal* brain death. The uncertainty relates not so much to the outlook as to the current status.

As discussed in Chapter 2, the distinction between whether an individual is already dead or is irreversibly brain-injured and certain to die has minimal prognostic significance. Continued efforts to resuscitate can not be justified in the patient's interests in either case. Any distinction between irreversibly brain-injured and already brain-dead may be effectively irrelevant if it is purely a question of whether the patient is to be submitted to further resuscitation. However, the distinction becomes of overwhelming importance when there is a question of the surgical removal of organs for transplantation. Thus, the significance of the case described above for management of infants manifesting similar symptoms lies not so much in whether to maintain supportive therapy but in the dubious legitimacy of classifying them as brain dead for purposes of organ removal. The hazards inherent in such a classification were sufficiently obvious to persuade the American Academy of Pediatrics to adhere, in its 1987 guidelines, to the position that clinical criteria of brain death were not of use in making this diagnosis in infants under 7 days of age.

It is clear that some paediatricians have been apprehensive that the difficulties inherent in diagnosis of neonatal brain death may be overlooked under the influence of pressure to facilitate transplantation. Freeman and Ferry wrote:

"The goals of improved clinical methods to obtain more donor organs for dying children are certainly laudable. But published 'guidelines' from prestigious physicians and groups have a way of becoming accepted dogma...Transplantation surgeons will pressure us to 'bend' the guidelines so that viable, well-perfused organs can be obtained to save lives of their patients."[3]

In the course of an exchange in the correspondence columns of the *New England Journal of Medicine* this potential conflict was well illustrated, as also was the manner in which professional affiliation can influence attitudes to a problem. Dr Alan Shewmon, a paediatric neurologist from the University of California stated that:

"There is no *a priori* reason why the state of the art of neurologic diagnosis should necessarily advance in phase with that of transplant surgery."[6]

In response, Dr Leonard Bailey, a paediatric cardiac surgeon from Loma Linda University argued for the use of neonatal organ donors in the following terms:

"We and others believe that brain death can be diagnosed with assurance in newborns and young infants, provided strict clinical criteria (as outlined) are fulfilled."[7]

The adoption of such diametrically opposed attitudes towards the use of neonates, especially if anencephalic, has commonly emerged in exchanges between paediatric surgeons seeking organs for transplantation and the physicians attending the potential donor.

The attitude of most paediatric neurologists to the diagnosis of brain death would appear to be that this diagnosis can be adequately made after observation and reflection over a period, provided the subject is not also under consideration as an organ donor. The contention by a surgeon from the Loma Linda team, referred to above, is interesting as it appears to be in conflict with earlier statements from this group. During the course of the intensive discussion which followed the transplantation of a baboon heart to Baby Fae in 1985, the difficulty in diagnosing brain death in neonates was advanced as one of the justifications for considering the use of a heart from a non-human source. Apart from the frequent lack of a reliable history of the extent and duration of anoxia *in utero* and the complicating effects of hypotension, referred to above, interpretation of the neonatal electroencephalogram (EEG) is difficult. The EEG of the normal infant younger than 30 weeks can exhibit periods of discontinuous low-amplitude activity. Following brain injury, the EEG trace can be isoelectric (flat) for a prolonged period. However, this can be followed by subsequent recovery of the subject, at least to a vegetative state. Such a clinical history emphasizes the differing requirements for decisions to discontinue life support and to designate an infant as a source of organs for transplantation. As Volpe indicated:

> "The two essential requirements for the diagnosis of brain death, i.e. the establishment of cessation of cerebral and brain stem functions and the demonstration of irreversibility are extraordinarily difficult in the newborn and young infant."[4]

He also noted that the criteria recommended for brain death diagnosis become useful "7 days after neurological insult".[4]

The use of anencephalic infants as a source of organs for transplantation has been advocated on several grounds. The first of these is the presently unfilled requirements for suitable organs. The estimates of organ requirements that have been formulated and the possible impact that anencephalic usage might make on these will be considered in Chapter 5. At this point, it is sufficient to note that substantial benefit from the use of anencephalic infants in heart, kidney and liver transplantation in infants has been foreshadowed.[8-10] A second case for anencephalic usage has been based on the premise that diagnosis of brain death is possible with greater certainty in these infants than is the case in the normally developed neonate. I believe that this proposition is scientifically unsupportable. The actual *recognition* of brain death in anencephalics (as distinct from formulation of a prognosis of its early occurrence) is unlikely to be significantly easier in an anencephalic infant than it is in neonates with intact cerebral hemispheres. A third ground for use of anencephalic infants as organ sources has been raised frequently as, for example, in one article under the succinct headline in a popular science magazine, "Surgeons want the organs of babies 'born brainless'."[11] The article indicated that the transplantation of organs from an anencephalic infant offered the only way in which something good could come out of something tragic. It described the reaction of the mother of an anencephalic girl who had unsuccessfully requested that her daughter be used as an organ donor. She lamented that, "It is a terrible waste to have the medical technology available to save a sick child's life and not be allowed to utilise it".

THE ANATOMICAL FEATURES OF ANENCEPHALY

The prevailing perceptions of the condition of anencephaly, and of infants affected by it, appear to have been strongly influenced by traditional accounts of its anatomical features. However, the anatomical descriptions that appear in most current non-medical, and some medical, commentaries are out of date. It would be more appropriate if current attitudes towards anencephalic infants and the treatment to be accorded them were to reflect contemporary understanding of the nature of the condition.

The first feature of anencephaly that should be stressed is that its nomenclature does not accurately describe it. A knowledge of the Greek origins of the term has not infrequently led commentators to assume that the anencephalic infant, by definition, lacks a brain. Whereas these infants suffer from gross disruption of brain development, incompatible with prolonged *ex utero* existence, they are certainly not brainless. The description of development and anatomical features of anencephaly that has been traditionally presented in textbooks may be summarized as follows.[12] During the first month of gestation of the normal embryo the brain and spinal cord are formed by the rearrangement of one structure, referred to as the neural plate, into another that is termed the neural tube. At approximately 3 weeks gestational age, this tissue rearrangement is followed by closure of the neural tube, throughout its length. The process by which the neural tube closes has attracted considerable attention in the non-medical literature recently because some scientists have advocated that it be adopted as the marker event up until which it would not be unethical to maintain human embryos in tissue culture. It has usually been stated by anatomists that anencephaly results from failure of the head (cephalic) end of the neural tube to close at this early stage of development. As a result, it is inferred that the brain has not proceeded to develop further forward than the brain stem. Accompanying this interruption of brain development is a failure of the cranial bones to enclose a cranial cavity. As a result, in the absence of the vault of the skull, the malformed brain and its membranes remain exposed. The shaping of the facial bones is also disturbed resulting in the production of a facial appearance that is typical of anencephaly.

The detailed nature of the anatomical deformation and of the pathological process which operates during foetal life to produce anencephaly might well appear, at first sight, to be esoteric information with no relevance to management of the anencephalic after birth. However, many of the arguments that have been advanced to support utilization of anencephalics as organ donors, under conditions that would be patently unacceptable if applied to other patients, have been based on assumptions about the development and characteristics of anencephaly that are substantially at variance with anatomical reality. The anatomical presumptions underlying these arguments are not usually spelt out explicitly, but this becomes necessary if they are to be evaluated. The first common contention is that the forebrain is completely absent and unrepresented in the anencephalic. (The forebrain includes the cerebral hemispheres and the cerebellum. It is the part of the brain that has developed to a disproportionate extent in man, in comparison with other species.) A second belief relates to the pathological events leading to anencephaly. It holds, in effect, that the forebrain has *never* developed, i.e. its absence represents a primary failure of development. A third proposition is that the resulting pathological state, categorized as anencephaly, is a highly discrete, clear-cut entity, and that other conditions similar to it do not occur. I believe that, whilst partially correct, all three arguments contain some substantial inaccuracies.

THE STATUS OF THE FOREBRAIN IN ANENCEPHALIC INFANTS

The presumption that the forebrain is lacking in anencephalics has been used to underpin contentions that these infants are either "not alive" or "not persons". Textbook accounts of the development and nature of anencephaly similar to that summarized above have remained substantially unchallenged for many years. However, recent reports suggest that they are fundamentally in error. For example, in discarding the traditional presumption, Chaurasia observed, in 1977, that:

> "present knowledge about the morbid anatomy of human anencephaly is erroneous and incomplete." [13]

In contrast with the previously established view that the anencephalic subject regularly lacks a forebrain, Chaurasia found that the forebrain is always present, albeit in a rudimentary form. This rejection of the conventional teaching in relation to anencephaly has been reinforced by the subsequent research of Bell and Green. [14] These authors also discarded the traditional view that anencephaly can be characterized as an absence of the forebrain. In its place, they described anencephaly as "that condition in which acrania [failure of cranial bones to develop and fuse] is associated with the presence of a dark vascular mass attached to an abnormal skull base and containing no grossly recognisable neural tissue". They undertook detailed microscopic examination of this mass. As a result of this examination, they reported that the vascular mass (the area cerebrovasculosa) was much less disorganized than had generally been inferred from its gross appearance. A cerebral vesicle, which they interpreted as a poorly developed equivalent of the normal cerebral hemisphere, was consistently present in this mass. Microscopically, the cerebral vesicle appeared to be a poorly organized example of neural differentiation.

Nature of the mechanisms of interference with forebrain development in anencephaly

The second, largely erroneous, presumption underlying much non-medical speculation on the status of the anencephalic infant is that development of the forebrain has been interrupted at its earliest stage, namely during the formation of the neural tube in the first month of gestation. As mentioned above, this event has been invested with considerable importance by some commentators as marking the end of the period in which human embryo experimentation should, at present, be acceptable (because of lack of a central nervous system).[15] For example, in response to the question, is there a time limit for research?, one reply was as follows:

> "Other proposals have been based on the ability of the embryo to experience pain, but at the present state of scientific knowledge, the exact point in time when this occurs is not known. Day 17, when the first signs of the formation of the nervous system are visible, has been proposed by the Royal College of Obstetricians and Gynaecologists. The birth of the brain is therefore considered to be a sign of the birth of the individual, just as brain death is recognized to be the absolute indication of death."[15]

Others have identified formation of the neural tube in discussion of the status of the anencephalic, as the time at which "brain life" begins.[16] The significance that has been placed on the traditional belief that anencephaly represents cessation of brain development at this stage lies in the conclusion drawn from it, namely that the anencephalic subject has never acquired even the earliest anatomical correlate of "personhood", i.e. the formation of a forebrain. Following this line of reasoning, Beller and Reeve have concluded of anencephalic infants that: "they do not at any time possess brain life".[16] Perhaps a similar belief influenced the determination of a West German court to the effect that anencephalics have never been alive. As Beller and Reeve noted:

> "In West Germany the corresponding paragraph in the commentaries of criminal law which states that an anencephalic is a stillbirth has been used to justify terminations of pregnancy after the 22nd week of gestation."[16]

Not only does anencephaly *not* represent a complete failure of the forebrain to develop, but it has become increasingly apparent that a number of different pathological processes occurring at different stages of development can lead to the same outcome, i.e. the clinical diagnosis of anencephaly does not necessarily correspond with the single sequence of pathological events that is usually assumed. For example, as early as 1934 a report described a foetus in which cerebral hemispheres had developed but in which the overlying tissues had failed to do so.[17] This condition of "exencephaly" has been observed only in young foetuses. It appears highly probable that subsequent deterioration of the exposed hemispheres in these foetuses leads to the development of an anencephalic state. Strong support for this hypothesis has been provided by observations reported in the last few years. It now appears, beyond reasonable doubt, that at least some cases of anencephaly result from *secondary* degeneration of the forebrain, after the formation of this structure, perhaps because of the loss of the protection normally afforded by surrounding skull and scalp tissues.[18]

Another pathological state that can lead to an outcome often regarded as anencephaly, but which nevertheless also supervenes secondarily following a period of normal development of the foetal forebrain, has been characterized as the "amniotic band syndrome". It is believed that, in this situation, a strangulating band of the amnion, one of the foetal membranes, constricts the head at a later stage of development. In a recent study of the amniotic band syndrome, it was concluded that the final outcome could be identical with that considered to represent typical anencephaly.[19] Further support for the interpretation that anencephaly can occur as readily after secondary degeneration of a previously formed (presumably) normal neural tube as from a primary failure of neural tube formation has been provided by observations of degenerating forebrains in fetuses in the third month of gestation.[20]

The significance of the recent evidence, which suggests that anencephaly can develop as a secondary event after the initial normal formation of the forebrain, is that explanations of the abnormality couched in terms that a forebrain has never developed are no longer biologically sound, i.e. the anencephalic cannot be dismissed in the category of "never has been".

The validity of regarding anencephaly as unique

The third presumption concerning anencephaly, namely that it can legitimately be classified as a unique condition without any similar forms of malformation of the cranial contents, has been increasingly called into question in recent years. There are three salient features of anencephaly. The feature that gives rise to assessments which question the vital status and the personhood of affected infants, and also to the hopeless prognosis of the condition, is the gross abnormality of the forebrain. Nevertheless, two associated features, namely failure of cranial bone development and interruption of development of the facial bones, provide important bases for identification of anencephaly as a distinct clinical entity. Diagnosis of anencephaly is dependent upon the recognition of these features.

I believe that the statement that anencephaly is a unique condition is subject to several different interpretations. In the first place, it can be taken to mean that development of the features of anencephaly results, in all cases, from a single pathological process. As indicated above, this is certainly not in accord with the facts. Secondly, it is sometimes implied that the extreme degree of brain disruption encountered is such as to render anencephaly unique in its severity. As will be indicated below, other cerebral catastrophes can produce equally severe degrees of brain malformation, albeit without accompanying skull and facial bony abnormality. As proposals for use of anencephalics in a manner not suggested for any other group of neonates are totally based on the *severity* of the brain malformation (the facial and cranial bony abnormalities being of no relevance to any of these proposals), arguments of "uniqueness" lack support. Thirdly, anencephaly has been described as unique in a diagnostic sense with the connotation that it is most unlikely that other conditions would be mistaken for it. As will be discussed later, two reports recently published by the US Task

Force on anencephaly and by Shewmon *et al.* noted that misdiagnosis by well-qualified physicians was not rare. Whichever of the three interpretations is chosen, description of anencephaly as "unique" may be successfully challenged.

The goals that can be achieved if anencephaly is accepted as a unique condition appear to me to be two-fold. In the first place, if the condition is considered to be unique as regards its causative process and its severity, it may be possible to propose strategies for dealing with anencephalics, which need not be subject to the objection that they may "spill over" and affect infants with other conditions. Secondly, if it is conceded that the "unique" features of anencephaly render misdiagnosis an impossibility, there is no risk that non-anencephalics could be accidentally lumped together with, and treated as it is proposed to deal with, anencephalics. I do not think that the first goal can be logically established, or that the second is medically accurate.

As if to complicate the question of the unique severity of anencephaly even further, if this was necessary, cases that are accurately diagnosed clinically as "anencephaly" have been found to encompass a range of conditions with *varying degrees of brain malformation*, i.e. not only do other conditions with degrees of cerebral malformation comparable with the "typical" case of anencephaly occur, but there are variations in severity of anencephaly itself corresponding with many of them. The heterogeneous nature of the anencephalic state is evident from comparison among the cases described in the monograph of Lemire, Beckwith and Warkanay on the subject.[21] A recent review of anencephaly conveys a similar message:

> "Indeed anencephaly is not an all-or-none phenomenon, but constitutes an imprecisely defined range of conditions toward one end of a spectrum of congenital malformations related to failure of closure of the neural tube or its later reopening."[22]

The term "anencephaly" does not delineate a tidy, homogeneous group of individuals, all with replicate abnormality. However, much of the discussion of the morality of subjecting anencephalics to organ harvesting under conditions not acceptable for other classes of subject has completely ignored this variation and elected to consider anencephaly as a clear-cut, easily diagnosable condition of uniform severity.

In considering other forms of congenital cerebral malformation, which can fall within the range of severity observed in anencephaly, the related condition of hydranencephaly requires attention. It differs from anencephaly in that infants with hydranencephaly may survive for considerably longer. However, as the extent of brain deformation can be comparable with that observed in anencephaly, observations made on hydranencephalic infants will be discussed on pp. 122–124 as an indication of what levels of function would be likely to be detectable in anencephalic infants if prolonged clinical testing was feasible. Hydranencephaly is a condition in which large portions of the cerebral hemispheres are replaced by fluid-filled membranous sacs enclosed within a cranium of relatively normal size.[23] Whereas anencephaly had, until recently, been considered to result exclusively from failure of normal differentiation during the first month of gestation, hydranencephaly is thought to result from abnormalities occurring later in foetal development, possibly as late as the third month of gestation. It is inferred that development of the brain may have proceeded normally until that stage.

Hydranencephaly is believed to result from a diverse group of pathological processes. As is the case with anencephaly, its severity is variable. Infants affected by the two conditions may retain similar quantities of cerebral tissue. Whilst the range of neurological development occurring in hydranencephalic infants can overlap with the spectrum of anencephaly, the closure of the cranium in the former obviates the risk of direct infection of the malformed nervous system. This is likely to account for more prolonged survival. Another factor that probably increases the chances of extended survival is the greater likelihood that those parts of the brain (hypothalamus and pituitary gland) which are concerned with temperature control and hormonal balance will remain functional in the hydranencephalic infant.

Another type of brain malformation comparable in severity with anencephaly but notable for cranial closure and relatively normal facial development has been described.[24] It is characterized by microcephaly, which has been interpreted as resulting from disturbances in the second and third months of gestation. Forebrain development is limited to the formation of cerebral vesicles. This condition has been tentatively described as microhydranencephaly. The discovery of these variant forms of foetal brain disruption has effectively blurred the classification of anencephaly. It is highly likely that further clinical and experimental observation of this group of malformations will necessitate re-classification of all. The precise form of the final classification is not relevant to our present interest; the plurality of forebrain disruption conditions is.

Anencephaly and acephaly

The significance of anencephaly, and the biological status of anencephalic subjects, have sometimes been obscured by confusion of this condition with that of *acephaly*. Unlike anencephaly, the term "acephaly" (meaning absence of the head) is literally accurate. Acephaly is a much rarer condition than anencephaly. However the major difference between the conditions is that the "acephalic foetus" is not a discrete individual, albeit malformed, like the anencephalic but is a "parasitic twin" attached to an otherwise intact foetus. As such, the acephalic twin consists of a body lacking a head and attached by its neck to its otherwise normal co-twin. The nature of this most severe of congenital anomalies is implied in the medical title of one form, namely "acardinacephalus". Acephalic parasitic twins invariably also lack a heart.[25-27] The blood circulation is provided by the heart of the co-twin. An acephalic twin is, in effect, no more than a malformed appendage of the co-twin. It can have no existence independent of the foetus to which it is attached and cannot in any sense be considered as analogous with the anencephalic infant.

Notwithstanding the major differences between the two conditions, the acephalic has, nevertheless, been misleadingly equated with the anencephalic in some instances of advocacy for use of the latter in organ transplantation. Consider, for example, the report by Holzgreve and Beller on the removal of kidneys from anencephalic infants without any regard for their vital status. In responding to criticism of their practice, these authors argued as follows that the presence of vital signs could be ignored in anencephalic infants:

> "Regarding organ donation, it seems to us somewhat artificial to consider true anencephaly, because of residual brain-stem activity, as substantially different from acephaly, which is complete lack of head and neck development resulting from an obliteration of the first and third branchial arch, when the body below the neck is also fully developed."[28]

This spurious and misleading analogy between acephaly and anencephaly was reiterated by Beller and Reeve in an article in the *Journal of Medicine and Philosophy*[16] Writing about acephaly, they observed that:

> "this malformation demonstrates that a foetus can show full development of the body, including a complete circulation (heart beat) despite the absence of the entire brain."[16]

Such a disingenuous statement, which is clearly at variance with the actual nature of the acephalic malformation, could scarcely be other than misleading for the non-medical readership at which it was directed. Rather than use acephaly as an analogy for anencephaly, I suggest that the very rare acephalic serves to demonstrate a state which genuinely lies outside personhood. An acephalic appendage to an intact foetus accords with many of the more florid categorizations that have been misapplied to anencephalics.

COMPARISON OF BRAIN FUNCTION IN NORMAL NEONATES, ANENCEPHALIC INFANTS AND INFANTS WITH RELATED DEFECTS

It may come as a surprise to anyone whose attitude to anencephalic infants has been conditioned by the dismissal of them as lacking a brain to discover that there is no shortage of reports of neurological functioning in anencephalics. Additionally, as mentioned above, infants with brain malformations similar in severity to anencephaly, but who have a closed cranium, are less likely to succumb to infection and so may survive postnatally for longer periods. Reports of their extended neurological and behavioural status, which reflect the longer survival, are more frequent than in the case of the typical anencephalic.

When reports of the functional capacity of anencephalic infants who survived beyond the typical short period are tendered as an indication of the possession of some of the abilities usually attributed to higher parts of the brain, they have commonly been dismissed as a reflection of misdiagnosis of the condition. This argument, however, necessarily cuts in both directions. If anencephaly was as clear-cut a condition as is maintained by those denying these infants the possession of neurological capacities (and frequently advocating procedural or legislative changes in their management, on the basis of that deficiency), then such mistakes would not occur. It is likely that some reports of prolonged observation of anencephalic infants may represent misdiagnosis. However, descriptions of behavioural capacity, both in surviving anencephalics and in infants with other brain malformations of comparable severity, such as hydranencephaly, are, I suggest, admissible as indications of the extent of their retained abilities, as distinct from their prognosis.

The scientific motivation for detailed observation of longer surviving infants with either anencephaly or with other equally severe malformations, albeit with a closed cranium, has generally been provided by the hope of defining the extent to which the establishment of the full range of higher cerebral functions is required for the typical behavioural pattern of the *normal* newborn. Because of the major differences that exist between the structure of the higher parts of the brain in man and any other animal, experimental study of this question in other species is impracticable. Study of infants with severe forebrain maldevelopment, with or without a closed cranium, has provided considerable insight into the extent to which the cerebral hemispheres contribute to the behavioural capacity of the *normal* human neonate.

The point that seems sometimes to have received inadequate emphasis in assessing neurological function in anencephalic infants is that their situation should be compared with that of the normal neonate, *not* of older subjects, in order to assess the contribution of the cerebral hemispheres to typical neonatal behaviour. There is no question that the anencephalic lacks any capacity for further development of the nervous system. However, study of infants with severe forebrain malformation, including anencephaly and, in particular, study of the range of neurological functions which they retain, has led inescapably to the conclusion that much of the behavioural pattern of the normal neonate is mediated by lower brain (subcortical) structures. For instance, the recent use of the new technique of positron emission tomography (PET) has strongly supported the contention that behavioural patterns in the *normal* neonate are substantially mediated by brain structures below the cerebral cortex. PET enables the level of activity of small, accurately localized structures in the brain of the fully conscious individual to be accurately measured. The study that formed the basis for these conclusions was undertaken in children ranging in age from 5 days to 15 years who were judged to be neurologically normal but who had previously suffered from transient interruptions of brain function.[29] (Selection of these children for inclusion in the study was undertaken on the basis that PET examination could be of direct prognostic value to them as individuals, whereas its use on entirely normal children could not be ethically justified.) The investigators concluded that their data were:

> "... congruous with the thesis that there is a relationship between a metabolic increase within neuroanatomical structures and the emergence of corresponding function. Neonatal behaviour is primarily dominated by subcortical brain structure activity. Intrinsic brainstem reflexes, such as the Moro, root, and grasp reflexes, are prominent. Visuomotor function is present only in rudimentary form and cortical function is mostly limited to primary sensory and motor areas."[29]

(In lay terms, their conclusion was that brain activity, in the normal neonate as objectively assessed and located by PET scanning, was predominantly confined to the lower parts of the brain.)

PET study of progressively older infants revealed increasing metabolic activity of the cerebral cortex relative to subcortical structures, with increasing development. This was equated with increasing "cortical suppression of brainstem reflexes". In essence, the interpretation was that much of the behaviour of both normal and anencephalic neonates does *not* require cerebral activity. This activity appears during the following months in normal infants and supplants the role of lower parts of the brain. A substantial increase in the activity of the frontal cortex of the normal infant by 8 months postnatally was considered to "coincide with the appearance of higher cortical and cognitive function". (No development of this type would be possible in the anencephalic.) The general conclusion now appears inescapable that subcortical structures subserve considerably more functions than hitherto assumed in both normal and cerebral-malformed neonates.

Comparison between the behavioural features of anencephalic and normal neonates has been the aim of a number of studies. The transmission of signals to the part of the brain influencing heart rate would conventionally be assumed to require participation of certain parts of the cerebral cortex. Graham *et al.*[30] studied the influence of noise upon the heart rate. They observed an anencephalic infant who responded to acoustic stimulation with the cardiac deceleration typical of normal, older infants.[30] In this respect, the infant's response pattern was typical of that of normal, awake subjects in excess of 2 months of age. However, paradoxically, following the death of this infant at 51 days of age, the abnormality of the brain appeared incompatible with this capacity. Post-mortem examination suggested that "cerebral microscopic as well as gross structure was so distorted as to preclude function". This notable divergence between observed function and the underlying structure of the nervous system (which would be regarded, on conventional understanding of the relationship between nervous tissue structure and function, as completely afunctional) prompted re-examination of the presumed relationship between structure and function.

Graham *et al.* suggested, as a result of their study of this case, that:

"in the normal infant, feedback from immature, higher centres may sometimes interfere with, rather than modulate, the functioning of lower centres."[30]

It seems probable that some of the functional capacities of the normal *neonate*, which make a substantial contribution to the impression that an observer forms of it, are mediated by parts of the brain that remain functional in anencephalics. Graham *et al.* suggested that the unusually well-developed response pattern demonstrated in the anencephalic subject whom they studied might be analogous to some unexpected competencies observed in experimental animals. In particular, it had been reported that experimentally damaging the brain of an animal in such a way as to sever some connections between the cerebral hemispheres and the remainder of the brain (the procedure of decerebration) could result in the appearance of new functional capacities on the part of the separated, lower brain. This led, in its turn, to the conclusion that some impulses originating in the higher centres could suppress activities generated in lower parts. This proposal is in accord with the suggestion from the PET studies of human neonates, discussed above, that an increasing "cortical suppression" of lower parts of the brain occurs during maturation of the nervous system in the normal infant. The observation, exemplified above, of considerable discrepancy between functional capacity of an anencephalic infant during life and the structural cerebral deficit in the same infant at post-mortem has been remarked upon on a number of occasions. Perhaps the most recent example of this was included in the report of Peabody *et al.*[31] on the Loma Linda transplant project. It was noted that:

"The correlation of behaviour with neuropathological features in the infants in our study clearly showed that behaviour and activity were not due to cortical or subcortical neuronal function but rather to some lower brain-stem response."[31]

Another attempt to distinguish the relative contributions of cerebral hemispheres and the remainder of the brain *in the normal neonate* by studying an anencephalic infant has been documented by Brackbill.[32] The subject of her study was an anencephalic boy who survived for 5 months. The response of this infant to repeated ringing of a bell was compared with that of normal infants. Whereas the normal infants, after responding initially, ignored the bell when it was repeatedly rung, the anencephalic continued to respond to repeated ringing by adjusting his position each time that the bell was rung, i.e. this "orienting reflex" was extinguished by repetition of the stimulus in the normal but not in the anencephalic neonate. Brackbill concluded that the inhibition of responses, which occurred in the normal neonate despite continued repetition of a stimulus, was a cortical function. This implied that normal neonatal cerebral function was responsible for extinction. This would be an example of immature, higher centres exerting a depressing effect on the functioning of lower centres as suggested above by Graham *et al*.

As discussed on pp. 40–43, the electroencephalogram (EEG) may be used either as a research technique or in monitoring the condition of individual patients. While it might seem reasonable to consider that the EEG could have no more than research application in relation to anencephaly, it has occasionally been used to support a diagnosis of death in anencephalic infants preparatory to their use as organ sources. Shewmon *et al*.[22] wrote critically of this practice, drawing attention to the great difficulty in knowing *how* an EEG might be recorded in an anencephalic infant in order to be comparable with tracings obtained from infants with intact cranial bones. They were also sceptical about the feasibility of interpreting an EEG from an anencephalic, regardless of how the tracing was taken.[22]

When used as a means of investigating the nature of the abnormality, rather than the clinical condition of individual patients, the EEG of anencephalic infants has been reported to retain some of the normal neonatal components despite the absence of normal cerebral function. Schenk *et al*.[33] reviewed earlier reports in the literature on this subject. A frequent feature of these reports was that, despite being of low voltage, the records were virtually identical with those of normal infants. For example, one infant in whom the cerebrum was represented only by a cyst, had a normal EEG at 3 months of age. Examination of two additional anencephalic infants by Schenk *et al*. revealed EEG patterns which were clearly different from those of normal infants of the same age. They speculated that the source of electrical activity in their subjects lay in the brain stem (medulla and distal pons).[33] EEG status should not be equated with neurological status. Nevertheless, EEG examination may be accorded some value as a means of assessing the infant's state, together with direct observation of neurological and behavioural capacity and post-mortem examination.

Measurement of neurological function in any individual will inevitably be affected by his or her general status. Depression of blood pressure, respiration and body temperature can all be expected to result in depression of the level of activity of the nervous system, so that it is likely to be assessed as being more impaired than would be the case if it was examined in an infant whose other organ systems were functioning normally. The very poor general physical condition of most anencephalic infants, and the frequency with which they have been already moribund when examined, can reasonably be expected to have compromised attempts to measure their neurological status. As will be discussed on pp. 125–128, there are strong indications that the early death of anencephalic infants may largely be attributable to cardiovascular failure. Poor performance when neurologically tested may well be similarly attributable.

For example, Brackbill reported that the response of the anencephalic infant to testing was frequently impaired by fatigue.[32] Limitations imposed by early onset of fatigue would probably be a regular complication of most attempts to undertake a thorough neurological examination. It might be anticipated that anencephalic infants would be unable to perform, even to the extent permitted by their neurological impairments, for more than short periods. Apart from those limitations imposed on any assessment of neurological capacity by the rapidity of onset of fatigue, other impediments are likely to ensure that under-estimation of capability readily occurs:

> "Some brain-stem functions may appear to be absent when they are not. Special sense organs and facial muscles are frequently malformed, impeding input and output from the nervous system; this may compromise the ability to measure intact reflexes of the central nervous system that depend on this input and output."[22]

That is, even if a particular part of the central nervous system retains some function, this may not be demonstrable if the peripheral organs responsible for detecting stimuli, or those that are normally observed in order to detect that function, are themselves inactive.

It may be feasible to make allowance for the depression of observable neuro-logical function attributable to these complications if one examines infants with other types of malformation that are comparable with anencephaly in the severity of their central nervous system abnormalities but which are not accompanied by the additional deficiencies in peripheral sensory and motor functions likely to occur in anencephalic infants. As already mentioned, when discussing the anatomical features of anencephaly, there are other conditions in which disturbance of brain development of comparable extent coexists with an intact cranium. In such disorders, there is much less risk of infection of the exposed nervous system and longer survival of the infant is likely. A number of infants with these malformations have been studied as a means of determining the contribution of cerebral hemispheres to behavioural patterns in the normal infant.

In view of the considerable overlap between anencephaly and hydranen-cephaly when the severity of disruption of forebrain development is compared, information gained from longer surviving infants with the latter condition cer-tainly has applicability to anencephalic infants. This close similarity in neuro-logical status and some likely implications of this were brought out by an experienced American paediatrician in the course of correspondence in *Pediatrics* on the subject of anencephalic use in transplantation:

> "From the narrow perspective of organ procurement policy, it is indeed tempting to ask whether the distinction between anencephaly and hydranencephaly is more than a fine neuropathologic nuance."[34]

Examination of the behavioural capacity of a hydranencephalic infant has been reported by Francis *et al.*.[35] Their conclusions were similar to those already mentioned as an outcome of the study of anencephaly by Graham et al.:[30]

"These observations suggest that the cerebral cortex does not play a central role in many behaviours that contribute to our perceptions of infants as social."[30]

Whilst the capacity to undertake some activities was markedly abnormal in this hydranencephalic infant, Francis et al. inferred that:

"it appears that some behaviours, particularly those that we tend to interpret as social, are possible as long as the brainstem and midbrain are intact."[35]

The preceding conclusion indirectly focuses attention on an important aspect of the subject. Any evaluation of an individual's capacity to participate in activities that are interpreted as "social" raises the question of the observer component in such assessments. Even if unrecognized, this may be substantial. Although not readily quantifiable, when it becomes a question of whether social behavioural activity or brain structure is to provide the benchmark for assessment of capacity for interaction with others, I suggest that the former should take precedence. Individuals create impressions and evoke responses, such as parenting, in others on the basis of appearance and behaviour rather than on the extent of development of their cerebral cortex. When the state of the brain, as demonstrated anatomically, is at variance with behavioural assessments, the latter should properly determine the issue. As indicated in Chapter 2, reliable correlation between structure and function of many parts of the brain remains very incomplete. It should again be emphasized that the activity of much of the brain cannot readily be tested. Consequently, it is not possible to determine the extent to which discrepancy between functional capacity and structural development reflects no more than our relative ignorance concerning this relationship.

Conclusions essentially similar to those of Francis et al.[35] concerning the importance of the contribution of brain-stem structures to behavioural characteristics were drawn by Tuber et al.[36] Their report concerned a pair of twins, one of whom was normal whilst the other was shown by means of pneumoencephalogram (an X-ray taken after introduction of air into the normal ventricular cavity of the brain) and computerized axial tomography (CAT) scan to be hydranencephalic with a virtual absence of cerebral hemispheres. The hydranencephalic twin was found to be as capable of associative learning in response to the application of paired stimuli as was the normal twin. The authors of the report drew attention to the similarity between the hydranencephalic twin and experimental animals that have been subjected to transection through the upper brain stem, in that both retained the capacity for associative learning. In discussing the behaviour of the hydranencephalic infant, Tuber et al. were led to reattribute some functions, generally considered to be mediated by the cerebral hemispheres, to other parts of the brain. It was noted that development of the human cerebral cortex during evolution has led to the elaboration of behavioural capacities that were previously mediated by centres lower in the brain. However, they considered that their results "bolstered the growing view that subcortical networks are capable of mediating complex behavioural processes". This led them to conclude that:

> Continued research into the neural mechanisms of behaviour has greatly expanded our appreciation of the capacity of lower brain structures to subserve many complex behavioural processes—processes which historically have been considered to be the domain of the cerebral hemispheres."[36]

Prolonged observation has been possible in the case of some infants in whom cerebral hemisphere development has failed but who, nevertheless, have had closed crania. Halsey et al.[23] reported that hydranencephalic infants surviving into the second year retained neurological features, such as the grasp and Moro reflexes, characteristic of the normal neonate. However, a major point of distinction from the normal infant was that no further functional development occurred in the brain-damaged infant. Barnet et al.[37] studied an infant who survived for 6 months after birth and was then found at post-mortem, despite having an intact cranium, to have only rudiments of the cerebral hemispheres. They also noted that normal neonatal reflex responses persisted in this infant without any indication of behavioural maturation. A greater range of these reflexes could be elicited than is the case in most anencephalics and this led the authors to suggest that:

> "Patients with anencephaly are often moribund and it is therefore difficult to derive conclusions from negative findings obtained in them."[37]

This conclusion is in accord with the hypothesis, already touched on, that the level of brain function usually *observed* in anencephalic infants may be depressed below that level which would otherwise be manifest. This would result from the failing state of other organ systems, retention of function in which is essential for brain activity.

Attention has been directed above to the functional capability of the nervous system of anencephalics for two reasons. The primary interest lies in determining the extent to which such infants manifest features usually associated with life. I suggest that the evidence emphatically supports a positive conclusion: such infants are neither dead nor "brain dead". When discussion shifts to utilization of these infants as an organ source, a secondary source of interest concerns the ability of the anencephalic to appreciate pain. It can easily be appreciated that this is a question to which the answer is unknowable if one relies on testimony of the subject (which is the only way in which an observer can confirm that a subject is feeling pain). Writers proposing the use of anencephalics as a source of organs for transplantation are usually dismissive of the possibility that an anencephalic could feel any form of noxious or unpleasant sensation. For example, discussion of this subject in one commentary pointedly included "painful" within inverted commas whenever the term was used in reference to procedures undertaken on these infants.[38] A typical sentence was:

> "Some anencephalics have grasping, sucking and vestibular activity and respond to 'painful' stimuli. However, the latter is best understood as a reflex pain response mediated by the brain stem."[38]

In contrast, a critique of anencephalic use in transplantation written by a paediatric neurologist expressed the opinion that:

> "it neither logically nor physiologically follows that anencephalic infants 'by definition...can neither feel nor experience pain'."[22]

This critique also concluded that:

> "Without question, decerebrate infants [that is, infants in whom a lesion has separated the cerebral hemispheres from the remainder of the brain] are neurologically much more similar to normal infants than they are to decerebrate adults, and it simply begs the question to apply adult-derived neurophysiological principles to this age group in support of a claim that a functioning cortex is necessary for consciousness or pain perception in newborns. Moreover, the phenomenon of developmental neuroplasticity could, in principle, allow brain-stem structures in the congenital absence of cerebral hemispheres to assume somewhat more complex integrative activity than would ordinarily be the case."[22]

CARDIOVASCULAR FUNCTION AND SURVIVAL

The anencephalic subject should not be regarded as an individual with a grossly malformed central nervous system in an otherwise normal body. It has already been indicated that the accuracy of any assessment of the capacity of the anencephalic infant's nervous system is likely to be compromised because of the deleterious effects exerted on its function as a result of deficiency in function of other organ systems. The degree of impairment of other systems, especially the cardiovascular system, will also determine the likely duration of postnatal survival. Equally important, when anencephalic infants are being evaluated as organ donors for transplantation, the efficiency of function of organ systems, such as the cardiovascular system, will substantially affect the value of tissues and organs for use in transplantation. It has been emphasized previously, when considering the pathological anatomy of anencephaly (see p. 115), that the term covers infants with malformations varying over a considerable range. The most severely affected individuals will most readily approach the requirements for a diagnosis of brain death. However, they are also, by virtue of the severity of their condition, the least likely to provide a source of organs of a quality that is suitable for transplantation. The implications of this paradox for utilization of anencephalics have been spelt out by Shewmon *et al*. and will be considered in Chapter 5.

Reports of the duration of postnatal survival of anencephalic infants have varied considerably. Baird *et al*.[39] reviewed records from British Columbia and found that of the 25–45% anencephalics who were liveborn in the province, over 40% survived for periods in excess of 24 h,[39] while 5% of liveborn infants remained alive on the seventh day. In contrast with this frequency of survival, Melnick *et al*.[40] reported that one-third of the anencephalics liveborn in California died within 15 min, while two-thirds had died within 3 h. The US Medical Task Force on Anencephaly considered the variable outcomes that have been reported in relation to postnatal survival of anencephalics. Whilst noting reports of longer survivals, they indicated that 2 months was the longest period that they could validate. Confounding factors were recognized as contributing both to underestimation and overestimation of survival time:

> "First, unusually long survival is often poorly documented with regard to the certainty of the diagnosis. Second, the early deaths involve varying degrees of withholding of medical treatment that might have prolonged survival. In most cases cardiorespiratory arrest apparently occurs before the cessation of brain-stem functions."[41]

While speculating on the length of time for which anencephalics might survive "with standard neonatal intensive care", the Task Force noted that of infants entered into the Loma Linda trial and receiving maximal support, "many became more vigorous and most survived at least one week without loss of brain stem functions".

Another source of information on the duration of postnatal survival of anencephalic infants is provided by accounts of experimentation on these infants. It will be recalled from Chapter 3 that the possibility of undertaking experimentation on brain dead-subjects has attracted attention and generated controversy in recent years. In contrast, anencephalic infants have been intermittently used in experiments without apparently attracting argument or even editorial comment, even though the subjects manifest spontaneous ongoing respiratory and cardiac function, i.e. by any criteria, they remained alive. Experimental interest in anencephalics has probably been aroused for at least two reasons. In the first place, these infants may provide an opportunity for studying function of the pituitary gland in the absence of the normal influence of the brain on this gland. Secondly, one suspects that they have been considered appropriate subjects for experiments that would be ethically unacceptable with normal infants. Anencephalic infants have been used, for example, in experiments to measure changes in blood hormone levels following the injection of other hormones into the rudimentary cerebrum of the subject. It would be inconceivable that similar procedures would be acceptable on non-anencephalic infants. In the circumstances of these experiments, which do not appear to have entailed provision of extraordinary resuscitative measures, most experimental infants seem to have survived for at least 12 h after birth. [42, 43]

The possibility of utilizing anencephalic infants as organ donors has led to considerable interest in the general physiology of the anencephalic infant. Before this possibility was recognized, there was little motivation to study the physiology of the anencephalic. Given the certainty that early death was inevitable, research on cardiovascular and respiratory function offered no promise of therapeutic application and could reasonably be viewed as an unjustified, and therefore unethical, intrusion on the patient.

However, when an anencephalic infant is deemed to be a candidate for organ harvesting, his or her physiological status becomes a most important consideration in determining the likelihood of recovering an organ in condition suitable for transfer. It is evident that, once the use of an anencephalic infant as the source of a transplanted organ is contemplated, the surgeon's duty of care to the prospective recipient requires that the organ be preserved in optimal condition. The other side of the coin is that, to the extent that continued functioning of other organ systems (especially the cardiovascular) results in the continued manifestation of sufficient signs of life, organ harvesting will have to be deferred. Reference in the literature to the state of preservation, and success as transplants, of organs obtained from anencephalics is confusing as a range of differing standards has been applied to determine when it is reasonable to excise the required organ. The question of the grounds that have been required for diagnosis, or presumption, of death in anencephalics will be considered in Chapter 5.

Quite recently, the considerable importance of circulatory inadequacy in anencephalic infants, both in magnifying their clinically observed neurological deficit and in curtailing duration of life, has been forcefully demonstrated. This recognition occurred, inadvertently, following the application of vigorous resuscitative measures from the time of birth with the aim of avoiding the detrimental effects of prolonged circulatory depression, in particular the curtailment of blood supply and oxygenation to organs destined for transplantation. Attempts at resuscitation *in the interests of the anencephalic infant* would, I believe, have been universally condemned as completely unjustified. Unexpectedly, resuscitation protocols intended to preserve transplantable organs by supporting the cardiovascular system have now been found, incidentally, to improve brain-stem function markedly and so to prevent deterioration of neurological status:

"We modified the medical care of 12 live-born anencephalic infants for one week to determine whether organ viability could be maintained and whether the criteria of total brain death could be met...Only two infants met the criteria for total brain death within one week, and no solid organs were procured [because biochemical tests undertaken on blood samples following brain death indicated that the livers of these two were too damaged to be transplanted]. Most organs were suitable for transplantation at birth"[31] (as assessed by biochemical blood tests). The conundrum to emerge was that:

> "When intensive care was provided from birth, organ function was maintained; however brain-stem activity ceased in only one infant within the first week."[31]

In the alternative procedure that was trialled:

> "When intensive care was delayed until death was imminent, most organs were damaged to an extent that made them no longer suitable for transplantation."[31]

These observations provide the best indication to date of the importance of circulatory impairment in both depressing brain function and shortening survival.

THE BIOLOGICAL STATUS OF ANENCEPHALICS

The biology of the anencephalic, which has been briefly considered in the preceding sections, is, I submit, essential background information in framing answers to questions about the status of these infants, which may appear primarily to be philosophical or legal issues. Discussion about anencephalics originally concentrated on the manner in which others should respond to and deal with them. I believe that a substantial part of this discussion was initiated, not necessarily because of problems posed by anencephalic infants *per se*, but because they were seen as examples of a class of subjects who could be separated from the general run of human beings. More recently, additional speculation and argument about the status of anencephalics have been triggered by the prospect of their use as a source of organs for transplantation. Whilst there will inevitably be some overlap between the specific issues raised when the anencephalic infant is considered in these two contexts, I propose to examine the more general issues now. Those raised by advocacy for the use of anencephalic infants in transplantation will be discussed in Chapter 5.

Are anencephalics alive?

This question has been raised in relation to anencephalics in whom spontaneous respiration persists. Clearly, anencephalics can ultimately become as dead as any other category of subject. The question of the vital status of the spontaneously breathing anencephalic is one that could be framed only after the introduction of the concept of brain death and the concurrent downgrading of "conventional" manifestations of life in organ systems other than the nervous system. Viewed from this perspective, two strategies have emerged as a result of which breathing anencephalics might be classified as dead.

When the existing, commonly accepted criteria for brain death are applied, the anencephalic infant presents many of the difficulties characterizing the diagnosis of brain death in any other neonate. The nature of these difficulties was discussed on pp. 106–110. The only feature of the anencephalic infant which may enable the requirements for diagnosis of brain death to be satisfied more readily than is the case with other infants is the accurate delineation of prognosis that a diagnosis of anencephaly permits. The *current* vital status can be as difficult to measure for the anencephalic as it often is for other neonates. (The Loma Linda protocols, to be discussed in Chapter 5, set out to measure this, albeit with some cutting of corners.) One possible solution to the difficulty inherent in recognition of irreversible cessation of brain-stem function in anencephalics could be to replace the currently accepted definition of brain death with a formulation of cerebral death. This could be undertaken as a generally applicable strategy to maintain a consistency between diagnosis of death in anencephalics and other subjects. An ambiguous statement on the subject of the anencephalic being alive was reported in 1986 from the President of the Royal College of Physicians, Sir Raymond Hoffenburg.[44] In indicating his approval for organ removal from anencephalics he noted that, "death is absolutely inevitable among babies born with anencephaly". Coupled with this seemingly unexceptionable statement, he was reported also as saying:

"There is no possibility of organs being taken from a patient who is still alive. This is an outmoded and idiosyncratic view held by a very small minority."[44]

An alternative approach, which has been suggested on a number of occasions would *automatically* define anencephalic neonates as dead, irrespective of their vital status. As will be discussed in Chapter 5, this has been proposed as a legislative tactic to facilitate anencephalic use for transplantation. On one hand a general change of criteria for brain death in order to implement a cerebral-death standard would envisage policy towards the anencephalic leading to the introduction of a cerebral-death standard for *all* categories of patient. Statutory definition of all anencephalics as automatically dead might quarantine anencephalics and retard a "flow on" from them to other classes of subject. The possibility that brain-death criteria in general might be amended so as to adopt a cerebral-death rather than a brain-stem or total-brain-death standard requires the community to consider whether it regards the existing criteria as appropriate. If this is so, there is little justification for change: if not, there may be a case for complete re-evaluation of the current definition. This should include adjustment of criteria either to contract or to expand the scope of operation of "brain death".

If the general requirements for categorization of individuals as "brain dead" are to be reassessed, it is necessary to recall the original reasons underlying its introduction. As outlined on pp. 7–9, the basis for the brain-death concept was to spare patients and their families the imposition of futile treatment. It may be appropriate to consider whether this primary objective has been overtaken by the more recent aim of facilitating the harvesting of organs for transplantation. As discussed on pp. 106–110 this is likely to have been the major consideration in introducing the concept of brain death in relation to neonates. It would seem to be a case of confounding loss of cognitive function with death if anencephalics were to be statutorily defined as dead. As indicated in discussing cerebral death, in Chapter 3, this change would effectively establish quite different definitions of death for humans and members of other species. The distinction between life and death would have become incontestably non-biological.

When the intentions underlying definition of death in the "typical" non-infant patient and in the anencephalic neonate are contrasted, it is clear that the latter is to be regarded as an exercise undertaken totally in the interests of others. There can be no justification, on the basis of the patient's interests, for either institution or maintenance of life-support measures in the anencephalic. There is no reason for placing an anencephalic on a respirator other than that of improving the chances of acquiring organs usable for transplantation. It is a completely contrived situation with no therapeutic basis for the subject. In contrast, full resuscitation with use of a respirator may be at least *initiated* in adult patients with the anticipation that it may be in their interest. This interest may take the form of gaining time to permit accurate diagnosis of irreversibility of loss of brain-stem function or of providing an opportunity for reversible lesions to resolve. (Prolonged *continuation* of resuscitation, as distinct from its initiation, may cease to be in the patient's interest.) To summarize the difference between anencephalic and other patients, resuscitation of the latter *may* be in the patient's best interests while resuscitation of the former *never* can be.

Are anencephalics persons?

The preceding question of whether anencephalics are dead is amenable to a scientific response, to the extent that there is societal agreement on what death is and what medical criteria are accepted for its recognition. However, it is immediately evident that questions of personhood can not be resolved in this way. The issue of whether an entity is alive or dead can be approached at the level of the cell, the organ or the whole organism. Uncertainty arises when one seeks to identify, and perhaps to seek agreement on, which of these levels is to be selected. However, this uncertainty becomes insignificant when one attempts to bring precision to bear on the question of whether a given organism is a person.

Initiatives to categorize anencephalic infants as non-persons have been based principally on two diverse contentions, one overtly trivial, the other, I suggest, lacking the objective basis that has been claimed for it. The first proposition would deny personhood for the reason that an anencephalic is not a member of the human species. I do not suggest that any biologically literate commentators have adopted this position but there is little doubt that it may have indirectly coloured the attitudes of some others. It is probable that an impression of non-human status has been derived, at least subconsciously, from traditional folk lore that infants with such severe malformations were not wholly human but were the product of cross-species fertilization. Confusion about the biological nature of anencephalics resulted in their designation, together with other classes of grossly deformed infants as "monsters" (see discussion of this subject in Chapter 1 of the monograph of Lemire *et al.*).[21] This term persisted unquestioned, in medical textbooks until the 1960s. A legacy of the interpretation that can be read into the term and its historical background, occurred in a monograph on legal attitudes towards human life which has since been quoted frequently.[45] In discussing anencephalic infants, its author, Glanville Williams opined:

> "There is, indeed, some kind of legal argument that a 'monster' is not protected even under the existing law...Yet the question still remains whether it is permissible both morally and legally so to define a human being as to exclude the grosser sports of nature...It seems probable...that a creature that is clearly a monster in the old-fashioned sense could lawfully be put to a merciful death."[45]

I have difficulty in envisaging any objective means by which one could decide on which of the "grosser sports of nature" are non-human.

More recent attempts to exclude severely deformed neonates from the legal provisions normally applying to them by the stratagem of typing them as "non-human" have sought to derive scientific bases for the distinction. An example of such a basis, provided by a legal discussion paper on the management of these infants, was to define humanness on the basis of chromosome number.[46] There does not appear to have been any serious support from practising scientists for this type of approach.

Some discussion of the status of anencephalics appears to adduce a combination of deficiency in both humanness and life in order to disqualify such infants from personhood. One prominent bioethicist who appeared to opt for such an "each way bet" was Paul Ramsey. He wrote:

> "I suggest that we can deal with the issue of anencephalic births by the definitional route: they are not alive human beings."[47]

That the writer based this opinion on a less than perfect knowledge of the nature of anencephaly is suggested by some of his other comments in this context:

> "an anencephalic baby, it could be argued, no more enters the human community to claim our care and protection than a patient remains in the human community when his brain death is only disguised behind a heart-lung machine."[47]

Similarly, his comment in relation to the anencephalic that "one should be willing to bury a reflexly reacting corpse (although other reasons override such an action) but not a terminal patient whose heart is still beating naturally, showing signs therefore that the brain is not wholly dead" suggests an incomplete understanding of the condition.

Perhaps an even better example of confusion about the biology of anencephaly was provided in an article by a philosopher. In writing of "hydrocephalic infants", Lachs affirmed that such a "child" is "not a person, and the fundamental error of our ways consists in thinking that it is one".[48] He continued:

"The hydrocephalic child is altogether without the cortical structures that make the development of such personhood possible."[48]

This will be recognized as *not* being a description of hydrocephaly. It is closer to some of the opinions that have been expressed about anencephaly. Careful reading of Lachs' paper, in which, among other attributes of his "hydrocephalic" non-person, he refers to the possibility that society may end up "saddled with a sad burden for 20 or 30 years", obviously also excludes anencephalics. Biological science has yet to recognize any medical condition that matches his impressions. Nevertheless, the failure of neuropathology to keep pace with his philosophy did not inhibit Lachs' categorization of the deficiencies of "hydrocephalic" infants. He indicated that, in comparison with them, "pigeons have more personality [and] the indigo bunting more intellect". In commenting upon the Lachs paper in the course of an extensive article on the anencephalic infant, Shewmon *et al.* drew attention to:

"The potential for diagnostic confusion that can invade attempts to draw lines of 'personhood' based on neurological deficit."[22]

Some neurologists, nevertheless, have remained undeterred in attempting to define the human person in terms of neurological capacity. For example, Julius Korein, who participated actively in the development and presentation of the original concept of brain death has subsequently suggested that the essential deficit in brain death is irreversible damage to those systems in the brain responsible for "sentience, mentation, emotions, memory, self-awareness, learning, attention and other forms of complex information processing including storage and analysis".[49] On this basis, he has claimed that:

"the development of structure and function...which defines a human being occurs after 20 weeks of fetal age. Brain life, and the life of the human being, can be said to begin between 20 to 30 weeks of fetal life."[49]

On this basis, the anencephalic would never have begun "brain life" nor become a human being. Korein placed his concept of "brain life" in context by considering it as the mirror image of "brain death" as generally recognized. A pithy response to Korein's attempt to define personhood on scientific grounds was not long in coming at the same meeting of the Transplantation Society at which it was presented:

> "Those who date life's beginnings with some other event or process—conception, for example, or birth—do not necessarily dispute any of Dr Korein's science: they simply deem it irrelevant."[50]

Any proposition to subdivide the human *species* into categories of person and non-person has, presumably, to identify first what is perceived as the basis for according to persons treatment which differs from that which is accorded other species. Again presumably, the qualities identified will vary with the background and beliefs of those who are surveyed. Further consideration of the attributes required before any individual member of the human species can qualify as a person is likely to lead to the conclusion that, whilst biological features are included within them, the ultimate grounds for making the decision may not be scientific. I assume that assessment of the personhood status of another individual will inevitably be heavily influenced by such subjective factors as the intuitive response of the observer to the subject. Subjectivity does not equate with non-reality. It may be difficult to identify precisely the factors which have influenced a subjective assessment, but that is a problem of their identification not of establishing their existence. Consider, for instance, the observations of the parent of an anencephalic:

> "As the father of an anencephalic boy I know that he could feel pain. He developed a clear personality showing pleasure by smiling, displeasure by becoming agitated; he could even follow you around the room with his eyes. The only time he cried was when he was dying—a really pitiful heart-rending sound, which clearly showed his pain and distress. I feel sick at the thought of babies like my son dying under the surgeon's scalpel."[51]

This parent was, presumably, not trained in neuropathology. As a result, his assessment of the anencephalic infant was necessarily based on his subjective impressions. I would find it difficult to discard these out of hand in favour of inferences based on the presumed degree of development of nervous system structure that was required for sentience.

To the extent that commentators take it upon themselves to arbitrate upon the claims of another individual to be considered and treated as a person, it is incumbent upon them to ensure that any scientifically verifiable inputs to their decision are indeed accurate. As already discussed, the anencephalic infant does have a brain, albeit one in which the forebrain component is grossly disorganized. It also now appears highly likely that development of the forebrain has been underway for some time before onset of the pathological process. Consequently, the notion that the upper part of the anencephalic's brain has never started to form is inaccurate. Neither argument should be admitted to a discussion of personhood.

The potential for extending conclusions about the status of the anencephalic to non-neonatal patients diagnosed as having sustained cerebral death was mentioned in Chapter 3. The idea that the beginning of "brain life" should have features resembling those accepted as characterizing brain death was mentioned above. In arguing for adoption of a cerebral-death standard, Cranford and Smith maintained:

> "We believe there are more similarities relating to consciousness between the end of life and the beginning of life than previously appreciated. If this is the case, the arguments concerning when human personhood ends will have significant impact on when human personhood begins during gestation."[52]

If this proposition was accepted, the features required to identify the onset of brain life might be queried. For instance, would the appearance of synaptic connections between neurons in the cerebral cortex by 8.5 weeks of gestation be significant?[53] Perhaps it is unjustified to accept the proposition of similarities between onset of "brain life" and "brain death". As Wikler[50] commented in responding to this proposal when framed by Korein,[49] many would not necessarily accept that "the measure of life's beginning ought to mirror the measure of life's end".

Is anencephaly a unique condition?

The extent to which anencephaly can be claimed to be unique has been considered on pp. 114–116. As implied then, this claim has connotations at both the diagnostic and the conceptual level. As a diagnostic contention, it implies that no other condition will be mistakenly diagnosed as anencephaly and, therefore, that there will be no risk of other classes of subjects being accidentally entrapped within the anencephalic donor net. As regards the uniqueness of anencephaly, considered as a diagnostic entity, it has been indicated that there *are* other conditions which resemble, and can be mistaken for, anencephaly. The scope for false positive diagnoses is well exemplified by the "long surviving cases" referred to by the US Task Force on Anencephaly.[41] Shewmon et al. also drew attention to the difficulty that could arise as "the least severe cases of meroanencephaly, in which the forebrain and overlying tissues are only partially absent are indistinguishable from the most severe cases of microcephaly with encephalocoele".[22] They noted that the scientific literature on this subject "is replete with both photographs and descriptions exemplifying the potential for confusion surrounding these two diagnoses".

Shewmon et al. illustrated the diagnostic confusion which can occur by means of the case of an infant in Dallas who was diagnosed by a neurologist and a geneticist as being anencephalic:

> "The parents were told that the infant would die within a few hours, but they eventually took her home and she lived for 14 months."[22]

Shewmon *et al.* concluded that:

> "because microcephaly with encephalocoele constitutes a spectrum of its own, at the other end of which are quite functional individuals, the danger of misapplication of a revised Uniform Determination of Death Act to living, nonvoluntary organ sources other than anencephalics is far from hypothetical."[22]

Whereas Shewmon *et al.* cited the ease with which anencephaly can be misdiagnosed as grounds for indicating that the condition was not the unique, clearcut diagnostic entity that others have claimed, Beller and Reeve sought to adjust their line of argument *after* the event to assure uniqueness of the condition, even in the face of misdiagnosis:

> "It must be concluded that those who live longer than a week were exencephalics, not true anencephalics."[16]

The argument in support of the unique nature of anencephaly has been heavily used in advocacy of use of anencephalics in transplantation as will be discussed in Chapter 5. I believe that it becomes a particularly circular and fragile argument when it seeks to maintain *both* that anencephaly is an unmistakable condition and that the diagnosis may be retrospectively revised on the basis that a mistake has been made in the event of an infant surviving for more than a week.

At the conceptual level, the unique nature of anencephaly has been invoked as a device to "quarantine" anencephalic usage. The purpose of this appears to be to establish that "unique conditions" justify "unique measures". A supplementary role of the contention that the condition is unique is to forestall any objections to implementation of the aforementioned unique measures. In particular, objectives based on the risk that designation as a donor could gradually extend to infants with other conditions could be deflected because of the unique nature of the condition. However, the contention fails as noticeably in relation to conceptual use as it does in the context of diagnostic use. As already noted, there *are* other types of malformation of the brain that are of a degree of severity comparable to anencephaly.

Do anencephalics lack sentience?

The possession of sentience has frequently been selected as the primary feature in determining the consideration to be shown to an organism. For example, it is hardly an oversimplification to suggest that the widespread movement to accord increased consideration to animals is based upon the perception of their sentient capacity. The degree of consideration that should be shown to an animal is proportional to that capacity. The reverse situation is that if sentience is to be the prime consideration and consistency is to be established, it is necessary to advocate that the level of rights to be accorded the severely disabled human should be diminished in proportion to the *estimated* diminution in his or her sentient capacity. When the extent of sentient capacity of individuals with malformation or injury of the brain is accepted as the guide to the course of management to be selected for them, there is often a tendency tacitly to equate diminution or loss of sentience with diminution or loss of life itself. As discussed on pp. 17–18 there is no logical reason for this equation. My preference would be decidedly to agree with the proposition of Hans Jonas on the subject that was noted at that stage, namely that the question of sentience is subsidiary. The real point of the argument turns on "the determinancy of the boundaries between *life* and *death*, not between sensitivity and insensitivity".[54]

Propositions that anencephalic infants are, by reason of their disability, incapable of feeling pain or of responding to those caring for them can only be inferred very indirectly in the light of their observed behaviour. It is both a conceptual and a practical impossibility to measure awareness on the part of an individual unable to communicate his or her experience. The comments of Shewmon *et al.* on the impossibility of determining the extent to which an anencephalic may experience some form of pain in response to various stimuli are, I believe, entirely relevant. With an admirable eye to the context in which the issue of sentience has been popularly raised, they concluded that:

> "both prudence and logical consistency demand that we attribute to anencephalic infants at least as much consciousness and capacity for suffering as we attribute to laboratory animals with even smaller brains which everyone seems to feel obliged to treat 'humanly'."[22]

It is interesting that, notwithstanding confident statements to the effect that anencephalics are known to lack sentience completely, physicians at the Loma Linda clinic adopted a protocol which entailed the administration of the analgesic pethidine to infants who had been entered into procedures during which the occurrence of brain death was to be assessed as a prelude to organ removal.[55] I find it difficult to construct a logical argument for this intervention. On the one hand, if the infants were, as advertised, totally incapable of appreciating pain, administration of an analgesic was quite superfluous. Furthermore, the selection of an agent as potent as pethidine, which possesses respiratory depressive side-effects, would predictably run the risk of vitiating the conditions prerequisite for diagnosis of cessation of spontaneous respiration. On the other hand, if analgesic use was indicated because there existed a reasonable possibility of retention of capacity to feel pain, the foundations of the argument for utilization of anencephalics as organ sources necessarily collapse.

As already indicated, the *normal* neonate is neurologically immature and it has increasingly become apparent that typical neonatal behaviour reflects subcortical functions to a much greater extent than was previously believed. On this basis, I have suggested that the actual nature of infant behaviour, rather than interpretations as to the part of the brain responsible, would be the appropriate parameter for assessing response to social contact. The likelihood that anencephalic infants can be accepted by their families, notwithstanding major abnormalities, is suggested by descriptions of behavioural capacity in individual infants. For example, Brackbill noted that the anencephalic infant studied on pp. 120–121 was apparently blind:

"He was sensitive to auditory stimuli; however auditory threshold, as measured by motor responses was higher and more variable than normal. Repeated administration of a standard set of odorants and gustatory substances indicated that although taste was probably present, olfaction was absent...Rooting and sucking responses were adequate. There was no evidence of smiling or babbling."[32]

The only state that could be clearly identified in this infant was rapid eye movement sleep:

"Whether the infant was 'awake' or asleep when not in rapid eye movement sleep could not be determined."[32]

The anencephalic infant studied by Graham et al.[30] between 3 and 6 weeks of age was observed, during periods of testing, to remain:

"in a state that approximated active sleep. The eyes were closed, but eye movement and lid twitching could be observed as well as small movements of head and mouth. Occasionally, gross body movement was observed."[30]

After a prolonged period of observation of a long-surviving group of hydranencephalics, Halsey et al. commented:

"During the early months of life these infants would typically be either asleep or crying with considerable spontaneous motor activity. The state of consciousness would frequently shift quickly from one extreme to the other without an intermediate period of quiet wakefulness. [In several infants] crying consistently appeared to be inhibited when the infant was held and cuddled or spoken to in a soft voice."[23]

Food preferences were apparent in some infants. These were indicated by "consistently frowning, grimacing and crying in response to certain foods placed on the lips and tongue."[23]

The US Medical Task Force on Anencephaly provided a composite description of possible anencephalic behaviour patterns. In doing so the authors drew some implications for normal infants:

"Many behaviours of newborns have been ascribed to cerebral hemispheric activity; however, the presence of these behaviours in infants with anencephaly indicates their brain-stem origin. These behaviours include responses to noxious stimuli (avoidance, withdrawal or crying), feeding reflexes (rooting, sucking or

swallowing), respiratory reflexes (breathing, coughing or hiccups), and many inter-
actions involving eye movements and facial expressions that are seen in newborns
with intact cerebral hemispheres."[41]

None of these four descriptions of the range of response of anencephalic infants
to their surroundings, and in particular to human contact, could be presented
as grounds to suggest that they were equivalent to normal infants with an intact
nervous system. As discussed earlier, the discrepancy between performance of
anencephalic and normal infants becomes even more pronounced with the efflux
of time, because of the failure of the central nervous system of the former to
undergo subsequent development. However, I believe that it can be deduced
with considerable confidence from such composite summaries of behavioural
patterns in anencephalics, as from the earlier descriptions of individual infants,
that they are far from the totally insentient masses of human tissue that they
have sometimes been claimed to be.

The allocation, in this reinterpretation, of functions that were previously considered to be of cortical origin to subcortical areas again serves to raise the question of whether the acceptance of an individual is to be based on the possession
of capacities that constitute a central feature of what is intuitively regarded as
normal infant behaviour. Alternatively, is the identity of those parts of the brain
responsible for particular behavioural features to be adopted as *the* crucial feature
in determining the significance to be attached to that behaviour? Is account to
be taken only of those capacities currently believed to be exclusively of cortical
origin? My impression is that the bulk of observers, medically trained or not,
would judge a subject as a live human infant on its behaviour and not on the
basis of what was currently believed as to the part of the brain mediating that
behaviour. If an anencephalic infant manifests features which, when they occur
in a normal infant, contribute substantially to development of empathy with it
on the part of others, then the precise neuro-anatomical location of those functions (or the currently accepted understanding of this) would not appear to me
to be of primary importance.

As implied from the preceding descriptions, individual infants with anencephaly and hydranencephaly have been observed to display a variable range of
capacities. This presumably represents the functional equivalent of the range of
variations in anatomical structure of the nervous system already referred to in
infants with these abnormalities. It is common for the manifestation by anencephalics of some of the behavioural characteristics of infants with an intact
nervous system to evoke parenting responses on the part of both natural and
adoptive parents. A well-documented example of such a case, in which the
accuracy of diagnosis of anencephaly can hardly be questioned, is provided by
an infant who passed through the Loma Linda "pre-donation program" (to be
described in Chapter 5).[56] Following her failure to meet the brain-death criteria,
the parents of the longest surviving of these infants, Baby Hope, took her home

to Knoxville, Tennessee, where her mother cared for her until Hope died about 2 months later.

The existence of strongly conflicting views between some transplant surgeons and paediatricians regarding the management of anencephalic infants has been mentioned earlier in this chapter. An instance of such a conflict provides an informative example of the different attitudes towards anencephalic infants which can be adopted. An article by a physician in *Pediatrics* suggested that:

> "Indeed, in consoling grief stricken parents and encouraging them to hold their baby, pediatricians will invariably point to the usually normal other body parts, having first placed a bonnet on the child's head."[57]

In response, a paediatric surgeon from Denver argued that anencephalic infants:

> "do not, as proposed by Milunsky, provide counsel to the grieving parents by holding the 'bonnetted' anencephalic newborn. To the contrary they can be an enormous source of guilt to the parents. They are no more 'living persons' than the heart-beating infant donor in the next bed with clinical brain death from meningitis."[58]

Subsequently, in defending parental holding of the bonnetted anencephalic, Dr Milunsky replied:

> "Dr Karrer wrote that this should not be done and that anencephalic infants can be an enormous source of guilt to parents. His comments reflect inexperience, lack of insight and a failure to consult with senior pediatricians versed in the subject in his own school. The compleat surgeon requires skills far beyond the use of the scalpel. Dr Karrer, it would seem, has much to learn."[59]

The attitudes of paediatric surgeons in relation to anencephalic infants will be considered further in the following chapter when the course of advocacy for the use of ancephalic infants in transplantation is considered.

REFERENCES

1. McMillan, S. A baby born to die. *The Sun*, (Melbourne), December 22, 1987.
2. Dawson, J. quoted in Anderson, I. Surgeons want the organs of babies born brainless. *New Scientist*, November 6, 1986, p. 20.
3. Freeman, J. M. and Ferry, P. C. (1988) New brain death guidelines in children: further confusion. *Pediatrics*, **81**, 301–303.
4. Volpe, J. J. (1987) Brain death determination in the new born. *Pediatrics*, **80**, 293–297.
5. Pasternak, J. F. and Volpe, J. J. (1979) Brief clinical and laboratory observations: full recovery from prolonged brainstem failure following intraventricular hemorrhage. *Journal of Pediatrics*, **95**, 1046–1049.

6. Shewmon, D. A. (1987) Cardiac allotransplantation in newborns. *New England Journal of Medicine*, **316**, 878.
7. Bailey, L. L. and Nehlsen-Cannarella, S. (1987) Cardiac allotransplantation in newborns. *New England Journal of Medicine*, **316**, 878–879.
8. Bailey, L. L., Jang, J., Johnson, W. and Jolley W. B. (1985) Orthotopic cardiac xenografting in the newborn goat. *Journal of Thoracic and Cardiovascular Surgery*, **89**, 242–247.
9. So, S. K. S., Nevins, T. E., Chang, P.-N., Mauer, S. M., Ascher, N. L., Fryd, D. S., Sutherland, D. E. R., Simmons, R. L. and Najarian, J. S. (1985) Preliminary results of renal transplantation in children under 1 year of age. *Transplantation Proceedings*, **17**, 182–183.
10. Gartner, J. C., Zitelli, B. J., Malatock, J. J., Shaw, B. W., Iwatsuki, S. and Starzl, T. E. (1984) Orthotopic liver transplantation. Two-year experience with 47 patients. *Pediatrics*, **74**, 140–145.
11. Anderson, I. Surgeons want the organs of babies 'born brainless'. *New Scientist*, November 6, 1986, p. 20.
12. Patten, B. M. (1956) *Human Embryology*. J & A Churchill, London.
13. Chaurasia, B. D. (1977) Forebrain in human anencephaly. *Anatomischer Anzeiger*, **142**, 471–478.
14. Bell, J. E. and Green, R. J. L. (1982) Studies on the area cerebrovasculosa of anencephalic fetuses. *Journal of Pathology*, **137**, 315–328.
15. Revillard, M. (1986) Responses to nine questions concerning research on human embryos. *Human Reproduction*, **1**, 265.
16. Beller, F. K. and Reeve, J. (1989) Brain life and brain death—the anencephalic as an explanatory example. A contribution to transplantation. *Journal of Medicine and Philosophy*, **14**, 5–23.
17. Hunter, R. H. (1934) Extroversion of the cerebral hemispheres in a human embryo. *Journal of Anatomy*, **69**, 82–85.
18. Papp, Z., Csecsei, Z., Toth, K., Polgar, K. and Szeifert, G. T. (1986) Exencephaly in human fetuses. *Clinical Genetics*, **30**, 440–444.
19. Urich, H. and Kaarsoo Herrick, M. (1985) The amniotic band sydrome as a cause of anencephaly. *Acta Neuropathologica (Berlin)*, **67**, 190–194.
20. Ganchrow, D. and Ornoy, A. (1979) Possible evidence for secondary degeneration of central nervous system in the pathogenesis of anencephaly and brain dysraphia. *Virchows Archives (A) Pathological Anatomy and Histology*, **384**, 285–294.
21. Lemire, R. J., Beckwith, J. B. and Warkanay, J. (1978) *Anencephaly*, New York, Raven Press.
22. Shewmon, D. A., Capron, A. M., Peacock, W. J. and Schulman, B. L. (1989) The use of anencephalic infants as organ sources. A critique. *Journal of the American Medical Association*, **261**, 1773–1781.
23. Halsey, J. H., Allen, N. and Chamberlin, H. R. (1968) Chronic decerebrate state in infancy. Neurologic observations in long surviving cases of hydranencephaly. *Archives of Neurology*, **19**, 339–346.
24. Russell, L. J., Weaver, D. D., Bull, M. J. and Weinbaum, M. (1984) *In utero* brain destruction resulting in collapse of the fetal skull, microcephaly, scalp rugae, and neurologic impairment: the fetal brain disruption sequence. *American Journal of Medical Genetics*, **17**, 509–521.
25. Benirschke, K. and Harper, V. D. R. (1977) The acardiac anomaly. *Teratology*, **15**, 311–316.
26. Simpson, P. C., Trudinger, B. J., Walker, A. and Baird, P. J. (1983) The intrauterine treatment of fetal cardiac failure in a twin pregnancy with an acardiac, acephalic monster. *American Journal of Obstetrics & Gynecology*, **147**, 842–844.

27. Robie, G. F., Payne, G. G. and Morgan, M. A. (1989) Selective delivery of an acardiac, acephalic twin. *New England Journal of Medicine*, **320**, 512–513.
28. Holzgreve, W. and Beller, F. K. (1987) Kidney transplantation from anencephalic donors. *New England Journal of Medicine*, **317**, 961.
29. Chugani, H. T., Phelps, M. E. and Mazziotta, J. C. (1987) Positron emission tomography study of human brain functional development. *Annals of Neurology*, **22**, 487–497.
30. Graham, F. K., Leavitt, L. A., Strock, B. D. and Brown, J. W. (1978) Precocious cardiac orienting in a human anencephalic infant. *Science*, **199**, 322–324.
31. Peabody, J. L., Emery, J. R. and Ashwal, S. (1989) Experience with anencephalic infants as prospective organ donors. *New England Journal of Medicine*, **321**, 344–350.
32. Brackbill, Y. (1971) The role of the cortex in orienting: orienting reflex in an anencephalic human infant. *Developmental Psychology*, **5**, 195–201.
33. Schenk, V. W. D., de Vlieger, M., Hamersma, K. and de Weerdt, J. (1968) Two rhombencephalic anencephalics. A clinicopathological and electroencephalographic study. *Brain*, **91**, 497–506.
34. Landwirth, J. (1989) The anencephalic controversy: in reply. *Pediatrics*, **83**, 642–643.
35. Francis, P. L., Self, P. A. and McCaffree, M. A. (1984) Behavioural Assessment of a hydranencephalic neonate. *Child Development*, **55**, 262–266.
36. Tuber, D. S., Berntson, G. G., Bachman, D. S. and Allen, J. N. (1980) Associative learning in premature hydranencephalic and normal twins. *Science*, **210**, 1035–1037.
37. Barnet, A., Bazelon, M. and Zapella, M. (1966) Visual and auditory function in an hydranencephalic infant. *Brain Research*, **2**, 351–360.
38. Cefalo, R. C. and Engelhardt, H. T. (1989) The use of fetal and anencephalic tissue for transplantation. *Journal of Medicine and Philosophy*, **14**, 25–43.
39. Baird, P. A. and Sadovnick, A. D. (1984) Survival in infants with anencephaly. *Clinical Pediatrics*, **23**, 268–271.
40. Melnick, M. and Myrianthopoulos, N. C. (1987) Studies in neural tube defects. II. Pathologic findings in a prospectively collected series of anencephalics. *American Journal of Medical Genetics*, **26**, 797–810.
41. Stumpf, D. A., Cranford, R. E., Elias, S., Fost, N. C., McQuillen, M. P., Myer, E. C., Poland, R. and Queenan, J. T. (1990) The infant with anencephaly. *New England Journal of Medicine*, **322**, 669–674.
42. Grasso, S., Filetti, S., Mazzone, D., Pezzino, V., Vigo, R. and Vigneri, R. (1980) Thyroid-pituitary function in eight anencephalic infants. *Acta Endocrinologica*, **93**, 396–401.
43. Pezzino, V., Distefano, G., Belfiore, A., Filetti, S., Mazzone, D. and Grasso, S. (1982) Role of thyrotrophin-releasing hormone in the development of pituitary–thyroid axis in four anencephalic infants. *Acta Endocrinologica*, **101**, 538–541.
44. *The Times*, (London), December 16, 1986.
45. Williams, G. (1958) *The Sanctity of Life and the Criminal Law*, p. 31. Faber & Faber, London.
46. Human Rights Commission (Australia) (1985) Legal and ethical aspects of the management of newborns with severe disabilities. *Occasional Paper, no. 10.* Australian Government Publishing Service, Canberra.
47. Ramsey, P. (1978) *Ethics at the Edges of Life: Medical and Legal Intersections*, p. 213. Yale University Press, New Haven.
48. Lachs, J. (1976) Humane treatment and the treatment of humans. *New England Journal of Medicine*, **294**, 838–840.

49. Korein, J. (1990) Ontogenesis of the fetal nervous system: the onset of brain life. *Transplantation Proceedings*, **22**, 982–983.
50. Wikler, D. (1990) Brain-related criteria for the beginning and end of life. *Transplantation Proceedings*, **22**, 989–990.
51. *Today*, (London) July 14, 1987.
52. Cranford, R. E. and Smith, D. R. (1978) Consciousness: the most critical moral (constitutional) standard for human personhood. *American Journal of Law and Medicine*, **13**, 233–248.
53. Molliver, M. E., Kostovic, S. and Van Der Loos, H. (1973) The development of synapses in cerebral cortex of the human fetus. *Brain Research*, **50**, 403–407.
54. Jonas, H. (1974) Against the stream: comments on the definition and redefinition of death. In *Philosophical Essays. From Ancient Creed to Technological Man*, p. 130. Prentice Hall, Englewood Cliffs.
55. Barinaga, M. (1987) Maintaining anencephalic babies causes consternation in U.S.A. *Nature*, **330**, 592.
56. Goldsmith, M. F. (1988) Anencephalic organ donor program suspended: Loma Linda report expected to detail findings. *Journal of the American Medical Association*, **260**, 1671–1672.
57. Milunsky, A. (1988) Harvesting organs for transplantation from dying anencephalic infants. *Pediatrics*, **82**, 274–276.
58. Karrer, F. M. (1989) The anencephalic controversy. *Pediatrics*, **83**, 641–642.
59. Milunsky, A. (1989) The anencephalic controversy: in reply. *Pediatrics*, **83**, 643.

5 Brain Absence: Use of the Anencephalic Infant in Transplantation

The nature of anencephaly and some of the features of anencephalic infants, in particular the requirements which would have to be met if they are to be diagnosed as brain dead in a manner consistent with the treatment of non-anencephalic individuals, were considered in the preceding chapter. The considerable difficulty inherent in the diagnosis of brain death in any infant was also discussed. The compounding effect, on the availability of organs suitable for transplantation to other neonates, of the relative scarcity of potential infant organ donors, together with this diagnostic difficulty, was noted.

This chapter will examine those factors likely to influence the suitability and availability of anencephalic infants as a source of transplantable organs. This will entail consideration of estimates of the magnitude of any organ supply likely to become available from anencephalics and also of the quality of those organs. The projected demand for neonatal organs for transplantation and the extent to which close matching of age between organ source and recipient is necessary likewise requires examination. Proposals for use of anencephalics and the reasons advanced in support of this practice in relation to the earlier history of anencephalic use will be reviewed. Finally, attention will be directed to the question of why this subject has recently become an issue, 30 years after transplantation of organs from anencephalics began.

BASIC REQUIREMENTS FOR TRANSPLANTABLE ORGANS FROM INFANTS: CAPACITY OF ANENCEPHALICS TO MEET THESE REQUIREMENTS

The organs that may be transplanted to infants and children in the first 2 years of life are the heart, liver and kidney. It has been estimated that the likely annual requirements for these organs in the USA is of the order of 400–600 (heart), 400–800 (liver) and 300–450 (kidney).[1] Estimates of comparable size have been made by Caplan.[2] Whilst the view is gaining ground that renal transplantation is more successful if it is deferred until the second year of life, it has been the transplantation procedure most frequently undertaken in neonates. Nevertheless, success rates have been noticeably variable when anencephalic kidneys have been transplanted.[3] Renal transplantation to the neonate differs from heart and liver transplantation in that similar constraints in matching the size of donor and recipient do not apply. In practice, considerable disparity in donor and host ages can be acceptable. On one hand, it is likely that kidneys which have been removed from newborn anencephalics have been transferred to adult recipients more commonly than to other infants. On the other hand, kidneys from adult donors have been successfully transplanted to neonatal recipients. An early (1970) account of renal transplantation to young children, indicated that approximately 50% of the cadaveric donors had been adults.[4] A report, published 15 years later, while acknowledging that previous renal transplantation undertaken before 2 years of age had achieved "dismal" results, reported nine cases of surgery on children under 1 year of age.[5] All of these infants had received kidneys from adult donors.

To some extent, the use of adult kidney donors for recipient infants reflected the scarcity of neonatal donors. However, quite apart from this question of limited availability, kidneys from neonates have been reported to be technically unsuitable for transplantation. This unsuitability has been attributed to a peculiarity of their blood vessels. Perfusion of the blood vessels of infant kidneys, that is flushing them with saline, as a routine aspect of preparation of organs for transplantation, is difficult to perform. In consequence, it has been suggested, from an early stage in the development of the technique, that newborn infants may be unsuitable as kidney donors.[6]

Assuming that kidneys from infants were readily useable as transplants, the extent to which the supply potentially available from anencephalics would be likely to satisfy the projected demand is essential information before the possible impact of organ harvesting from anencephalics can be estimated. In some localities, this impact has been estimated to be substantial. For instance, half of the potential donors under the age of 3 months referred to transplant units in Southern California are said to be anencephalic.[7] The extent of this anencephalic supply in terms of annual numbers was not indicated. Calculations bearing directly on the question of likely supply have been made by Shewmon et al.[8] Having made notional reductions in the numbers of anencephalics likely to be available for organ harvesting by adjusting the prevalence rate to allow for abortion of anencephalic foetuses detected by ultrasound (an increasingly frequent occurrence) and for stillbirths, they suggested an annual yield of approximately 300 was realistic in the USA. It was also assumed that 60% of liveborn anencephalics would be "too small to provide transplantable organs", so that approximately 120 infants would remain available. This total was further reduced by applying the existing figure that only "around 25% of vital organs (all ages combined) are found acceptable by established organ-sharing networks, and the figure for hearts is even less".[8] Their estimates would suggest that use of anencephalics as an organ source would exert no more than an imperceptible impact on waiting lists. In commenting upon an incident in which an anencephalic neonate was flown from Canada to California in order to be used in transplantation, Annas commented:

> "This was not a case of a dying child in search of an organ, but of a dying organ in search of a child."[9]

Other accounts of programmed attempts to employ anencephalic donors suggest that difficulty in finding an appropriate recipient have not been uncommon.

THE RELATIVE SUITABILITY OF ORGANS FROM ANENCEPHALICS FOR TRANSPLANTATION

Apart from the quantitative aspect of anencephalic organ supply, divergent views have been expressed about the *quality* of organs from anencephalic infants in general. (This is additional to the general reservation already mentioned concerning the usefulness of kidneys from *any* neonate.) Thus, the growth pattern of all organs in anencephalics, has been described as "abnormal and retarded". More specifically, it has been claimed that there is a relative deficiency of parenchymal cells in organs from anencephalics.[10] (Parenchymal cells are the specialized cells which undertake the functions of an organ. Their structure is peculiar to each organ as distinct from that of the cells which comprise the connective tissue "packing" which all organs also contain.)

Organs from anencephalics have been reported to be liable to especially rapid deterioration. For example, Iitaka *et al.* considered that, "only a fraction of anencephalic newborn infants can be employed as donors" for renal transplantation.[11] They expanded on this conclusion:

> "Even in the absence of congenital malformations, the kidneys of anencephalic infants cannot be considered normal."[11]

Melnick and Myrianthopoulos reported that minor malformations were quite common in other organs in addition to the nervous system with 25% of available kidneys being affected.[12] In contrast with this assessment, Spees *et al.* believed that:

> "a high proportion of liveborn anencephalics could have been considered as renal donors on anatomic grounds."[3]

It is hardly surprising that the more severe the anencephalic malformation in any infant, the less likely is that infant to be born alive and, hence, to be useable as a source of transplantable organs. However, this association necessarily creates a paradox. The likelihood that any individual anencephalic will meet the criteria for brain death will *increase* as the probable transplantation value of that individual *decreases*. In discussing the frequent contention that anencephalic infants "are incapable of experiencing consciousness or pain and therefore have no interests and cannot be harmed" (part of the grounds traditionally presented to justify using them), Shewmon *et al*. have specifically identified this paradox:

> "Although this is undoubtedly true for those with complete craniorachischisis [i.e. malformation affecting brain stem and spinal cord in addition to cerebral hemispheres] such infants are of little interest *vis-à-vis* their organs, because they are almost invariably stillborn."[8]

The wide range of severity of brain malformations that is a characteristic of anencephaly was stressed in Chapter 4. The range that can be encompassed within the term "anencephaly" has been attested by the US Medical Task force on Anencephaly, a widely representative group which produced, in 1990, an authoritative report on the medical issues raised by anencephaly:

> "The amount and extent of disruption of neural tissue other than the cerebral cortex vary from little or none to the complete disruption of all levels of the brain and occasionally the spinal cord."[13]

Liver transplantation is now becoming a recognized method of treatment of children.[14] Technically, it is considered to be essential that liver donors have a beating heart at the time of removal of the organ and that they are of approximately similar size to the prospective recipient. There appear to be divergent opinions on whether livers from neonates are required for transplantation to other neonates. If transplantation is to be undertaken in the first year of life:

> "infant donors less than one year old are highly desirable. However, it is felt that neonatal livers (including those from anencephalic donors) are untested and therefore less suitable."[14]

In practice, liver transplantation in the first year of life has been rare until recently. For example, in reviewing the progress of liver transplantation in the initial period up to 1982, Iwatsuki *et al*. noted that 119 out of 126 paediatric recipients did not receive their transplant until after the first year of life.[15]

Irrespective of the question of whether neonates *as a class* are suitable as a source of livers for transplantation, some specific concerns have been expressed about the quality of anencephalic livers. It has been speculated that the viability of livers transplanted from anencephalics may be impaired because of reduction of the levels of glycogen stored in the organ. An additional reservation that may apply to organs removed from anencephalic infants was raised by Holzgreve and Beller:

> "Rapid deterioration of vital signs makes most anencephalic infants unsuitable as donors after death...the compensating step proposed recently of 'gradual cooling of the body of the newly delivered anencephalic to save the organs from ischaemia' does not yield viable organs."[16]

As discussed in Chapter 4, death of the anencephalic infant is frequently attributable to cardiac failure. In the absence of vigorous resuscitation, failure usually follows a period of increasing impairment of cardiac function. The liver is probably the organ most susceptible to damage under these circumstances.

A recent development, which may have implications for paediatric liver transplantation, involves the removal of one lobe of the liver from a living adult donor and its transfer to the infant recipient. It is certainly too early to determine the ultimate value of this measure, although the initial results appear promising.[17] However, it is already apparent that the degree of success of the procedure may be only one of the factors determining its ultimate acceptability. This is because the ethical issues raised by submitting a healthy donor to major surgery are likely to be considerable. One important issue is whether the donor can make a reasonable, free decision under the crisis conditions associated with a rapidly deteriorating prospective infant recipient. The likely urgency of the situation is conveyed by a report from a group from the University of Chicago who were preparing to undertake liver transplantation from living donors. They estimated that up to 50% of infants awaiting liver transplantation in the USA died before operation. Their proposed solution to the ethical problem of obtaining valid consent from the donor was to commence transplantation to recipients who had not yet become critically ill. It was hoped that this would remove pressure on the prospective donor and so permit time for their thorough evaluation (including psychiatric assessment).[18]

Heart transplantation to infant recipients is still regarded (at the time of writing) as an experimental procedure. The principal indication for undertaking it is provided by "the recurring, virtually hopeless entity of hypoplastic left heart disease".[19] Alternatives to replacement of the recipient's damaged heart with a transplanted organ include transplantation of an additional heart to assist the recipient's own heart, either for a limited period or indefinitely,[20] and staged reconstructive procedures on the diseased organ.[21] Another option, which has received a very limited trial, entailed the transplantation of a baboon heart to an infant.[22] This procedure, which proved to be equally disastrous from the point of view of both recipient and donor, attracted considerable criticism at the time it was undertaken principally on the grounds that the procedure was so experimental as to render its clinical application ethically unjustifiable.[2, 23] One ethicist queried whether the infant involved, Baby Fae, had been "the unconsenting subject of an experiment on a human being that had no therapeutic justification".[24] Subsequent to this episode, unfavorable clinical and ethical assessments of xenografting (transplantation of an organ between different species) have proved to be among the most forcefully presented arguments marshalled in favour of the use of anencephalic infants.[25] This aspect, which will be discussed on pp. 166–167, recalls the manner in which the potential risk of development of a trade in organs from live, unrelated donors has emerged as a major point in arguments for the use of the alternative of beating-heart donors.

As is the case when kidneys and livers are transplanted from anencephalics.

there is a possibility that a heart from an anencephalic infant may be subnormal. For example, 45% of anencephalics had hearts that were more than one standard deviation below average size.[12] It may be especially relevant to proposals for transplantation of anencephalic hearts to recall the recent finding, mentioned above, that cardiac failure is likely to be a frequent, immediate cause of death in anencephalic infants. Information about the immediate cause of death has usually been obtained in relation to other disease processes by the practical expedient of attempting to treat the patient and, in the course of this, finding out which therapeutic measures avert deterioration and death. This measure had not been adopted in the case of the anencephalic as the possibility of longer term survival and development is non-existent.

For this reason, it has been regarded as unconscionable, in the interests of the patient, to adopt any vigorous measures to prolong life. However, recent experience, inadvertently gained in the course of intensive resuscitation of anencephalics in order that they could be used as a source of organs for others (see pp. 154–157), strongly suggests that cardiac function may be impaired in these infants. Intensive cardiovascular resuscitation of a series of anencephalic infants consistently produced marked improvement and extended survival. The implication of this is that cardiac decompensation probably accounts, to a large extent, for the rapid deterioration and death, which usually occurs in the absence of intervention.[26]

Irrespective of their quality as transplants, the extent to which anencephalic organs will continue to be available for this purpose remains an open question. The incidence of anencephaly has been declining in locations as diverse as Australia,[27] the Netherlands[28] and the USA.[29] This decrease was well advanced in each instance before the widespread availability of prenatal screening for neural tube defects and abortion of affected foetuses. (The report from the Netherlands actually drew attention to the likely adverse effect of the *spontaneous* decrease in incidence of anencephaly on the cost-effectiveness of screening programmes.) In addition to this spontaneous decrease in incidence, increasing use of prenatal diagnosis with selective abortion seems certain to result in a decreasing supply of anencephalics suitable for use as a source of organs. One paediatrician noted in 1988 that the majority of anencephalic foetuses in Canada and the USA could be expected at that time to be diagnosed prior to 20 weeks.[30] Very recently, it has been confirmed that appropriate dietary supplementation can effect reduction in the incidence of anencephaly to even lower levels.[31] Hence, vigorous advocacy of anencephalic use in the face of their inevitable decrease in availability appears paradoxical.

HISTORY OF THE USE OF ANENCEPHALICS AS A SOURCE OF ORGANS FOR TRANSPLANTATION

Some insight into the present controversy relating to the use of anencephalics in transplantation can be gained by reviewing the history of this subject.

Perhaps, the first point to be grasped is that there *is* an extended history of anencephalic usage. This is surprising in view of the considerable publicity that the subject has attracted in the late 1980s. It raises the question of why the use of anencephalic infants has only become a major issue now. A claim to have been the first to report (in 1962) the transplantation of a kidney from an anencephalic infant was made more than a quarter of a century later.[32] The retired surgeon responsible reminisced, "It never occurred to us that there would be any moral or ethical problems associated with that". One of the first attempts to perform cardiac transplantation (in 1968) utilized an anencephalic infant.[33]

The question of how a subject is transformed into an "issue" is one which has relevance to each of the topics considered in this monograph. In general terms, one might suggest that significant changes in the subject itself, for example, in this case in donor management practices or in transplant success rates, might have such an effect. Changes in the perception or awareness of the subject on the part of others could be similarly effective. Concerted attempts to publicize the subject, in this case either to promote or prevent the practice, could be important. In addition to any of the preceding, the potential for interest and attention on the part of the media when a saleable topic appears cannot be underestimated.

Examples of news items concerning the use of anencephalics, which attracted considerable attention to the subject, include the transplant operations undertaken at the Harefield (UK) and Loma Linda (USA) hospitals that are to be discussed in this section. Active discussion in the media of anencephalic use has also been encouraged by explicit advocacy of the proposition that the anencephalic should be submitted to surgery to remove the required organs *before* death, or brain death, had occurred. It is frequently not clear from examination of published reports of transplantation of organs from anencephalics whether organ removal had been deferred until after death. However, there are a number of indications that removal has been undertaken before death with increasing frequency.

An attempt to reconstruct earlier practice in the timing of organ removal in relation to death has been made by Shewmon *et al.*[8] For example, referring to a 1968 account of a heart transplantation from an anencephalic, they expressed doubts about the value of the reportedly flat electroencephalogram (EEG), noting that "it is unclear how even to perform an EEG on these patients". The interpretation of EEG tracings from anencephalics remains subject to great difficulty. The EEG may have some value as a research tool in the anencephalic: it certainly has none as a diagnostic measure for brain death. In commenting upon the time selected for excision of the heart in one of these cases, Shewmon *et al.* observed that:

"cessation of heart beat...happened to take place conveniently in the operating room after heparinisation and cooling"

(a technique that was routinely employed to inactivate the heart reversibly before surgical correction of cardiac lesions). This raised "further questions as to whether the donor's death was entirely spontaneous". Reconstruction of the events surrounding a 1973 kidney transplantation in which the organs were removed immediately after caesarean section, at 37 weeks gestation, led them to conclude that "plainly the source of the kidneys was a live-born infant". From the description of another renal transplantation reported in 1978, Shewmon *et al.* judged that:

> "determinations of death appear to have been made that would have been unacceptable in non-anencephalic patients."[8]

Attempts to reconstruct the management procedures that have been applied in the past to anencephalics, whom it was intended to use as a source of organs, have necessarily had to be confined to instances in which reports of these procedures were published. However, cases in which a description was published may constitute a minority of the actual number of cases. In this context, a disconcerting note was introduced by Ronald Cranford, Chairman of the Ethics and Humanities Committee of the American Academy of Neurology. He acknowledged in a 1986 interview that the harvesting of organs from anencephalic infants was already taking place around the USA "surreptitiously".[34]

Paradoxically, a 1985 report, which has been responsible for directing much attention to the subject of anencephalic usage, did *not* deal with the use of anencephalics. It nevertheless provides a good example of the way in which recoil from one option may provide an effective stimulus to the ready adoption of another. This report, already mentioned, came from the Loma Linda University Medical Centre in California and described the transplantation of the heart from a baboon into an infant with hypoplastic left-heart syndrome.[22] The outlook for survival of infants with this condition is as certain and as negative as is that for anencephalic infants with most victims dying during the first month of life, irrespective of any therapy. In electing to use a baboon as donor, the surgical team had reportedly been influenced by the difficulty inherent in defining brain death in infants.[35]

The aftermath of this episode of xenotransplantation (i.e. the transfer of grafts *between species*) entailed vigorous criticism directed especially to the inadequacy of the immunological techniques employed in matching donor and recipient for histocompatibility.[2] Following this response, the Loma Linda surgical team became vigorous proponents of the trial of anencephalic infants as heart donors in preference to xenografting. However, the obstacles to diagnosis of brain death in normal neonates that were outlined in Chapter 4 remain applicable to anencephalics. Whilst it is possible to arrive readily at the conclusion that the underlying cause of the brain disability is both identifiable and irreversible, it is no easier to guarantee that irreversible cessation of brain-stem function *has already occurred* in the anencephalic infant. This reality was identified in a *New Scientist* report. In a headline which almost said it all ("Surgeons want the organs of babies born brainless") the question of removal of organs from subjects who retain spontaneous respiration and heart beat was addressed:

> "The dilemma is that although anencephalics are doomed to die shortly after birth, they are alive when born. Removing their organs would quicken their death." [34]

As the "donors" would rapidly succumb to exsanguination following organ removal, the last proposition contains a substantial element of understatement.

As if in recognition of the reality that brain death can be as difficult to diagnose in an anencephalic as in an intact neonate, bills intended to expedite diagnosis of death in anencephalics have been introduced into three USA State legislatures in recent years. Whilst the basis of these bills, which were intended to legitimize usage of anencephalics, will be discussed later, the direction of some of the supporting medical comments is worth noting now. For example, one surgeon cited the wish of parents of anencephalic infants "to see some good come out of a tragic situation". Another stressed that the application of any new law could be confined to anencephalics because of the reliability and ease of diagnosis of the condition: "There is no blurring at the edges". [2]

A major input to the debate about anencephalic use was provided, 2 years after transplantation of the baboon heart, by a report from the Federal Republic of Germany describing transplantation of kidneys from anencephalic infants. [36] As already mentioned, the use of anencephalics' kidneys as transplants had been underway for some 25 years. The reason for the impact of the article by Holzgreve *et al.* in the widely read *New England Journal of Medicine* lay not in the report of use of this procedure but in the explicit details provided of donor management (or mismanagement) and the arguments provided to justify that course of management. To summarize that course, *in utero* diagnosis of anencephaly was followed by elective delivery of the infant undertaken at a time suitable for organ collection. Intensive resuscitation of the infant was commenced immediately after delivery, followed within an hour by removal of the required organs without any reference to the status of the infant's vital signs. The latter were clearly considered to be irrelevant to management of the patient. Beller identified the reason for the attention given this report quite explicitly in a subsequent article:

> "Kidney transplantations from anencephalics have already been described eleven times in the world literature. However these were all transplantations from cadavers as opposed to the life-related donors in Munster." [37]

Apart from the general claim that benefits would accrue to recipients, two specific arguments to justify intervention to remove organs from anencephalics, without reference to their clinical status, were advanced by Holzgreve *et al.* The first argument was based on an earlier article in the *New England Journal of Medicine*, the second on a ruling from a West German court.

The earlier article, by Chervenak *et al.*, concerned possible grounds for termination of pregnancy in the third trimester.[38] It has been cited on a number of occasions in discussion of the utilization of anencephalics as a source of transplantable organs. However, in a notable inconsistency, many of those citing it have aligned themselves with its conclusion but have then felt free to pursue a line of argument and practice quite contrary to that of the arguments underlying that conclusion. Chervenak *et al.* concluded that there were two valid criteria for identifying foetuses who could justifiably be aborted as late as the third trimester. These were a "total or virtual absence of cognitive function" occurring in a condition for which "highly reliable diagnostic procedures were available".

Chervenak's argument to justify a third-trimester abortion in cases meeting these two requirements was firmly based on a "principle of beneficence." It was argued that:

> "In comparison to these alternatives [namely neonatal death or a near vegetative existence], prenatal death does not constitute a harm."[38]

The argument proceeded:

> "Conversely allowing foetal or neonatal life to continue in such circumstances—or even intervening vigorously to prolong foetal or infant life—does not benefit the foetus or infant in any customary sense of the term 'benefit'."[38]

Paradoxically, Chervenak's phrase, "intervening vigorously to prolong infant life", appears to be the most apt description that could be applied to the procedure subsequently adopted by Holzgreve *et al.* for management of the newly delivered anencephalic infant. It appears quite inconsistent to argue that third-trimester abortion of anencephalic infants, in order to spare them from the infliction of non-beneficial experiences, can provide a supporting case for inflicting on them precisely those experiences, in the form of vigorous resuscitation, in the interests of others.

The second argument adduced by Holzgreve *et al.* for early intervention to collect organs from anencephalic infants regardless of their vital status, was based on a decision of a West German court. The point which they advanced to justify their action was that:

> "The concept that the anencephalic fetus, because of the absence of brain development, has never been alive despite the presence of a heart beat is now accepted in the courts of the Federal Republic of Germany and allows termination of pregnancy involving an anencephalic fetus at any time of gestation."[36]

Holzgreve's paper provoked discussion. In the course of a response to criticism of their actions, Holzgreve *et al.* advanced what appears to me to be a remarkably inaccurate analogy:

> "It seems to us somewhat artificial to consider true anencephaly because of residual brain-stem activity, as substantially different from acephaly, which is a complete lack of head and neck development."[16]

However, as discussed on pp. 116–117, the term "acephaly" refers to a form of parasitic twinning. An acephalic "foetus" is no more than a parasitic appendage lacking head and heart and attached to an intact individual on whose blood circulation it is dependent. To classify an anencephalic infant who breaths spontaneously and can cry and swallow, withdraw from a needle and behave in a number of respects as a normal neonate, and who may survive independently for days or weeks, in the same category as an appendage lacking head and heart does seem to be drawing a very long bow.

Before returning to description of the history of anencephalic usage in the USA, a case which arose in the UK in 1986 deserves mention because of the attention which it drew to the subject. This case involved a high-profile cardiac surgeon, Dr Magdi Yacoub. The procedure was undertaken at the Harefield Hospital in London. Interestingly, in view of the practice mentioned in Chapter 4 of popular media reference to anencephalics as "brainless", the hospital statement, released to the lay press, noted that "the donor was an anencephalic child—a baby without a brain".[39] Despite the inaccurate description of this anencephalic infant released by the hospital, a major controversy rapidly erupted. The headlines on the following day reflected this response: "Anger at baby kept alive for transplant",[40] "Heart swap enquiry"[41] and "Police alerted in controversy over heart transplant".[42] After a further 2 days, the headlines persisted, "A miracle—but is it right"[43] and the key issue was being vigorously canvassed:

> "The rumpus is over the state of the first baby. Although it had no brain was it, in fact, dead?"[43]

> "The operation was strongly criticized by the Opposition health spokesman in the following terms: "He said the public had doubts and revulsion against spare-parts breeding, and rightly so".[44]

An authoritative response on the subject came from Dr John Dawson, secretary of the British Medical Association's ethical committee. After pointing out that the then existing code of ethics for diagnosis of brain death as a prerequisite to organ removal was not applicable to an anencephalic, he suggested that:

> "Taking an organ from an anencephalic child was more like taking cells from an embryo and developing them."[45]

This represented a substantial change in response on the part of this spokesman in view of his statement 6 weeks previously (already noted on p. 106) that:

> "The legal definition of brain death in Britain is the irreversible cessation of function in the brain stem and that is the same at 70 years or two hours."[34]

An even more substantial change in the attitude of medical authorities in the UK became apparent when, 2 years later, the British Medical Royal Colleges decided that the absence of spontaneous respiration would suffice to signify death in anencephalic infants.[46] It should be noted that the imputation that death has occurred in these cases related to infants who have been maintained on respirators. As will be discussed below, the placement of an anencephalic infant on a respirator does not necessarily imply that spontaneous respiration had ceased. For example, the practice of Holzgreve *et al.* included the *routine* placement of newly delivered anencephalic infants on a respirator. To designate loss of spontaneous respirations as "death" as the Medical Royal Colleges recommended, represents a substantial shift from the existing UK recommendations for non-anencephalic subjects. These still require, not just suspension of spontaneous respiration, but positive recognition that *irreversible cessation of brain-stem function* has already occurred. The extent of the inconsistency created by selecting this standard for anencephalics will be evident if it is compared with the generally accepted attitude, that organs should not be removed from non-anencephalic neonates with beating hearts within 7 days of birth even if they satisfy the brain-stem death criteria for older children and adults. As discussed on pp. 106–110, this cautionary approach reflects widespread uncertainty among paediatric neurologists as to whether brain death can be reliably diagnosed in the first week of life. By adopting a standard for death that would be quite unacceptable for its diagnosis in any other class of subject, there is a risk that doubts may arise in the general community about the fairness of the rules for designation of individuals as a potential organ source. The possibility of adverse general effects had been raised by the British Labour Health spokesman, Mr Frank Dobson, after the Harefield Hospital incident. He cautioned that the case brought transplants into disrepute and "would damage the chances of attracting more potential kidney donors".[47]

Whilst the Harefield case was attracting attention to anencephalic use in the UK, the Loma Linda University Medical Center in California was proceeding to implement a new policy for the use of anencephalic infants. This consisted essentially of routine placement on a respirator from the time of birth of any infant who was considered to be a potential donor. Placement on a respirator was to occur irrespective of whether the infant was breathing spontaneously, i.e. there was no suggestion that it was being undertaken in the interests of the infant. This support was to be maintained, together with drug therapy as necessary to maintain blood pressure, until the required organs had been harvested. In describing this protocol, which was initiated in late 1987, the report in

Nature noted that:

> "The procedure will provide respectful treatment of the infant, including traditional provisions for comfort and pain relief, although anencephalics lack the capability to experience or interpret pain."[48]

The Loma Linda protocol proposed the administration of a strong synthetic opiate drug, Demerol (pethidine), if an anencephalic infant exhibited any signs of distress. This administration of pethidine to relieve "non-existent" pain inevitably raised the question of the capacity of these infants to feel pain.

In discussing the question of whether anencephalics have any capacity to appreciate pain, it was indicated that dogmatic denials of this possibility had been based on the belief that adequate development of those parts of the brain thought to be responsible for this function had not occurred in these infants. However, if the possibility is admitted that the present state of knowledge concerning the specific parts of the brain required to receive unpleasant sensations remains incomplete, the question necessarily arises as to where the burden of proof should fall. As already indicated, it is impossible to prove inability to feel pain or other forms of unpleasant sensation in any subject who is incapable of communication. It is interesting that some non-medical observers have raised the possibility that categorical assurances of the absence of sentience in anencephalics might be inaccurate. For instance, a lawyer advocating exemption of anencephalics from "brain death" legislation in order to facilitate their use remarked that:

> "The grimaces and crying of these children have convinced some physicians that they can feel pain, even though they are missing the portions of the brain that apparently respond to pain stimuli."[49]

The writer, nevertheless, obtained swift reassurance with the reasoning that:

> "Since they have no brain, they have no perception of pain, no hunger, no suffering."[49]

Unfortunately, this reflects the quality of much of the logic supporting the conviction that anencephalic infants lack anything resembling sentience as we know it. It would be of interest to obtain this writer's response to the parental description of an anencephalic infant that was quoted on p. 133.

Apart from raising some questions about the certainty of the medical and nursing staff concerning the anencephalic infant's inability to feel pain, the use of pethidine introduced another major complication into the Loma Linda project. In addition to its capacity to alleviate pain, this drug has sedative and respiratory depressive side-effects. However, one of the conditions which categorically precludes reliable diagnosis of brain death is the presence of sedative drugs in the patient's body. Such agents may invalidate one of the procedures invariably used in making the diagnosis of loss of spontaneous respiration, namely testing for the absence of spontaneous respiratory efforts when the ventilator is disconnected. In an attempt to overcome the potentially invalidating effect of use of pethidine, on the diagnosis of brain death, the Loma Linda protocol made provision for the use of another drug, antagonistic to the respiratory depression effects of pethidine. This was to be administered before testing for the cessation of spontaneous respiration was to be undertaken. (It has been reported that one of the physicians responsible for the preparation of anencephalics for organ removal had indicated in a press interview that the then current (third in the series) infant had received pethidine twice but had not received any drug to counteract its respiratory depressant effect.)[50]

The report on the Loma Linda protocol in *Nature* also noted that no infant was to remain on resuscitation beyond 7 days, "because of the consensus that indefinite maintenance of an anencephalic would be immoral".[48] A decision to proceed to organ removal was to be made if spontaneous respiration failed to resume on three successive occasions after the respirator was disconnected. This test was to be repeated at 12 h-intervals. In the course of the press interview referred to above, the chief neonatologist at Loma Linda made an interesting comment:

> "Speaking some 16 hours after the baby had been declared 'brain dead', Peabody said in answer to one question that if John's heart or liver were removed, 'the baby would totally die'."[50]

The University of California, San Francisco also adopted the Loma Linda procedures from May 1988.

The original Loma Linda protocol for maintenance of anencephalic infants was to be instituted as soon as each infant became available, irrespective of whether spontaneous respiration was adequate. However, the outcome of instituting resuscitation of anencephalic infants immediately after birth in this way was unexpected. None of the first six infants entered into this procedure in preparation for organ transplantation qualified to be used as a source of organs, i.e. none satisfied the prerequisite criterion for organ transplantation, namely of loss of the capacity for spontaneous respiration after disconnection of the ventilator, within the 7 days allowed.[51] In reviewing the trial, Peabody *et al.* concluded that, in the infants studied:

> "it is likely that the heart, liver and kidneys are initially suitable for donation in most live-born infants with anencephaly."[26]

They identified as an objective of the exercise the determination of whether the protocol would permit maintenance of organ viability until the criteria for total brain death could be met. Their conclusion was that the institution of intensive care sufficiently vigorous to maintain organ viability concurrently resulted in the maintenance of brain-stem activity, i.e. the infant was likely to retain the capacity for spontaneous respiration.

To summarize the Loma Linda trial, the motivation for placing infants on full resuscitation had been exclusively that of preserving organs destined for transplantation until their removal could be sanctioned under the guidelines for brain death. The unexpected and unintended incidental effect of the procedure was to support brain-stem function, so that those guidelines could not be met. So successfully was the unintended consequence achieved that one of the six infants in the trial left hospital and was adopted out for the remaining 2 months of its life.

Following the failure of the first protocol (institution of resuscitation at birth) to provide any anencephalic infants suitable for organ harvesting, a variation was introduced. This was to defer the initiation of resuscitation until death of the infant was thought to be imminent. However, even with this modification, the resuscitation that was required in order to forestall organ deterioration caused by circulatory failure still had the unintended consequence of interrupting the process of dying. As a result, none of the six infants who were entered into the second protocol became available for organ harvesting. Peabody *et al.* observed that deferral of placement on a respirator until brain stem failure was occurring permitted a degree of deterioration in the infant's organs incompatible with their use for transplantation.

A different protocol for the management of anencephalic infants in preparation for organ removal was developed at a Canadian hospital:

> " [The] objectives of the protocol were to avoid intervention and prolongation of the dying process of the anencephalic infant and to reduce the time the parents and their infant with anencephaly might have to spend apart." [52]

This protocol entailed waiting until the heart beat was no longer audible before instituting life-support measures. The report of this protocol noted incidentally that of five liveborn infants referred to the hospital as anencephalics, 2 represented misdiagnoses. [52]

The Loma Linda trial produced some further, unexpected results. Referring to an interview with Dr Peabody published by the *Los Angeles Times*, Shewmon *et al.* drew attention to the reported referral by "good physicians" of infants with less severe anomalies. [8] They noted that these referring physicians "could not understand the difference between such newborns and anencephalics". The experience of the trial appeared to have influenced Dr Peabody. A report of September 1988 from a hospital spokesman indicated that she was "sequestered, seeking time and space in which to prepare a report for the scientific community". [51] Furthermore, the *Los Angeles Times* was reported as quoting her to the effect that, "I have become educated by the experience...The slippery slope is real". [8]

The courses of management reported for anencephalic infants appear to me to raise the question of applicability of *Article 10* of the *Declaration of the Rights of Disabled Persons* adopted in 1975 by the United Nations General Assembly:

"disabled persons shall be protected against all exploitation, all regulations and all treatment of a discriminatory, or abusive or degrading nature".[53]

Removal of organs from any incompetent individual could be argued to be exploitative. Application to anencephalics of treatment which would not be applied to any other class of individual is undoubtedly discriminatory. Infliction of life support on a patient for whom it can predictably have no benefit is certainly abusive. Presumably, the response to these charges would be that the anencephalic was not a person and was therefore outside the scope of the Declaration.

Similar considerations were identified in the protocols for use of anencephalics (albeit without explicit reference to the United Nations Declaration) by Arras and Shinnar in their critique of the practice:

"The question is whether prolonging the infant's life by mechanical ventilation and then abruptly terminating it by harvesting vital organs is compatible with the minimum respect due to all persons...even a dying person is still a person and is entitled to a full measure of dignity and respect as discussed above."[54]

ARGUMENTS ADVOCATING ANENCEPHALIC USAGE IN TRANSPLANTATION

The first of the arguments advanced to support the use of anencephalics in transplantation that I wish to consider is based on the needs of organ recipients and of the families of anencephalic infants that would thereby be met. A second argument, namely that anencephalic infants are not persons, has been discussed on pp. 130–134. Another point of view has been that the rights, which individuals have in relation to their bodies, rest with others in the case of anencephalics. Finally, the use of anencephalics has been claimed as a course that is preferable to some undesirable alternatives.

As was the case with beating-heart donors, discussed in Chapter 2, the role of advocacy in shaping the transformation of biological data into issues to be discussed in the community deserves attention. The distinction between reporting or commenting on a subject and advocating a position on it is not always clear. However, the outcome of discussion on issues such as anencephalic usage may be considerably influenced by overt advocacy and its impact on reporting.

Needs that may be met by the use of anencephalics in transplantation

Two distinct needs have been identified as likely to be satisfied by harvesting of organs from anencephalic infants. The more immediately evident of these is represented by the potential benefits accruing to the recipient from organ transplantation. The quantitative extent of the contribution that anencephalic usage could reasonably be expected to make to paediatric transplantation has been considered on p. 144. Estimates vary widely but the most thoroughly argued appear to be so low as to suggest that any impact on waiting lists for paediatric transplantation would be negligible.[8]

The other need, which might be met if anencephalics were incorporated in organ transplantation programmes, has been expressed as follows:

"Second, there is the need of the parents of an anencephalic infant to salvage some good from a tragic situation. Allowing the infant to be used as an organ donor may help satisfy this need."[54]

The "salvage" value for the family of anencephalic use in transplantation has been stressed on a number of occasions. It has, for instance, been described "as seeking to redeem the pregnancy".[55] In a 1986 article in the *Lancet*, which advocated the use of anencephalics as organ sources, Harrison observed of families with anencephalic infants that they would "clutch at any possibility that something good may be salvaged from a seemingly wasted pregnancy".[56] This line of argument developed to the point where he speculated that:

"The ability to transplant foetal organs may now give us the chance to recognize the contribution of this doomed foetus to mankind."[56]

The premise underlying his advocacy was that the anguish of parents of anencephalics might be alleviated, at least in the short term, by harvesting of the infants' organs.

If the use of anencephalics as a source of transplantable organs is to be advocated seriously as a means of assuaging the distress occasioned by the birth of a disabled infant, it is legitimate to seek scientific support for the proposition that such use does produce a beneficial effect on the infant's parents. In particular, the relief which it is argued will be afforded by organ transplantation needs to be demonstrated. It should then be balanced against the possible disadvantages to the parents of deprivation of participation in both the living and dying of their infant as a result of the mandatory relocation of these events to intensive-care ward and operating theatre, respectively. As discussed in Chapter 3, remarkably little information has been published on the impact of the removal of organs from brain-dead subjects on surviving family members. The few published reports are derived from studies undertaken within a relatively short time after the episode. No estimate is possible of any impact that the inevitable realization within the community of what organ removal from beating-heart donors entails will have on the attitudes of surviving family members. Whilst there have

been reports of parents and prospective parents of anencephalics wishing to have
these infants used as organ sources, I am not aware of any longer term follow-up
studies *after* such use. To form a decision on the issue of whether use as an organ
source is likely to relieve the distress of parents after an anencephalic birth will
require information on at least two subjects. These are the impact on a family
of the birth and death of a severely disabled infant and the effects of organ donation on the donor's family.

The first point to note in relation to the former is the change that has occurred
in assessing the implications of a perinatal death for the infant's family. The
reversal of medical attitudes was summarized in the introduction to a 1987
article on the subject in the journal *Clinical Obstetrics and Gynecology*.[57] The
attitude that prevailed in the past was described in this article as follows:

> "Until fairly recently, it was commonly believed that although the death of a baby
> before or shortly after birth represented a loss, it was emotionally less significant
> than other forms of death, a medical misfortune rather than a human tragedy.
> Medical response was geared accordingly: the mother was discouraged from seeing
> her infant (so she would not 'get attached') and consoled with platitudes such as
> 'you can always have another'."[57]

This perception of the situation, and its relationship to reality, was commented upon succinctly in a leading article in the *Medical Journal of Australia*:

> "It was once thought that a woman would rapidly 'get over' a still birth or a
> neonatal death, because she had not 'known' the baby or known it for very long.
> Nothing, of course, could be further from the truth, as every woman who has
> experienced such a loss would well recognize."[58]

Whilst the transformation in medical attitudes to the impact of perinatal death
that was described in these two articles had occurred over the preceding decade,
its impact upon practitioners in different medical specialties had clearly been
variable. For example, the article by Chervenak *et al.*, referred to earlier in this
chapter, had advocated third-trimester abortion of anencephalic foetuses "in
order to shorten the inter-pregnancy interval".[38] However, it has been increasingly recognized that infants conceived soon after the perinatal death of a sibling
are at increased risk of parental neglect.

The traditional downgrading of the significance of perinatal death was probably attributable to a failure to recognize the strength, or even the existence, of
parent–infant bonding. A frequent consequence of such downgrading is likely
to have been the failure of the family of the deceased infant to complete an adequate grieving process. Psychologists studying grieving in response to perinatal
loss have concluded on more than one occasion that:

> "the loss of a baby may have at least as severe an effect on a woman as the death
> of her husband."[59]

The effects of incomplete grieving of a perinatal loss are likely to be compounded by its frequently unexpected occurrence. This can lead to an ongoing denial of the death by the parents and a consequent inability to accept it. Such a sequence has been reported following not only stillbirth or the death of a neonate, but also the neonatal loss of one twin, spontaneous abortion and midtrimester termination undertaken because of foetal abnormality.[57] It has been observed that the "shadow" of a perinatal death may linger with the mother throughout her lifetime.[58]

In view of this change in understanding, the advice that has been given, on occasion, to the parents following the birth of a lethally malformed infant to forget it and to go away and have another child to compensate is now recognized to have the possible consequence that there will be substantial impairment of the relationship between the mother and that subsequent child. Nevertheless, advocacy continues for the adoption of this course of action. For instance, in developing proposals for the management of newborns with severe disabilities, a 1985 paper from the Australian Human Rights Commission described the painless killing of an extremely deformed neonate and its replacement the following year by a normal birth to the mother as:

> "the ultimate form of the quality of life argument that the creation of a new worthwhile life is to be preferred to maintenance of a highly imperfect life."[60]

Irrespective of the morality of the proposal, there can be little doubt about the scientifically shoddy nature of the advice.

Is the likelihood of inadequate grieving in response to perinatal death relevant to consideration of use of anencephalic infants as organ donors? I believe that acknowledgement of the connection necessarily becomes inescapable once the argument is pressed that the use of these neonates as a source of organs will offer *positive benefit* to their parents. If a decision is taken to use an anencephalic infant as an organ source, the removal of the affected infant to a paediatric transplant centre to become the subject of intensive resuscitation is essential as a preliminary to organ collection. This course of action abruptly and effectively terminates any association of the infant with its family. Participation by the family in an intensive-care experience, in which highly intrusive management techniques are imposed on the infant in order that it may serve as a better source of organs, would be equally damaging. There is general agreement among those responsible for the care of the parents of infants dying in the perinatal period that the best chance of avoiding pathological grieving lies in maximizing the opportunity for the parents to know and to remember their child. This would seem to be no more than a natural response to recognition of the difficulty of grieving for a poorly known individual.

In practical terms, a strategy to facilitate effective grieving is likely to entail encouragement of the parents to see and hold the baby, to name it, to be with it during its life, however brief, and to remain there during its dying.

Malformations such as anencephaly would not be regarded by paediatricians as contradicting this policy. A reflection of this is the advice, mentioned on p. 139, of passing the bonnetted infant to the parents. Psychological studies of the mothers of dead infants have suggested that "maternal grief is relative to the length of the baby's life".[61] The importance of parental contact with dying neonates has been stressed:

> "They may see or touch their baby even when the infant is critically ill and receiving respirator support. This approach to care is believed optimal for families to facilitate adjustment irrespective of whether the child lives or dies."[62]

The interposition of intensive resuscitation techniques followed by surgical removal of the organs to be transplanted, as discussed in Chapter 2, certainly intrudes on family participation in the process of dying in adult patients. This intrusion would seem to be much more of a problem in the case of a dying infant than in that of the brain-dead adult. In the case of the former, the family not only has to come to terms with the reality of loss but is abruptly required to learn to know the infant. In view of what is done in the course of protocols already practised for handling anencephalic infants in preparation for organ donation (see pp. 154–158) the total separation of parents from infant at an early stage would be expected.

If claims that organ donation from anencephalics can provide parental consolation for loss of the infant are to be substantiated, it will be essential to establish that the benefits flowing to the parents from the donation significantly outweigh the disadvantages of abrupt removal of the infant from its parents. There are a number of anecdotal reports of requests from the parents of anencephalics for their infant to be used as a source of organs for transplantation.[45] The extent to which parents professing this view have had a thorough understanding of the technicalities of anencephalic maintenance and subsequent organ removal is unknown. There is no reason to doubt that some parents of anencephalics would wish to see an outcome of value that could be offset against the loss of the infant. This response may be compared with that observed among the families of suicide victims who are reported to be keen for the affected individual to be used as a multi-organ donor. However, apart from the initial wishes of the family, it would be necessary to have reliable information on the ultimate attitudes of families who have had an anencephalic infant used as an organ source. As previously indicated, there is a complete lack of data in relation to the long-term impact on the families of infant organ donors and, surprisingly, there is only minimal information on this subject for adult donors. An investigation of the impact of heart donation on the family of the donor written in 1985 by a social worker with a heart transplant programme reported that only two previous publications on the subject had been located. Examination of the medical literature of the succeeding 5 years does not disclose additional articles. The author of the 1985 article emphasizes the point that the family of a prospective donor should not "be led to expect that their grieving will be lessened by the donation of an organ".[63] Taking account of the substantial body of information available in relation to the progress of grieving, it would seem likely that any attempt to introduce other substitute considerations as a means of lessening grief would be counterproductive. On the basis of her experience with a heart transplant programme, Pittman raised the possibility that a donor family may regard heart donation as a means of reinforcing their denial of the donor's death.[63] She reported instances of the transfer of family attachment from donor to recipient:

"Some families of donors have expressed distress at the lack of news of 'their recipient'."[63]

An interesting comment on the processes that can underlie decision on organ donation relates to the families of suicide patients mentioned above. Pittman noted that, in contrast with the families of other classes of donor, families of suicide patients were not selective in deciding upon organs to be donated. Their tendency to donate all tissues was interpreted as an expression of "anger, distress and confusion". It also raises the question of the extent to which rational processes play a part in family decision-making in relation to organ donation. This in itself should justifiably raise some doubts about the favourable nature of long-term impact on the surviving family. At the present time, the only valid assessment of the emotional outcome of organ donation for the family of the anencephalic infant is that this remains entirely conjectural.

"Non-personhood" as grounds for anencephalic use

The question of the personhood status of anencephalics has been considered on pp. 130–134. However, it is appropriate in any discussion of the course of advocacy of anencephalic use to indicate the extent to which highly emotive claims for non-personhood have been presented. Few presentations of this argument have been as emotive and as intolerant of alternative positions as those of the paediatric cardiac surgeon L. L. Bailey from Loma Linda. Bailey dismissed the anencephalic as:

"a nonperson human derivative, a resource we should be able to capitalize on."[51]

On another occasion, he claimed that:

"the anencephalic infant, while human, has never been a person and has no possibility for personhood."[7]

He also observed with reference to anencephalic infants that:

> "all are grotesque in appearance and all die."[7]

In supporting his opinions, Bailey readily dismisses alternative positions:

> "Bioethicists, right-to-life groups and others who oppose the use of anencephalic
> infants as organ donors seem unable to come to grips with a clear medical defi-
> nition of what anencephaly really is."[7]

It is difficult not to come away with the impression that he believes that none
other than medical personnel, perhaps none other than cardiac surgeons, have
the right to present a view on the subject. For instance, he believes that:

> "most of the things that are considered psychosocial or ethical issues, and so forth,
> can be *made* to become medical criteria."[7] (my italics).

Whilst Dr Bailey appears to have provided the most florid comments on the
subject, his has not been a lone voice. For example, two practitioners writing
to the *Canadian Medical Association Journal* in support of the Loma Linda program juxtaposed recommendations for the treatment of anencephalic infants
with propositions of non-personhood:

> "Anencephalic infants do not meet the legal criteria for brain death: they are simply
> brain absent. By most commonly used criteria they are not human."[64]

The other asserted:

> "That normal criteria for brain death need hardly be applied in the case of anen-
> cephalic infants will no doubt be officially recognized in due course."[65]

The right to "donate" an anencephalic infant for transplantation

A conclusion which those advocating the exclusion of anencephalics from personhood often feel entitled to draw is that those rights which might otherwise
attach to the anencephalic should be automatically transferred to others:

> "The parents and families of anencephalics are, after all, the real persons at stake."[7]

Several commentators have responded unfavorably to the proposition that anencephalics lack the rights of normal infants because of their gross disability and
hopeless outlook. An interesting, and more balanced, response to arguments for
automatic classification of anencephalics as equivalent to dead because of "brain
absence" or "non-personhood" came from the Committee on Bioethical Issues

of the Medical Society of New York:

> "On the other hand, babies born with hypoplastic lungs or hypoplastic hearts are also doomed to die without lung or heart transplants, but nobody has proposed lung absence or heart absence to constitute a new definition of death."[66]

The innate inconsistency of separating anencephalics as automatic donors primarily on the basis of their hopeless prognosis, has attracted comment from other authors. For example:

> "If the crucial issue is uniform early mortality, then a number of other conditions, such as Potter's syndrome and trisomy 13, would qualify."[54]

Taking the argument for designation as an organ source on the basis of transient life expectancy a step further, Shewmon *et al.* inferred what could be its logical extension:

> "Specifically, using this kind of logic, half of all the infants who die of congenital kidney, heart and liver disease would better be used as organ sources to preserve the lives of the other half, rather than letting them all die along with their transplantable organs."[8]

The theme that the anencephalic lacks any rights has been used to advocate de-restriction of the use of these infants. This outcome has been validated by proposing the transfer to the infant's parents of "ownership" of any commodity that can be derived from the anencephalic. The phraseology used in discussing this subject often provides a very clear insight into the view that is being presented:

> "If the parents of an anencephalic infant *wish to donate their child as a tissue or organ source*, and if this can be accomplished in a manner that does not violate the sensibilities and values of the medical profession or society concerning the treatment of *human materials*, then it would seem desirable to amend existing laws governing organ procurement to include anencephalics as possible organ and tissue sources"[67] (my italics).

The attitude embodied in the preceding approach to the anencephalic assumes that there is no distinction between the actions of donation and expropriation. I do not accept this assumption. I believe that, if the term "donation" is to be used accurately, its implication is indisputably that of the gift of something from one individual to another as a result of a decision freely taken by the former. Whilst parents in some societies have been considered to "own" their children, in the sense that they can exercise rights of life and death over them, the attitude prevailing in most contemporary communities is to regard the parental role as one of guardianship rather than ownership. An attitude which regards anencephalic infants as "human materials" to be disposed of at the wish of the parents runs counter to the course of evolving recognition of individual human rights during the present century. Recourse to jargon in describing the management of the anencephalic infant in terms such as "the protocol-designated predonation life of the deformed infant"[51] does not, to my mind, disguise the nature of the proposal.

The manner in which use of the term "donor" has become established and then extended is in itself a good illustration of the way in which selection and repeated usage of particular terminology can, imperceptibly, shape attitudes. The earliest donors to participate in clinical transplantation were, in fact, just that. They were most commonly relatives of patients with renal failure who, after opportunity for reflection, elected to donate a kidney. As the use of conventionally dead and brain-dead subjects to provide organs was introduced, the term donor was retained, with tacit recognition that donation, being an action, could not logically be attributed to a cadaver. Description of such a subject as a donor might be sustainable on the basis that the decision to remove an organ was construed to be the one which that individual, given their previous views on the subject, might reasonably have been expected to take. Such considerations can scarcely be claimed to apply to the anencephalic. As it is impossible to know what the infant's wishes might have been, assuming the malformation was not inconsistent with their formulation or expression, it becomes ridiculous for a parent or anyone else to construe those wishes. Under these circumstances, the term "donor" is being used as a synonym for "supplier. Altruism is being conveniently imputed on behalf of others. The alternative approach quoted above[66] of attributing the action of donation to parents of the anencephalic rather than to the infant, however, raises the question of how one can donate that which one does not also own. One of the few contributions to the subject of use of anencephalic infants to have appreciated and responded to the incongruity introduced by their description as donors was the critique of Shewmon *et al.* to which reference has already been made.[8] The title referred to the use of anencephalics as "organ sources" and the term "donors" when first used in the text was placed between inverted commas.

Anencephalic usage may obviate the need for less acceptable approaches to the problem of organ procurement

One of the most potent arguments that has been advanced to support the use of beating-heart (non-neonatal) organ donors was that this would forestall the development of a commercial market in transplantable organs. The strategy of raising the spectre of alternatives that will be perceived as less desirable than the course which is being advocated has also been used to promote anencephalic utilization. The selected alternative in this case has been the use of non-human organ donors. The approach of arguing from a less acceptable alternative is well illustrated in an article entitled, "Primates and anencephalics as sources for pediatric organ transplants," by Fletcher et al..[68] The authors adopted the well-recognized difficulty of obtaining cadaver organs from children as the starting point for discussion. They then proceeded to canvass the question of using xenografts from non-human primates as an alternative to human organs. The improbability, on immunological grounds, that xenografting could be successfully undertaken was noted as also was the dubious ethical status of submitting recipients to such experimental procedures. Scarcity and expense of chimpanzees were additional arguments against xenografting. All of these arguments against the use of organs from non-human primates appear to me to have some validity. Nor should an additional argument, namely that the use of animals as organ sources represents an unreasonable imposition upon them, be dismissed out of hand. However, I believe that statements such as that of Dr Leonard Bailey on the relative appropriateness of the two organ sources lack a sense of proportion. As one of the few individuals to have used both anencephalic infants and non-human primates for cardiac transplantation he concluded:

> "For me, I have much more difficulty taking the heart out of a living baboon than I would from an anencephalic."[69]

Whilst the various arguments against xenografts have merit, I do not accept that any of them thereby becomes a valid argument for the use of anencephalic infants instead of animals as organ sources. Recitation of the unfavorable aspects of an alternative procedure can be a very effective tactic for diverting attention away from negative features of one's preferred course of action. However, it can not serve as a means of enhancing the positive features of that course other than in a relative way. Irrespective of the potential attractiveness of success with organ transplantation to neonates, this procedure is not an imperative for the community. However, the vigor of the advocacy of anencephalic usage, exemplified by Fletcher et al.,[68] might well lead one to accept that an unquestionable imperative exists to develop transplantation programmes.

SOME LEGISLATIVE APPROACHES TO ANENCEPHALIC USAGE

The ultimate goal of advocacy of any objective is often its incorporation in legislation. A number of legal commentators have made proposals for legislative changes to facilitate the use of anencephalics as an organ source. Paediatric surgeons have issued similar calls. At least one German court has effectively ruled that anencephalics may be treated as though already dead, irrespective of their vital signs. Legislation to facilitate the use of anencephalics as organ donors has been introduced into the legislatures of several American states.

The first attempt to facilitate access to anencephalics by legislative means appears to have been a bill introduced into the California legislature in 1986 by

State Senator Milton Marks. This bill would have allowed considerable latitude in the use of anencephalics. Its specific purpose was to supplement the *Uniform Determination of Death Act* with a provision that, "an individual born with the condition of anencephaly is dead", without any regard to the infant's vital signs.[49] If accepted, its consequence would certainly have been to ensure that the process of organ removal could soon enable any anencephalic to qualify as dead according to any set of criteria. The pointed response of one ethicist to the bill ran along the lines that:

> "Calling them 'dead' will not change physiologic reality or otherwise cause them to resemble those (cold and non-respiring) bodies that are considered appropriate for post-mortem examinations and burial."[70]

Classification as "dead" will not cause an anencephalic who is breathing to cease doing so. As has been remarked on a number of occasions in discussion of the subject, one would be required also to accept the burial of a spontaneously breathing patient if the anencephalic is to be treated as dead.

A second bill seeking to facilitate use of anencephalic infants as organ sources was presented in October 1986 by New Jersey Assemblyman Walter Kern Jr.[49] Its provisions were such that organ transplantation from an anencephalic infant would become permissible, provided the parents submitted a written request for use of the infant in this way. Physiological impediments, which might give the impression of persistent life, were not to be allowed to stand in the way of this variety of organ "donation". Organ removal would be legitimate,

> "regardless of whether the infant has sustained an irreversible cessation of circulatory and respiratory functions or an irreversible cessation of all functions of the brain stem."[49]

Whereas the bill already mentioned and a subsequent version from Ohio, to be discussed below, sought to extend the current definition of death so as to include anencephalic infants, the Kern bill overcame any obstacle seemingly presented by a spontaneously breathing donor by the expedient of legitimizing organ removal, irrespective of vital status. The bill read:

> "Section 2(a) of the Uniform Anatomical Gift Act specifies that any gift of organs takes effect on the death of the donor. The proposed statute would eliminate this requirement in the case of anencephalics."[49]

The controversy engendered by this bill was such that its sponsor eliminated the changes proposed in the determination-of-death law. In its place, a bill was passed to authorize an examination of the legal, medical and ethical aspects of the original proposal.

A third legislative initiative was entitled the "respirator brain death" bill by its proposer when introduced into the Ohio legislature. Under its provisions, anencephalic infants could be automatically placed on a respirator and tested for the absence of spontaneous respiration every 6 h. Failure to resume spontaneous respiration on three successive occasions would suffice for diagnosis of death. The proposed legislation would confine the use of this diagnostic protocol to infants with anencephaly. Existing Ohio law, which would remain applicable to all non-anencephalic members of the community, required the "total and permanent cessation of all brain function including the brain stem".

The Ohio respirator brain death bill attracted severe criticism from Dr Alan Shewmon, a paediatric neurologist at the University of Southern California.[71] He pointed out that patients with a variety of other conditions would also satisfy the bill's requirements for diagnosis of death. Anyone losing the ability to breathe spontaneously over a period of 12 h would become eligible. This would include not only patients with progressive neurological diseases, such as amyo-trophic lateral sclerosis and myasthenia gravis, but also those with conditions producing transient loss such as Guillain–Barre syndrome, botulism and curare poisoning. The bill's requirements for diagnosis of death could also apply with equal validity to many patients on the first day of coma (produced by a variety of causes) even though they could be capable of subsequent recovery. Shewmon described proposals to remove organs from anencephalic infants as,

"a legal gimmick aimed at circumventing the law. They can't take the organs from live people so they want anencephalics to be declared dead".[34]

This response recalls the earlier comments of a French paediatrician, Professor Minkowski, reported in *Nature*, that valid diagnosis of brain death in foetuses scheduled to provide tissues and organs for transplantation was not possible.[72]

Following the initial criticism, which it attracted, the respirator brain death bill was withdrawn only to be reintroduced in 1989 by Representative Tom Watkins. In its amended form, diagnosis of death required that the infant be an anencephalic who had failed the spontaneous breathing test and who did not have a significant (but undefined) degree of hypotension or hypothermia. (Lowering of blood pressure and/or body temperature may result in reversible depression of brain-stem activity.) Despite these modifications, the reintroduced bill, if enacted, would legitimize the removal of organs from infants retaining a gag reflex, pupillary reactions to light and spontaneous body movements.[73]

A recent ruling from a USA court indicated an accurate grasp of the legal issues involved in anencephalic usage. Judge Estella Moriarty, of the circuit court in Fort Lauderdale, Florida:

"ruled doctors could take any transplant organs from the terminally ill six-day-old [anencephalic] infant as long as they didn't kill her in the process."[74]

A transplant expert from the University of Miami was reported as commenting after the decision was handed down that:

> "the decision clears the way for one kidney to be taken, but it is questionable whether doctors could perform the operation without killing Theresa."[74]

The response from the lawyer responsible for presenting the case for organ removal gave the impression that the infant had no rights requiring representation:

> "the state had invaded the family's constitutional right to make a private decision with a doctor."[75]

Apart from the direct introduction of legislation to authorize the use of anencephalic infants as organ sources, there have been calls from medical personnel, primarily with an interest in transplantation, for such changes to be made. One Australian headline ran:

> "A leading Melbourne doctor has urged the Government to change organ transplant legislation. Cardiologist Dr Brian Edis of Melbourne's Royal Children's Hospital said the Hospital might seek special dispensation from the current ruling which prevents transplants being taken from dying rather than legally dead donors, in a bid to save the life of a 7-month old baby with a diseased heart."[76]

The conclusion of Arras and Shinnar to the effect that, "Admirable goals should not be advanced by improper means"[54] appears to be a most appropriate response.

Some 2 years later, in August 1991, another specialist from the same hospital took up the running:

> "The law should be changed to allow permanently comatose people to be declared legally dead according to a Melbourne hospital director. The director of the Melbourne Royal Children's Hospital's intensive care unit, Dr Frank Shann... said doctors tested only the brain stem to determine death, but the higher part of the brain should be the decider of whether a patient was legally dead. Dr Shann said changing the legal definition would prevent cruelty to relatives of patients left in a vegetative state."[77]

Almost as an afterthought, he added:

> "Also, more organs would be available for donation."[77]

Whilst the context of this advocacy appears to relate to anencephalic infants, its wording is strongly reminiscent of the calls, discussed in Chapter 3, for adoption of a cerebral death standard for *any* patient exhibiting permanent loss of consciousness. In leaving the argument in a form which would apply to either type of patient, this Australian approach differed from the USA attempts at legislation which sought, at least in the first instance, to restrict its area of operation to anencephalics.

THE IMPACT OF RESPONSIBILITIES TOWARDS POTENTIAL RECIPIENTS ON MANAGEMENT OF ANENCEPHALICS

Discussion of anencephaly in the preceeding and in this chapter has touched on its anatomical and physiological features, the requirements for paediatric organ transplantation and the various forms taken by advocacy of the use of anencephalics for this purpose. Before completing this chapter, I wish to summarize the ways in which the requirement for fair treatment of potential recipients of organs from anencephalic infants may impact on the management of these infants. Some questions, which bear directly on attributes of the anencephalic infant, have already been considered in Chapter 4. These include the questions of whether any individual anencephalic infant is alive or dead and whether anencephalics, as a class, are to be regarded as human persons. Should one believe that anencephalics lack personhood, the question of whether an anencephalic infant is alive or dead might be considered irrelevant in determining his or her treatment. In that event, conditions governing use of the anencephalic might reduce to those applicable to similar usage of living members of non-human species.

As regards the diagnosis of death, it has already been emphasized that this is equally difficult in anencephalic and normal neonates if it is required rapidly in order to permit use as an organ source. As emphasized at the beginning of Chapter 4, diagnosis of irreversible brain-stem failure is often considered to be an unreliable procedure during the first 7 days of life. Whilst a diagnosis of anencephaly guarantees irreversibility, it does not render recognition that total cessation of brain function has *already* occurred any simpler than it is in other neonates. To achieve this diagnosis sufficiently early to permit recovery of organs in suitable condition for transplantation can be as difficult in the anencephalic as in the non-anencephalic infant. One suggested solution to this impasse, that was noted above, has been to define anencephalics as automatically dead so as to avoid the provisions for diagnosis of death before organ removal.

Apart from scientific objections to the use of legislation to promulgate biological untruth, proposals to declare anencephalics as brain dead irrespective of their actual clinical status raise difficulties on other grounds. Brain-death provisions, which applied exclusively to anencephalic infants, would breach the perception of consistency of donor treatment that has been fostered during promotion of the concept of organ collection. Furthermore, it is likely that failure to respond to concerns about fair-dealing with subjects from whom it is intended to remove organs could lead to erosion of general community confidence in the role of medical personnel in management of subjects who are potentially organ sources. The assessment of this issue by the ethicist and lawyer, Ian Kennedy, remains relevant 20 years after it was written:

> "if this surgery is to become acceptable, and the voluntary supply of organs from cadavers is to be increased, every effort is needed to persuade the general public that such operations are being conducted in a responsible and humane way, that the law, in other words, is not being re-written in favour of the potential recipient and against the interests of the moribund donor."[78]

The duty of care owed to recipients of organ transplants is a major factor in considering transplantation procedures that are highly experimental or entail substantial risks. The likely course of the prospective recipient's disease, if left untreated, must be taken into account in considering organ transplantation. Questions of duty of care to the recipient may be raised in relation both to the experimental nature of some transplantation techniques and to the extent to which it is permissible to transfer organs that are in suboptimal condition. In the first instance, the legitimacy of subjecting patients to therapy that is so experimental as to afford minimal chance of success must be decided. For example, cardiac xenografts from non-human primates to infants with left-ventricular hypoplasia would currently be considered by most commentators to lie beyond the pale because of their highly experimental nature. Even the hopeless prognosis of untreated left-ventricular hypoplasia is unlikely to justify recourse to xenografts, which could be regarded as a burdensome imposition. In contrast with the totally experimental nature of transferring xenografts from baboons, the results of transplantation of hearts from human infants have probably been sufficiently encouraging to establish this as a reasonable risk to impose on the recipient. Liver transplantation to the neonate could also be regarded as offering sufficient chance of improvement in the recipient's condition to justify its use.

Apart from the intrinsic risk associated with transplantation. the second question concerning duty of care towards neonatal recipients of hearts and livers from anencephalic infants relates to the possibility that modifications of donor management may be indicated in the interest of the prospective recipient. To what extent does transplantation of an organ in suboptimal condition represent unfair treatment of the recipient? On the other hand, to what extent is it permissible to manipulate the circumstances surrounding organ acquisition, in the interests of the recipient, before one can be accused of unfairly treating the subject who is to provide the organ? When the interests of the recipient are considered, the choice may lie between undertaking such modifications of donor management or refraining from transplantation because an organ can not legitimately be obtained in optimal condition.

The types of modification of management of an organ donor that are considered necessary in order to optimize the outcome for the recipient may concurrently interfere with the diagnosis of donor death and also impose burdensome treatment on the donor. An example of the former effect may be provided by measures undertaken to improve the state of preservation of organs from anencephalic infants. Cooling of the anencephalic infant in order to retard organ deterioration may not only expedite the attainment of signs required for the diagnosis of death but may also effectively simulate these. As hypothermia is likely to mask evidence of spontaneous respiration and cardiac action it should invalidate any diagnosis of death.

THE IMPACT OF ANENCEPHALIC USAGE ON OTHERS

The potential effects of organ harvesting from brain-dead, beating-heart donors on others has been considered in Chapter 3. As indicated by Dr Leonard Bailey, the surgeon with the most experience of extended resuscitation of anencephalic infants for subsequent use as an organ source, a major limiting influence on the extent to which this practice can be used will be the tolerance of the staff, rather than that of the infant, towards it. Assuming nursing staff are "educated" to become comfortable with prolonged maintenance of anencephalic infants on life-support systems from birth solely to provide a source of human material for transplantation to others, to what extent may their attitudes and conduct towards other groups of patients be influenced? Is it unnecessarily alarmist to question whether attitudes towards severely disabled infants with *other* conditions may also be altered? On the other hand, will concern about this risk promote the tendency, already noted, to construct factitious classifications that differentiate anencephalics from other classes of human subject?

A second category of subjects likely to be affected by programmes for using anencephalic infants as a source of organs are the families of these infants. Advocacy for such programmes has frequently placed considerable emphasis on the consolatory effect that the usage of an anencephalic infant for the benefit of others may have on the parents. It has been claimed that this course of action may help to "redeem" the pregnancy. Nevertheless, the extent of this beneficial effect appears to remain largely anecdotal. Certainly the question of its duration is totally speculative as no extended studies of the families of anencephalic (or other groups of) infant donors has been undertaken. It has been suggested, by the very few surveys of the families of adult heart donors that this event may provide a positive experience in the short term. The extent to which the responses of these families would reflect the response of the surviving members of the families of infant donors is questionable. However, as discussed on pp. 159–163 the extent of interference with the grieving process might be expected to be much greater in response to the abrupt removal of a neonate whom the parents had not learnt to know. At the very least, the argument that parental compensation is an advantage accruing after use as an organ source of an anencephalic infant should be considered as dubious.

It appears very likely that, irrespective of any "redeeming" effects of infant usage on the family, the separation of parents from the infant during the dying process which this entails may produce long-term adverse consequences. (Parental involvement in the "no holds barred" resuscitation indicated to preserve the infant's tissues in optimal condition for transplantation would be equally unconducive to development of an acceptable recollection of the infant and its last days.) It is also uncertain whether the positive aspects of organ donation on the surviving family (irrespective of the age of the subject) are dependent upon the success of the transplant operation. There appears to have been a tendency among donor families to retain an interest in the identity and later progress of the recipients of organs from their family member. The very limited evidence available on this aspect suggests that donorship, or the death of a transplant *recipient*, do not lengthen the period of grieving experienced by the donor family.[79] However. as this information was produced by surveying families of non-infant donors and takes no account of the additional difficulties likely to be experienced in grieving for an infant (pp. 160–161), it may not be possible to extrapolate confidently to the situation of the parents of an anencephalic infant. There appears to be considerable need for detailed consideration of this aspect if a community decides to endorse developments of programmes of paediatric transplantation based on the use of anencephalics.

REFERENCES

1. Landwirth, J. (1988) Should anencephalic infants be used as organ donors? *Pediatrics*, **82**, 257–259.
2. Caplan, A. L. (1985) Ethical issues raised by research involving xenografts. *Journal of the American Medical Association*, **254**, 3339–3343.
3. Spees, E. K., Clark, G. B. and Smith, M. T. (1984) Are anencephalic neonates suitable as kidney and pancreas donors: *Transplantation Proceedings*, **16**, 57–60.
4. Fine, R. N., Korsch, B. M., Stiles, Q., Riddell, H., Edelbrock, H. H., Brennan, L. P., Grushkin, C. M. and Lieberman, E. (1970) Renal homotransplantation in children. *Journal of Pediatrics*, **76**, 347–357.
5. So. S. K. S., Nevins, T. E., Chang, P.-N., Mauer, S. M., Ascher, N. L., Fryd, D. S., Sutherland, D. E. R., Simmons, R. L. and Najarian, J. S. (1985) Preliminary results of renal transplantation in children under 1 year of age. *Transplantation Proceedings*, **17**, 182–183.
6. Potter, D., Belzer, F. O., Rames, L., Holliday, M. A., Kountz, S. L. and Najarian, J. S. (1970) The treatment of chronic uremia in childhood. I. Transplantation. *Pediatrics*, **45**, 432–443.
7. Bailey, L. L. (1988) Donor organs from human anencephalics: a salutory (sic) resource for infant heart transplantation. *Transplantation Proceedings*, **20**, (Suppl. 5), 35–41.
8. Shewmon, D. A., Capron, A. M., Peacock, W. J. and Schulman, B. L. (1989) The use of anencephalic infants as organ sources. A critique. *Journal of the American Medical Association*, **261**, 1772–1781.
9. Annas, G. J. (1987) From Canada with love: anencephalic newborns as organ donors? *Hastings Center Report*, **17**(6), 36–38.

10. Naeye, R. L. and Blanc, W. A. (1971) Organ and body growth in anencephaly. A quantitative morphological study. *Archives of Pathology*, **91**, 140–147.
11. Iitaka, K., Martin, L. W., Cox, J. A., McEnery, P. T. and West, C. D. (1978) Transplantation of cadaver kidneys from anencephalic donors. *Journal of Pediatrics*, **93**, 216–220.
12. Melnick, M. and Myrianthopoulos, N. C. (1987) Studies in neural tube defects. II. Pathologic findings in a prospectively collected series of anencephalics. *American Journal of Medical Genetics*, **26**, 797–810.
13. Stumpf, D. A., Cranford, R. E., Elias, S., Fost, N. C., McQuillen, M. P., Myer, E. C., Poland, R. and Queenan, J. T. (1990) The infant with anencephaly. *New England Journal of Medicine*, **322**, 669–674.
14. Lum, C. T., Wassner, S. J. and Martin, D. E. (1985) Current thinking in transplantation in infants and children. *Pediatric Clinics of North America*, **32**, 1203–1232.
15. Iwatsuki, S., Shaw, B. W. and Starzyl, T. E. (1984) Liver transplantation for biliary atresia. *World Journal of Surgery*, **8**, 51–56.
16. Holzgreve, W. and Beller, F. K. (1987) Kidney transplantation from anencephalic donors. *New England Journal of Medicine*, **317**, 961.
17. Raia, S., Nery, J. R. and Mies, S. (1989) Liver transplantation from live donors. *Lancet*, **2**, 497.
18. Singer, P. A., Siegler, M., Whitington, P. F., Lantos, J. D., Emond, J. C., Thistlethwaite, J. R. and Broelsch, C. E. (1989) Ethics of liver transplantation with living donors. *New England Journal of Medicine*, **321**, 620–622.
19. Bailey, L. L., Jang, J., Johnson, W. and Jolley, W. B. (1985) Orthotopic cardiac xenografting in the newborn goat. *Journal of Thoracic and Cardiovascular Surgery*, **89**, 242–247.
20. Barnard, C. N. and Cooper, D. K. C. (1984) Heterotopic versus orthotopic heart transplantation. *Transplantation Proceedings*, **16**, 886–892.
21. Norwood, W. I., Kirklin, J. K. and Sanders, S. P. (1980) Hypoplastic left heart syndrome: experience with palliative surgery. *American Journal of Cardiology*, **45**, 87–91.
22. Bailey, L. L., Nehlsen-Cannarella, S. L., Concepcion, W. and Jolley, W. B. (1985) Baboon-to-human cardiac xenotransplantation in a neonate. *Journal of the American Medical Association*, **254**, 3321–3329.
23. Jonasson, A. and Hardy, M. A. (1985) The case of baby Fae. *Journal of the American Medical Association*, **254**, 3358–3359.
24. Knoll, E. and Lundberg, G. D. (1985) Informed consent and baby Fae. *Journal of the American Medical Association*, **254**, 3359–3360.
25. Veatch, R. M. (1986) The ethics of xenografts. *Transplantation Proceedings*, **18**, (Suppl. 2), 93–97.
26. Peabody, J. L., Emery, J. R. and Ashwal, S. (1989) Experience with anencephalic infants as prospective organ donors. *New England Journal of Medicine*, **321**, 344–350.
27. Danks, D. M. and Halliday, J. L. (1983) Incidence of neural tube defects in Victoria, Australia. *Lancet*, **i**, 65.
28. Romijn, J. A. and Treffers, P. E. (1983) Anencephaly in the Netherlands: a remarkable decline. *Lancet*, **i**, 64.
29. Windham, G. C. and Edmonds, L. D. (1982) Current trends in the incidence of neural tube defects. *Pediatrics*, **70**, 333–337.
30. McGillivray, B. C. (1988) Anencephaly—the potential for survival. *Transplantation Proceedings*, **20**, (Suppl. 5), 9–16.
31. Wald, N. (1991) Prevention of neural tube defects: results of the Medical Research Council Vitamin Study. *Lancet*, **338**, 131–137.

32. Goodwin, W. E. (1989) The anencephalic controversy. *Pediatrics*, **83**, 641.
33. Kantrowitz, A., Haller, J. D., Joos, H., Cerutti, M. M. and Carstensen, H. E. (1968) Transplantation of the heart in an infant and an adult. *American Journal of Cardiology*, **22**, 782–790.
34. Anderson, I. Surgeons want the organs of babies born brainless. *New Scientist*, p. 20, November 6, 1986.
35. *Australian Doctor*, p. 27, May 22, 1985.
36. Holzgreve, W., Beller, F. K., Buchholz, B., Hansmann, M. and Kohler, K. (1987) Kidney transplantation from anencephalic donors. *New England Journal of Medicine*, **316**, 1069–1070.
37. Beller, F. and Reeve, J. (1989) Brain life and brain death—the anencephalic as an explanatory example. A contribution to transplantation. *Journal of Medicine and Philosophy*, **14**, 5–23.
38. Chervenak, F. A., Farley, M. A., Walters, L., Hobbins, J. C. and Mahoney, M. J. (1984) When is termination of pregnancy during the third trimester morally justifiable? *New England Journal of Medicine*, **310**, 501–504.
39. Fraser, L. Storm over 'kept alive' donor baby. *The Mail on Sunday*, (London), December 14, 1986.
40. Anger at baby kept alive for transplant. *The Daily Post*, December 15, 1986.
41. Heart swap enquiry. *The Courier & Advertiser* (Dundee), December 15, 1986.
42. Gillie, O. Police alerted in controversy over heart transplant. *The Independent*, (London), December 15, 1986.
43. A miracle—but is it right? *The Star*, (London), December 17, 1986.
44. "Baby transplant leads to inquiry", *Yorkshire Post*, December 15, 1986.
45. Sherman, J. Baby with no brain used as heart donor tests medical ethics. *The Times*, (London), December 15, 1986.
46. Salaman, J. R. (1989) Anencephalic organ donors. Guidelines available from Britain and North America. *British Medical Journal*, **298**, 622–623.
47. Ethics study on baby kept alive for transplant. *The Scotsman* (Edinburgh), December 15, 1986.
48. Barinaga, M. (1987) Maintaining anencephalic babies causes consternation in U.S.A. *Nature*, **330**, 592.
49. Friedman, J. A. (1990) Taking the camel by the nose: the anencephalic as a source for pediatric organ transplants. *Columbia Law Review*, **90**, 917–978.
50. Bond, L. and Andrusko, D. (1988) "Harvesting" anencephalic babies controversy grows in intensity. *U.S. National Right to Life News*, February 25, 1988.
51. Goldsmith, M. F. (1988) Anencephalic organ donor program suspended: Loma Linda report expected to detail findings. *Journal of the American Medical Association*, **260**, 1671–1672.
52. Frewen, T. C., Kronick, J. B., Kissoon, N., Lee, R., Lynch, A., Green, R., Whittall, S., Casier, S., Sommerauer, J. F., Silcox, J., Burke-Tremblay, C. and Stiller, C. R. (1990) Anencephalic infants and organ donation: the Children's Hospital of Western Ontario experience. *Transplantation Proceedings*, **22**, 1033–1036.
53. Tay, A. E.-S. (1986) *Human Rights for Australia*. Australian Government Publishing Service, Canberra.
54. Arras, J. D. and Shinnar, S. (1988) Anencephalic newborns as organ donors: a critique. *Journal of the American Medical Association*, **259**, 2284–2285.
55. Stiller, C. R. (1988) International consensus conference on anencephalic donors. Foreword. *Transplantation Proceedings*, **20**, (Suppl. 5), 1.
56. Harrison, M. R. (1986) Organ procurement for children: the anencephalic fetus as donor. *Lancet*, **2**, 1383–1386.

57. Stierman, E. D. (1987)   Emotional aspects of perinatal death. *Clinical Obstetrics and Gynecology*, **30**, 352–361.
58. Raphael, B. (1986)   Grieving over the loss of a baby. *Medical Journal of Australia*, **144**, 281–282.
59. Nicol, M. T., Tompkins, J. R., Campbell, N. A. and Syme, G. J. (1986) Maternal grieving response after perinatal death. *Medical Journal of Australia*, **144**, 287–289.
60. Human Rights Commission (Australia) (1985)   Legal and ethical aspects of the management of newborns with severe disabilities. *Occasional Paper, no. 10*, p. 13. Australian Governement Publishing Service, Canberra.
61. Peppers, L. G. and Knapp, R. J. (1980)   Maternal reactions to involuntary fetal/infant death. *Psychiatry*, **43**, 155–159.
62. Benfield, D. G., Leib, S. A. and Vollman, J. H. (1978)   Grief response of parents to neonatal death and parent participation in deciding care. *Pediatrics*, **62**, 171–177.
63. Pittman, S. J. (1985)   Alpha and omega: the grief of the heart donor family. *Medical Journal of Australia*, **143**, 568–570.
64. Laberge, J.-M. (1987)   Transplanting organs from anencephalic infants. *Canadian Medical Association Journal*, **137**, 473–474.
65. Tuttle, M. J. (1987)   Transplanting organs from anencephalic infants. *Canadian Medical Association Journal*, **136**, 797–798.
66. Rosner, F., Risemberg, H. M., Bennett, A. J., Cassell, E. J., Farnsworth, P. B., Landoldt, A. B., Loeb, L., Numann, P. J., Ona, F. V., Sechzer, P. H. and Sordillo, P. P. (1988)   The anencephalic fetus and newborn as organ donors. *New York State Journal of Medicine*, **88**, 360–366.
67. Caplan, A. L. (1988)   Ethical issues in the use of anencephalic infants as a source of organs and tissues for transplantation. *Transplantation Proceedings, 20*, (Suppl. 5), 42–49.
68. Fletcher, J. C., Robertson, J. A. and Harrison, M. R. (1986)   Primates and anencephalics as sources for pediatric organ transplants: medical, legal and ethical issues. *Fetal Therapy*, **1**, 150–164.
69. Bailey, L. (1988)   Anencephalic donors. Discussion of other issues. *Transplantation Proceedings*, **20** (Suppl. 5), 73.
70. Capron, A. M. (1987)   Anencephalic donors: separate the dead from the dying. *Hastings Center Report*, February, 1987, 5–9.
71. Wilkie, J. C. (1988)   A devastating critique. *U.S. National Right to Life News*, April 21, 1988, p. 3.
72. Walgate, R. (1983)   Human embryo research. INSERM to ponder ethics. *Nature*, **302**, 4–5.
73. Bond, L. (1989)   Lawmaker's attempt to 'harvest' organs from anencephalic babies stirs strong opposition. *U.S. National Right to Life News*, March 23, 1989, p. 4.
74. *The Canberra Times*, 'Solomon-like' ruling on organs of 'no-brain' baby. March 28, 1992.
75. *The Canberra Times*, Baby Theresa on a ventilator. March 30, 1992.
76. *Australian Dr. Weekly*, p. 7, July 14, 1989.
77. Comatose changes sought. *Australian Dr. Weekly*, p. 22, August 23, 1991.
78. Kennedy, I. M. (1971)   The Kansas statute on death—an appraisal. *New England Journal of Medicine*, **285**, 946–950.
79. Christopherson, L. K. and Lunde, D. T. (1971)   Heart transplant donors and their families. *Seminars in Psychiatry*, **3**, 26–35.

6 The Transplantation of Brain Tissue

The preceeding four chapters have considered the biological and clinical aspects of transplantation of organs other than the brain—principally kidneys, liver and heart. This chapter is concerned with the transplantation of tissue removed from the brain, predominantly with the transfer of parts of the brain of the foetus to the brain of patients with Parkinson's disease. In the late 1980s, this procedure evolved from being an experimental protocol in animals to one to be trialled as a therapeutic practice in humans.

The difference which is readily apparent between transplantation of other organs and transplantation of tissue from the brain is that procedures in the former group have been accepted on the basis that they are undertaken only *after* brain death has been diagnosed in the organ donor. As discussed in Chapter 2, brain death was originally envisaged as a state in which the brain, in its entirety, had ceased to function. Subsequent investigation of patients diagnosed as brain dead has increasingly suggested that cessation of function has only been established in, and may be confined to, those parts of the brain, the function of which can be assessed clinically. As discussed in Chapter 2, a range of techniques for examining brain function have suggested that residual function may persist in some parts of the brain after a diagnosis of brain death has been made on the accepted grounds. It appears logically inescapable that the nominal requirement applying to the removal of other organs, namely brain death, would constitute a contraindication to the use of foetal brain tissue for transplantation. If irreversible inactivation of the brain has already occurred, then transplantation of part of that organ would be an unjustifiable procedure because it would be certain to fail. On the contrary, if transplantation of portion of the brain is contemplated, it is necessary that irreversible inactivation of this organ has *not* already occurred, i.e. the subject to be used as a source of tissue should *not* be brain dead.

Whilst this point appears to have been immediately appreciated in the lay press, and attention drawn to it, informed responses to that concern do not appear to have been forthcoming. For example, within a week of the outbreak of publicity concerning foetal brain transplantation in the UK one columnist wrote in *The Guardian*:

> "these foetuses, aged between six and nine weeks gestation are said to be dead when their brain cells are transplanted. Yet by definition the brain cells are alive or else the transplant would be useless. So how can the foetus be dead? When heart

surgeons need a donor, death is when the brain (or part of it) dies. When neurologists need foetal brain tissue, death is when the heart dies. The goalposts are not just moving but flying back and forth."[1]

A consultant anaesthetist from Birmingham raised the question of whether the criteria generally accepted for brain-stem death would be applied to foetal brain-tissue donors:

"I very much doubt it, and I would be interested to know how the tests are done."[2]

The other side of the coin, namely the potential difficulties raised in *other* areas of transplantation practice by ignoring brain-death criteria in the case of foetal brain-tissue donors was raised in a letter to the *Daily Telegraph* from Dr Boultbee:

"It is also worth noting that brain tissue transplantation has the long-term potential of undermining the concept of 'brain death' as at present defined (newspeak for brain-stem damage with loss of function assumed to be irreversible) by rendering some cases treatable."[3]

Transplantation of the *whole* brain, as distinct from portions of brain tissue, has been undertaken in animals as an experimental procedure. It has been discussed as a possibility in humans but there do not appear to have been any reliable reports of its having been attempted. A 1971 report of transplantation of the head, undertaken in rhesus monkeys, purported to be relevant to application of this procedure in a clinical setting.[4] The authors dismissed the possibility of surgical connection of the brain *alone* to another body as being of little import because such a brain would be deprived of any means of sensory input or motor output. However, they suggested that:

"cephalic transplantation, on the other hand, would obviate this major problem by providing external environmental contact with information gathering and expression through the preservation of the cranial nerves."[4]

Two decades later, an American author was moved to publish a book with the title, "If we can keep a severed head alive...Discorporation and U.S. patent 4 666 425". It was asserted by a reviewer,[5] that the author had taken out a patent on the maintenance of severed heads, with a view to preventing further development of the technology. The author's response to the reviewer[6] was that the proposal "has important potential advantages, for research and for prolonging life in a conscious and communicative state with, probably, less pain than many dying people suffer today". He also claimed to have been contacted by half-a-dozen people, some dying others paralysed, inquiring about the operation:

"Most said that if the mind remains clear and the head can still think, remember, see, read, hear and talk and if the operation leads to numbness rather than pain below the neck then they would want it."[6]

There would appear to be a strong case for arguing that, in the situation described above, the transplanted entity would be whatever was connected to the head rather than the head itself. Whilst the extracorporeal maintenance of a severed head or its transplantation to a body might be expected to be successful for a limited period, it would appear improbable that any surgical team would invite the opprobrium likely to be generated by undertaking this experiment. In view of the increased sensitivity that has developed in relation to the treatment of experimental animals, especially primates, since 1971, the transplantation of an animal's head would now be regarded in most places as completely unacceptable and unjustifiable. Nevertheless, recent consideration of the propriety of transplanting tissue from the human foetal brain appears to have been influenced by the prospect of whole-brain transplantation to the extent that the transfer of other than very small fragments has been proscribed. The basis given for this has been to avoid the possibility of transfer of "a part of the brain which was sufficiently large to function as a neuroanatomical structure".[7]

Responding specifically to this contention by a spokesman for the British Medical Association, Professor Elizabeth Anscombe wrote that it:

> "shows that those important doctors, like many of my own colleagues [philosophers] are bitten by modern superstition about the brain. The brain, together with the central nervous system, says a well known philosopher, is the 'core person'. Others: if we were to swap brains, you'd be me and I'd be you. The BMA says: 'Nervous tissue may only be used as isolated neurones or tissue fragments for transplantation. Other foetal organs may be used as either complete or partial organs for transplantation'."[8]

An example of the outlook described by Anscombe, concurrently presented in the British press, came from Professor Pat Wall, a neurophysiologist at University College, London:

> "Could transplanting from one brain to another cause the transferral of behavioural characteristics? The answer is definitely yes...These are nerve cells that are being transplanted—they're not just producing chicken soup...What kind of effects might occur then—behavioural, clinical psychological? The works...You are highly likely to get unexpected results. That's one of the reasons for being cautious."[9]

In view of the unique features of transplantation of brain tissue, principally that the tissue is likely to be required before brain death has occurred and that any possibility of transfer of "personality" must be avoided, it is not surprising that the subject has readily attracted publicity. The circumstances surrounding the introduction of any newly developed procedure, and its manner of presentation, are as likely to determine the impact that it has on the community as is its substance. The recent history of the introduction of transplantation of foetal brain cells as an alternative form of treatment for Parkinson's disease illustrates this point. Use of the procedure of transplantation of a variety of structures from the foetal brain to the brain of other animals as an experimental tool to probe the potential of the graft for growth and function became increasingly frequent during the 1970s and 1980s. However, there was little indication in the scientific literature that application of this technique to human subjects was imminent.

THE INTRODUCTION OF FOETAL BRAIN-CELL TRANSPLANTATION AS A THERAPEUTIC MEASURE

"Professor Edward Hitchcock's recent announcement that he had implanted aborted foetal tissue into the brains of two patients suffering from Parkinson's disease must earn the dubious distinction of stirring up more media and professional controversies than any other single event in U.K. medicine since the 'brain-stem death' debate at the end of the 1970s."[10]

Whilst it was not the first occasion on which the procedure was used, the event which attracted the widest attention to foetal brain-cell transplantation, and from which an ongoing controversy surrounding it can be dated, was the disclosure of its use by a British neurosurgeon in April 1988. While a number of reasons probably account for the impact of this event, the most significant was its presentation by the British press. The two operations that had been performed immediately became front page news. The headlines over the following month indicate the press response; "My story, by brain transplant wife",[11] "I watched mother come out of hell"[12] and "New life plan by brain op. woman".[13] Not content with maximizing the impact of the new procedure in relation to Parkinson's disease, one paper saw fit to interview the parents of a child who had died from measles-induced encephalitis and elicit the comment, "This operation would have given us hope, where before we had none".[10] As there has not been any suggestion that foetal brain transplantation would have anything to offer in reversing damage produced by this form of encephalitis, this could be considered as a particularly insensitive journalistic intrusion.

The performance of the two British operations which triggered these media responses had been first reported at a meeting of the Society of British Neurological Surgeons by Professor Edward Hitchcock of the Midland Centre for Neurosurgery and Neurology in Smethwick, Birmingham. In probing the background to these two operations, the magazine *New Scientist*[14] implied that there could have been more to them than met the eye:

"But the timing of the operations, and the way in which he handled their disclosure, left almost everything to be desired. It cannot have escaped Hitchcock's notice that the British Medical Association had set up a working party on ethical aspects of the therapeutic use of fetal tissue which is due to report this summer. The publication of the guidelines would have been the cue for extensive public debate on the issue, before any operations were carried out. What possible reason could there be for operating in advance of the publication of the guide-lines— except to pre-empt the possibility that the ethical debate might go against his pro- ceeding? ...The sensible scientific course to take at that point would have been to describe the purpose of the operation but say, as the Swedes have done, that it is far too early to judge whether it has been effective in reducing the symptoms of Parkinson's disease. But once his cover was blown, Hitchcock apparently threw scientific caution to the winds. He claimed that both patients 'were better than they were'." [14]

To place the Smethwick operations in context it is helpful to trace the earlier, albeit less widely publicized, history of transplantation as a form of treatment for Parkinson's disease.

The first acknowledged transplantation of tissue into the brain of patients with Parkinson's disease was reported from the Karolinska Institute in Stockholm in 1985. Two patients with severe parkinsonism had fragments from the medulla of their own adrenal glands implanted in the caudate nucleus, a collection of nerve cells deep within the brain. In a report published 2 years after surgery had been performed on the first patient, Backlund and his co-workers noted that "the clinical effects were seemingly poor". However, the operation, as per- formed at the Karolinska Institute, was without significant risks. [15] An article published a year later reviewed both clinical cases and related experiments in animals, and reported results of operations on two further patients. [16] The second two cases differed slightly from the original two in that the site of implan- tation was the putamen, a different aggregation of nerve cells close to the cau- date nucleus. [17] It was noted that these patients had experienced some short-term benefits and no disabilities as a result of the operation.

There were no further accounts of attempts to transplant cells to the brain as a treatment for Parkinson's disease until 1987 when it was reported from Mexico City by Madrazo et al. [18] that dramatic improvements had been achieved in the condition of two Parkinson's disease patients following transplantation of their own adrenal tissues into their brains. Videotapes of patients from the Mexican clinic were shown at a series of scientific meetings and attracted enthusiastic acknowledgement for the clinicians managing the cases.

Although the only publication of results from Mexico City for a substantial period remained the original skimpy report in the New England Journal of Medicine, a host of clinics, mostly in North America, proceeded to attempt to emulate the Mexicans. An estimate, presented by Marsden to a meeting of the British Parkinson's Disease Society, of the number of patients submitted to sur- gery by mid-1988, was 300. [19] Whilst very few, if any, of the results of these operations were formally published in orthodox journals, the impression that all was not well rapidly gained currency.

The denouement came in March 1988 at a meeting of the United Parkinson

Foundation, held in Chicago. As reported subsequently in *Science*:

> "During the past year Madrazo and his colleagues carried out more than 40 adrenal-to-brain transplants, the great majority of which have been anecdotally represented to be as successful as those in the initial report. Meanwhile, 85 patients were similarly treated in clinics in the United States, the outcomes of which have been disappointing by comparison with Madrazo's results."[20]

Questioning of Madrazo at the Chicago meeting was reported to have produced "little in the way of satisfactory explanation". It was suggested that, "some of the Mexican patients had not suffered from Parkinson's disease but from some other movement disorder". It was also hinted that some of the patients who had received implants in Mexico City were in "extremely poor" clinical condition when examined in the USA.

The precise number of patients submitted to surgical implantation of their own adrenal tissue in the brain is not known: negative results of such procedures run a high risk of not being published. As already indicated, Marsden has estimated the total to mid-1988 at around 300. It is unlikely that many of these operations have been performed since then. He considered, on the basis of reports at conferences, that the risk of serious brain injury to the patient from the procedure was in excess of 25%. There was often an alteration of mental state together with sleepiness for some weeks post-operatively. Furthermore, the abdominal surgery required to harvest adrenal tissue was more hazardous in Parkinsonian patients. The large numbers of adrenal transplant operations undertaken in a relatively short period is consistent with the assessment provided in mid-1987 by John Sladek, one of those to have researched animal equivalents of the procedure: "Any competent neurosurgical team can do this operation".[20]

By early 1988, it was becoming increasingly clear that the procedure of adrenal autotransplantation described by Madrazo and his colleagues was both ineffective and dangerous. However, its extensive and indiscriminate use had encouraged expectations that relief for Parkinson's disease, in the form of transplantation of cells into the brain, *was* at hand. Clearly, circumstances were propitious for a trial of alternative transplantation procedures. Adrenal autotransplantation would be an easy act to follow.

Three events followed almost simultaneously. As already described, Hitchcock and his group at Smethwick implanted foetal brain cells into two patients and presented the outcome of these and subsequent cases in a very positive manner in the media. We will take up this sequence of events later. Bjorklund had undertaken a similar procedure, 2 or 3 months earlier, on two patients with the intention of observing and assessing them over an extended period.[20] Finally, Madrazo and his colleagues announced the earlier transfer (in September 1987) of foetal brain cells and foetal adrenal cells to the brains of two patients with Parkinson's disease.[21] They claimed that, at the time of publication (1988), there had been "an evident objective improvement in the symptoms of Parkinson's disease in both cases".

By mid-1988, as a result of the preceding experience with adrenal autotransplantation, the report of the Mexican group on adrenal autotransplantation had come to be generally regarded with considerable scepticism. Not only did the procedure appear to be ineffective, but it appeared increasingly likely that it was also potentially dangerous. A range of adverse behavioural side-effects had been observed in recipients of adrenal autotransplants. [22]

Subsequent letters to the *New England Journal of Medicine* from other laboratories hardly engendered confidence in the likely success of the two most recent Mexican patients who had received foetal brain and adrenal medulla, respectively. For example, it was claimed that, if attention was paid to the detail of earlier reports of transplantation of foetal animal tissue, neither of the Mexican cases could be expected to benefit from the procedure as reported. Specifically, it was suggested that the foetal source of brain tissue had been of an inappropriate gestational age, 13 weeks rather than the predicted optimum of 9 weeks. [23] Additionally, it was claimed that Madrazo and his colleagues had been mistaken in their understanding of the nature of the adrenal tissue transplanted. [24] The Swedish neurosurgical group had indicated that no report on the post-operative course of their two patients would be available before independent assessment of their condition later in 1988. Meanwhile, the British group was prepared not only to provide reports on their patients from an immediately post-operative stage but indicated to the press that further operations would be forthcoming. The construction placed on this course of action by *New Scientist* has been mentioned earlier. It is instructive to consider the response of the British medical community to the operations undertaken at Smethwick, as well as the response of the Smethwick group to published comments on the procedure and the implications of these events for patients with Parkinson's disease and their families.

Commentary on foetal brain-cell transplantation appeared in *The Lancet* and the *British Medical Journal* in response to the press reports on the operations at Smethwick. Both urged the adoption of caution, the latter quoting Lord Cohen to the effect that "the feasibility of an operation is no indication for its performance". [25] *The Lancet* noted the Smethwick reports of immediate improvement and commented:

> "Surely what is needed now is not more operations, but careful long-term follow-up, with positron emission tomographic scanning and neurophysiological and clinical evaluation, of patients who have already received grafts. Such a programme is already underway in Lund and London; these results should be known before any further surgery is contemplated." [26]

Apart from these editorial comments, little adverse comment from medical sources on the Smethwick group was published. One exception was the medical correspondent of *The Sunday Telegraph*, Dr James Le Fanu:

> "The results of the first operations in Sweden have never been published in a widely-circulated medical journal, so it is not possible to judge. This unethical secrecy is impossible to justify and raises the possibility that they were not entirely successful. Now it seems as though it could be a similar story with the British experiments. The public deserves better."[27]

A more muted criticism of the neurosurgeons was provided by Professor Marsden:

> "One of the sadnesses of this whole event is how most of our data that people have had to deal with in advising their patients has been presented informally through the newspapers, rather than though the scientific press."[19]

These comments might be read in the context of the *New Scientist* background article:

> "Professor Marsden, of London's Institute of Neurology, who is a member of the international team working with the Swedish patients, has frequently stated that we cannot say whether such operations are a practical possibility in Britain until we know the results of the Swedish study."[14]

Noting that in the same week in which Marsden issued this prediction, Hitchcock announced that he had started to use the procedure, the *New Scientist* queried:

> "Could it really be that two British neurologists with common interests in a highly sensitive area had failed to cooperate, even to the extent of exchanging information?"[14]

My impression is that, whereas few if any other British neurosurgeons have opted to follow the Smethwick group in its repeated use of foetal brain cell transplantation procedures, very few have broken ranks and criticized their colleagues.

The release of clinical reports of the outcome of an experimental procedure directly to the lay press, rather than submitting them for publication to an adequately refereed scientific journal, is at variance with traditional medical practice. Nevertheless, in this instance, it has provided some insights in relation to foetal brain-cell transplantation that might not otherwise have become generally available. Published interviews with post-operative patients from the Midland Centre has revealed the sequence of changes in response to surgery with remarkable clarity. In particular, these newspaper reports have stressed the rapidity of improvement in the patient's condition. For example, consider the following description of the operation (performed under local anaesthesia) by the third patient in the series:

> "There I was strapped in a chair with half my head drilled open and surrounded
> by doctors. Then I suddenly realized I could move my arm for the first time in
> ages...Millions of cells were implanted in just a few seconds. And as they went in
> I immediately felt relief."[28]

Such explicit descriptions inevitably raise the question of whether the changes
represent effects entirely attributable to mechanical interference with the brain,
which would have occurred *irrespective* of whether any cells had been injected.
This possibility will be discussed more fully when the effects on parkinsonism
of neurosurgery *per se* are discussed on pp. 193–194. However, the point that
should be identified now, before considering proposed modes of action of foetal
cell implants (pp. 203–204), is the strong similarity between the descriptions of
relief of their symptoms by the Smethwick patients and the consequences of
surgical intervention *alone*. As will be discussed on pp. 193–194, there are
adequate reports of immediate (albeit temporary) alleviation of parkinsonian
symptoms by surgical interference alone. Furthermore there is nothing to
suggest that, if any beneficial effects were produced by implanted cells, these
would be observed before some weeks (or, more likely, months) had elapsed.

The response of the British Medical Association to Professor Hitchcock's
operations has been interesting. As mentioned above, the Association had established a working party to examine ethical aspects of the therapeutic use of foetal
tissue before the announcement that this procedure had been adopted at
Smethwick. The initial response of the Association to the announcement was
guarded. Dr Dawson, the head of its professional division, stated on the day
after the story broke in the newspapers that:

> "There is a good general principle that you should do things with a patient's
> knowledge, understanding and consent. There may be occasions when you can't,
> but that is the position from which you start and its a good rule to follow."[29]

His comments were made in relation to the absence of any referral of the possible use of brain tissue to the mother of the aborted foetus. On this subject,
Professor Hitchcock was quoted to the effect that:

> "in the U.K. a woman undergoing an abortion is asked whether she has any special
> wishes 'for disposal of the pregnancy product'. If the woman says she does not,
> 'I assume it means you can do anything you like'."[30]

A medico-legal commentary on the significance of the form of question
addressed to women in the UK before abortion, expressed the opinion that:

> "the present forms in use frequently employ wording on the lines of, 'I have no
> special wishes concerning the disposal of material from my pregnancy' which is
> arguably so vague as to be virtually meaningless".[10]

The BMA guide-lines were released on May 6, 1988. They were welcomed by Professor Hitchcock as being the ones that he had been following already, based on the 1972 Peel Report.[31] Reading of the 1988 guide-lines alongside the Peel Report certainly indicates that little had been added to the earlier paper. The one noticeable addition was a proscription on transplantation of the whole brain or a substantial part thereof. In explaining this point to *The Times*, Dr Vivienne Nathanson, an executive of the BMA with special responsibility for ethics, provided an interesting insight into the thought processes of the working party with the biologically remarkable statement that:

> "The whole brain contains genetic memory which makes it completely different from any other organ."[32]

This does not appear to have been a misrepresentation of her views as other newspapers (for example, *The Independent*) carried specific reference to the brain's importance in "genetic memory". In extending the scope of this section of the report, Dr Dawson excluded transplantation of the whole cerebellum or hypothalamus and of frontal lobe tissue other than as small fragments to correct chemical defects.[7]

The response of the Smethwick neurosurgical team to any criticism of its use of transplantation as a form of treatment for Parkinson's disease remained remarkably consistent throughout. When speaking with reporters from *The Daily Telegraph* at the start of the saga, Professor Hitchcock had indicated that he was not worried about the discussions on ethics and had received total support and no criticism from the medical profession: "he described those who had complained about his 'cavalier' attitude as 'rude'."[33]

The Lancet editorial, already cited, which called for longer follow-up of patients already operated on rather than undertaking more operations, was firmly rebuffed.[26] The Smethwick group responded 3 days later by performing its third transplantation.

> "Britain's pioneering brain transplant doctors vowed this weekend to keep performing the controversial operations until long-term results become known. Professor Edward Hitchcock, whose third operation was announced last week, rejected calls for a moratorium until the effects on patients who have already received foetal brain cell implants are fully known."[34]

Writing to *The Lancet*, Hitchcock and his colleagues claimed that:

> "most scientists would not accept that no more operations should be done merely because the numbers are too small to say whether the procedure is useful or not."[35]

Whilst the possibility that some or all of the reported improvements could re-present placebo effects does not appear to have been considered by the Smethwick group, the rapid onset of these improvements might suggest this. Earlier discussion of the pattern to be expected if tissue implants were relieving parkinsonism had implied that *immediate* improvement, as detailed in some of the press reports (see, for example, reference 28) would be more suggestive of a placebo effect.[36]

Apart from responding to criticism, the Smethwick group was notable for its advocacy of future extension of the range of diseases to which the technique of foetal brain cell transplantation could be applied. When indicating that the group intended to proceed with transplant surgery on Parkinson's disease patients at the rate of "one-a-month", Dr Rod Hughes, a neurologist associated with the programme, predicted that, when a clearer picture of the success of this application was available, the technique could be extended to other degenerative conditions like Alzheimer's disease and Huntington's chorea.[37] This possibility had been already presented to the press:

> "Dr Gordon Wilcock, Professor of Care of the Elderly at Bristol said that transplanting a small amount of foetal tissue could be of great value to 400,000 people with Alzheimer's disease, as well as sufferers from Parkinson's disease."[38]

In view of its disregard for scientific practicability and its emotive implications, this claim appears to me to be lacking in responsibility. An appropriate response by an unidentified clinician was published 2 days later in *The Times*:

> "some doctors have expressed concern at the implication that the techniques used in these two operations might provide a ready and easy answer to Alzheimer's disease. There is a tenuous link between the two complaints: in both there is a shortage of a chemical essential to the proper functioning of the brain, but as one neurologist said, to extrapolate from the surgical treatment of one to the other is not so much a step as a gigantic leap."[39]

Six months after the beginning of the programme, releases from the neurosurgical group to the media retained a distinctly expansionist outlook. Under the headline, "Heartbreak of brain-op queue", it was revealed that the Midland Centre for Neurosurgery and Neurology had thousands of men and women

> "forming a heartbreak queue for revolutionary brain-cell transplants...The tragedy is that the operations, available only in the Midlands, are being carried out at the rate of just over one a month. [A solution was suggested,] But last night the professor who has pioneered the technique in Britain revealed hopes for a network of hospitals to help deal with the backlog."[40]

It may help to retain some perspective on the subject, to point out that, at the time of the newspaper interview, the individual responsible had yet to publish a refereed report on the subject in a scientific journal.

Shortly after the preceding report, by which time the score of operations at Smethwick stood at 12, the detailed assessments of the two Parkinson's disease patients treated by foetal brain transplantation in Sweden some 9 months earlier were published. The principal conclusion of the group of 20 assessors was that, "no improvements of therapeutic value to the patients have been observed up to 6 months postoperatively"[41] At a similar time, one of the regional newspapers from the British Midlands—an area in which foetal brain-cell transplantation had by then assumed a very high profile—reported on the "first United States transplantation of brain cells from an aborted foetus".[42] The operation had been performed at the Colorado University's health sciences centre on a 52-year-old man who was reported to be in good condition. The paper proceeded to quote the surgeon to the effect that "it will be 3 to 6 months before they expect to see any signs of improvement". The contrast with the local practice of immediate post-operative description was not noted.

Has the Midland Centre programme and its associated media presentation had any discernible impact on the community? Recent reports suggest that both the mothers of potential foetal cell donors and prospective recipients, and their families, have been affected. As already indicated, the topic of provision, of information concerning the possibility of transplanting foetal brain cells to the mothers of prospective foetal donors, at the time of abortion became an issue with the first announcement that the procedure had been used at Smethwick. It was pointed out by one British newspaper at the time of the first foetal brain-tissue transplant that the apparent failure to consult the mother about subsequent usage of the foetus in the UK would be in conflict with regulations currently in force in Sweden.[29]

The question of informing, and consulting with, the mothers of prospective foetal donors was subsequently considered to have implications not only in relation to obtaining informed consent but also in the context of donor recruitment. Dr Nathanson of the BMA said that:

> "the Swedish experience with brain implants suggested women would be more willing to donate their babies' tissue if they knew it might help other people."[7]

When asked if the material could be used for research, only 50% of women agreed, whereas more than 90% agreed if it was to be used for therapy.[7] Shortly afterwards, an indication of a strong positive response to foetal use in research on transplantation was forthcoming from England. A report in *The Nursing Times and Nursing Mirror* referred to a leaflet, which was provided to women presenting for abortions at the Elizabeth Garrett Anderson Hospital in London:

> "At the beginning we were very worried and the nursing staff anticipated this could cause great distress. But the response has been positive and the vast majority are happy to help...Some women say they are glad something positive can come from a negative experience."[43]

The effects of the positive presentation, which has generally been accorded foetal brain-cell transplantation, on the attitudes of women undergoing abortion remain to be thoroughly documented. However, there are some disquieting indications that the British style of presentation of the subject may have contributed to the manipulation of prospective transplant *recipients* and their families. Once again, published interviews with patients are a revealing source:

"The future was just not very rosy at all...When I agreed to have the operation I felt there was no choice. Psychologically I feel a better person because I am sure I'm going to get better."[44]

The British Parkinson's Disease Society, which represents the interests of patients and their families, displayed considerably more caution than the press in assessing the prospects of transplantation. At an early stage in proceedings, the Society called for a public debate on the ethics of using tissue from aborted foetuses.[45] In its *Newsletter* of September 1988, the Society reiterated its cautious appraisal of the value of the procedures. It nevertheless decided to provide some assistance to the Smethwick group and, in selecting a way in which to do this, gave an insight into its perceptions of the group's requirements:

"The value of Professor Hitchcock's experimental procedure has yet to be proven. However the Parkinson's Disease Society closes its eyes to no possibility and in an even-handed gesture has sent £5000 to his Birmingham unit to provide extra secretarial help to deal with the pressure from both the media and the public."[46]

In the face of ongoing controversy about the transplantation of foetal cells, the British Government announced an inquiry into the subject in June 1988. Several months earlier, the US Department of Health and Human Services had initiated an inquiry in response to requests for funding from American scientists to undertake research on foetal brain cell transplantation: the form of these inquiries, the recommendations that arose from them and the implications of these will be considered on pp. 211–218.

Practice in relation to the use of foetal brain-tissue implants to treat Parkinson's disease seems to have conformed to the alternative patterns of performing as many operations as possible, in the case of the Smethwick and Mexico City groups or of undertaking a limited number of operations with careful follow-up. A report, published in November 1991, summarized the progress as disclosed at the annual meeting of the Society for Neuroscience in New Orleans.[47] There were said to have been approximately 100 instances of foetal brain-tissue transplantation. Of six Swedish patients, the first two in which the donor/recipient ratio was unity, had not shown any improvement. The remaining four had each received tissue from four foetuses and, after an initial lack of response, had shown improvement. This time-scale of response is unequivocally at variance with that described in Smethwick press releases. In contrast with these modest case numbers, the Smethwick group reported that 48 patients had received implants. It was noted of Dr Hitchcock that "although he has not published many details about these experiments", a third of his patients were said to be doing "remarkably well" and another quarter had shown "measurable improvement". As previously, the Madrazo group at the New Orleans meeting reported procedures not undertaken elsewhere. In November 1991, these reports entailed foetal brain-cell transplantation to a patient with Huntington's chorea, which was said to have produced "some improvement". Nevertheless, other participants at the meeting did not consider that this procedure was warranted. Critical comments said of Madrazo that: "he tended to overstate his results, contending that patients make miraculous recoveries that later prove false".

Before proceeding to consider some of the scientific background to this clinical transplantation activity, and its implications for clinical practice, I will outline briefly the principal clinical features of Parkinson's disease.

CLINICAL ASPECTS OF PARKINSON'S DISEASE

Whilst the causation of most cases remains in doubt and its treatment is often unsatisfactory, parkinsonism is a common and well-characterized condition. Many thorough descriptions are available. To summarize one of these, the characteristic features include trembling and stiffness of the limbs and paucity of movement.[48] Its onset, which occurs with increasing frequency after middle age, is usually gradual and, consequently, recognition and diagnosis of the condition may be delayed. The disease is usually progressive and may be associated with mental deterioration. It can be expected to shorten the patient's life appreciably. Apart from the major neurological features, the disease may be associated with a variety of symptoms, which add to the patient's discomfort. Depression is common and, as the disease progresses, mental deterioration may occur. The relative extent to which this results from the disease itself or from drugs used in its therapy will vary.

At different periods, the treatment of parkinsonism has been based on drug therapy, neurosurgery or a combination of these. One of the difficulties in assessing the response to treatment, whether it be in the course of management of the individual patient or in conducting trials of the relative efficacy of different approaches, lies in the need to measure accurately the patient's current status. Measurement of the severity of a condition such as Parkinson's disease and of any improvement as a result of treatment is dependent upon semi-quantitative or qualitative observations that are liable to considerable subjectivity, Consequently, assessment of the effectiveness of treatment cannot be made with anything approaching the accuracy attainable in following a disease such as diabetes in which precise measurements of the blood levels of glucose and insulin are possible.

A second factor which can complicate assessment of Parkinson's disease is the innate variability in severity of its manifestations. Substantial fluctuations in symptoms can occur in the course of the day:

> "Variation in the severity of symptoms has always been one of the most charac-
> teristic features of Parkinson's disease."[49]

The rapid swings from mobility to immobility that may occur over a short
period are referred to as the "on-off effect". Two further confounding factors
that may interfere with assessment of a patient's status are the influence of psychological changes and the possibility of placebo effects produced by therapy.
As regards the former, remission in depression may lead the patient to take a
more optimistic view of his or her symptoms. Secondly, any modification of
therapy may appear to produce changes that are more marked than expected,
if it acts as a placebo:

> "As to the question of placebo responses to what is a very major surgical event,
> everybody who treats Parkinson's disease knows that you can get something in the
> order of a 30% improvement simply by a placebo response on entering into a
> clinical trial."[19]

> "Even at a late stage it is often surprising how much improvement results from a
> short period of hospital admission, simplification of treatment, and attention to
> detail in the domestic arrangements and mental attitudes to the patient's
> management."[50]

Therapy of Parkinson's disease in recent years has usually entailed use of the
drug levodopa with very infrequent recourse to surgery. When levodopa therapy
is first commenced, approximately one-third of patients show a moderate
improvement and the remaining two-thirds are unaffected.[51] However, after
several years of continued use, the response to levodopa often declines. Before
levodopa became available, and much less frequently since then, surgery has
been undertaken on a minority of those patients who were unresponsive to drug
therapy. The most effective form of therapy entailed the production of lesions
in the basal ganglia of the brain. In a review of the results of operation on 1035
parkinsonian patients, compiled in 1964 (when surgery was much more commonly used), 86% of patients were noted to have improved immediately after
the operation.[52]
A most dramatic indication of the instantaneous nature of this improvement
is provided in the original report of surgical removal of the caudate nucleus in
November 1939:

> "The entire head of the caudate nucleus was extirpated. As soon as this was
> accomplished a striking improvement in the tremors of the left-sided limbs
> occurred."[53]

In another case, again operated on under local anaesthesia to the scalp, it was noted that as soon as the caudate head was removed:

"the tremors promptly and completely disappeared from the limb at rest."[54]

A feature of this form of surgical treatment of parkinsonism, almost as constant as the immediacy of response, was the variability of its persistence. For example, in the first case referred to above, it was recorded that by mid-1940, the patient had completely relapsed.

In recalling these early experiences of neurosurgery in the light of the use of adrenal transplantation for the same condition half a century later, Sladek and Shoulson observed in June 1988 that "perhaps scientific history repeats itself".[55] In the course of their article, entitled "Neural transplantation: a call for patience rather than patients", these authors discussed the future of foetal brain-cell transplantation. They warned that:

"We should not repeat the experience of the adrenal autograft experiments wherein far more humans than nonhuman primates were operated upon as a result of a single unconfirmed report of two patients."[55]

Their recollection of the 1939 descriptions of caudate nucleus surgery on a parkinsonian patient and the occurrence of immediate improvement in response to this single manoeuvre bears an uncanny resemblance to the account (mentioned on p. 187) of the experience of the third Smethwick recipient of a foetal brain-cell implant. It raises, or should raise, the question of the extent to which the immediate lessening of symptoms following surgery and cell implantation might be fully attributable to the surgical intervention alone. Perhaps the tissue implantation is irrelevant. Sladek and Shoulson advocated the thorough investigation of foetal brain-cell transplantation using experimental animals. This would seem to be an appropriate stage at which to examine the results of animal experimentation on the subject.

THE PLACE OF ANIMAL EXPERIMENTATION IN DEVELOPMENT OF FOETAL BRAIN TRANSPLANTATION FOR PARKINSON'S DISEASE

The development of an animal analogue of a human disease provides one of the most useful means of forming a preliminary assessment of the likely efficacy of new therapeutic measures in that disease. The use of animal models frequently raises implications for management of those diseases. An experimental model of a disease may provide a means to test both the likely effectiveness and the safety of any new forms of therapy before they are clinically applied. It may, for instance, afford an early warning about possible complications which should be anticipated. It may also assist in understanding the mechanisms underlying both the symptoms of a disease and their alleviation by treatment. As a consequence, more rational approaches to the clinical management of individuals with the disease may be suggested.

A large body of information is now available about the possible consequences of transplantation of foetal brain cells to experimental animals and the influence on the outcome of the circumstances surrounding transplantation. This subject has been one of the most intensively researched fields in neurobiology during the past decade. Recognizing this, the outline presented in this section is not intended to do any more than provide a brief summary sufficient to enable the relationship between experiments with animals and clinical events to be considered. As in any field of science that suddenly becomes fashionable, much of the published research has been repetitive, doing little more than recapitulating with small procedural variations earlier experiments that were genuinely original when first performed. There is a tendency for experiments which provide the expected result to be replicated many times. (This feature is certainly not peculiar to foetal brain transplantation.) The intention of the following review is to highlight a very limited number of reports, which have been selected from an extensive literature specifically because I believe that they raise points that need to be taken into account when assessing possible application of the technology to human medicine.

The principal topics to be considered include the validity of animal models of human Parkinson's disease and of the criteria employed to assess disease progress and remission in experimental animals. This will be followed by consideration of some specific technical details of brain-cell transplantation in experimental animals and their implications for human therapy. One especially important technical aspect concerns the immunological response of the recipient. Speculation about possible mechanisms of action of foetal brain grafts in recipient animals will be followed by an outline of some adverse effects that have been observed in experimental recipients. Finally, the status of some suggested alternative methods of treatment will be indicated.

Experimental animal models of Parkinson's disease

Doubt about the accuracy with which experimental models of parkinsonism mimic the human disease could arise for at least two reasons. These are uncertainty about the precise nature of the experimental lesions produced and uncertainty about the comparability between man and the species of experimental animal used. The experimental model that has been most commonly employed until quite recently entailed the injection of 6-hydroxydopamine (6-OHDA) into the brain of the rat. This chemical, which achieves its effects by interfering with the action of the normal neurotransmitter dopamine, is likely to be replaced, in future research, by another substance, the abbreviated name for which is MPTP. MPTP produces effects resembling those of parkinsonism when injected into monkeys. It now appears increasingly likely that the extensively used model, in which brain lesions were produced in rats by means of 6-OHDA, may have had only a superficial resemblance to human parkinsonism, when compared with the effects that can be produced by MPTP. MPTP came to clinical attention as a cause of experimental parkinsonism following the inadvertent self-administration by drug addicts of this substance, present as a contaminant in pethidine. A substantial number of affected individuals were observed to develop the typical features of Parkinson's disease during the following weeks. The use of MPTP in primates produces what is currently believed to be the best model of the human disease. Apart from chemically produced brain injury, the other technique used to produce a condition resembling parkinsonism has been surgical interference with the brain of rats and monkeys.

The second experimental stage in each of these animal models of parkinsonism has entailed attempts, using implantation of foetal brain cells, to correct the behavioural abnormality produced by earlier damage to the brain. One detail of such models in relation to which it remains very difficult, if not impossible, to define a valid human equivalent is the time allowed to elapse between the infliction of injury and the remedial transplantation of foetal brain tissue. The duration of observation of experimental graft recipients that is required before final assessment of the efficacy of the procedure can be made also remains unclear but is likely to be in years rather than in months. Human parkinsonism (with the single exception of the disease that occurs in those exposed to MPTP) invariably results from a pathological process that has been present, and gradually progressing, for an extended period of many years. However, in the experimental models using animals. transplantation has been used to ameliorate the experimental injury within weeks or months of its infliction. As a generalization, it is reasonable to anticipate that the ease of reversal of any lesion, experimental or clinical, is likely to decrease as its duration lengthens.

The duration of observation of experimental animals that would be required to ensure that relapse is not going to occur following reversal of lesions by brain cell grafting, is unknown. It is possible that any secondary curtailment of graft function, for example, as a result of interference produced by chronic graft rejection or involvement in the original, ongoing disease process, may well appear after similar lengths of time in different species. Consequently, the maintenance of improvement in a rat for 6 months or even in a monkey for 12 months after transplantation, provides no guarantee that deterioration will not have occurred by 18 months in the human recipient. It is not possible to extrapolate reliably from the response to treatment of an experimental animal with an acutely produced lesion to the response of a human patient with a chronically developing disease. Specifically, there is little justification for assuming that the period after transplantation that elapses before deterioration in an experimental animal, if expressed as a fraction of total life span, can be anticipated also in human patients. Additionally, in view of the earlier clinical experience that immediate, but transient, improvement could occur in patients with Parkinson's disease following neurosurgery, *without the implantation of any graft,* the question of the persistence of improvements is of major importance. It is a question that appears not to have been acknowledged by the Smethwick neurosurgery group.

Apart from these difficulties in relating experimental animal models of Parkinson's disease to the human condition, the other cause for reservation in extrapolating from observations in animals to the human situation is the very limited number of experiments that have been performed in primates. For instance, when calling for restraint in the clinical application of foetal brain-cell transplantation, Sladek and Shoulson noted that adrenal autotransplantation, a procedure of dubious value for the relief of parkinsonism, had been performed more often in humans than in monkeys.[55]

Criteria for assessing experimental models of Parkinson's disease and their response to therapy

Apart from doubt about the accuracy with which experimental animal models of parkinsonism mirror the human disease, the value of the tests used to measure the severity of the experimental disease, and the extent of any remission of it following transplantation of foetal brain cells, is unclear. The nature of these tests is worth noting. For example, one of the commonest tests to have been applied to rats, which have sustained brain damage as a result of injection of the chemical 6-OHDA, measures the occurrence of spontaneous and drug-induced asymmetrical body movements. However, it is disconcerting that some reports have suggested that foetal brain-cell transplants may improve the performance of these rats in simple, but not in more complex, functional tests. Indeed, it has been queried whether the functional effects of foetal brain-cell grafts are generalized or restricted to improvement in the response to a limited number of tests:[56]

> "The reliability of dopamine-rich grafts to ameliorate some functional deficits induced by dopamine-depleting lesions on the one hand, and to have no effect on other, in some senses more complex, measures has implications for the clinical potential of neural transplantation...It is apparent that a simple functional measure such as rotation in rodents is insufficient to demonstrate the general viability of the graft procedure."[56]

A report from another laboratory suggested a similar conclusion:

> "In sharp contrast to the marked compensation in amphetamine-induced rotation, the transplanted rats showed no tendency to recover in a number of regulatory and sensorimotor tests."[57]

Even the most superficial comparison between the tests used in assessment of rats with "experimental parkinsonism" and the tests used in human patients with this disease indicates that the latter are much more complex and rely upon measurements for which no simple animal equivalent exists. It may mean very little that the tests used to assess behaviour in treated animals are the best available if their outcome cannot be interpreted in relation to the human situation. Nevertheless, reference in the lay press to the results of such experimental treatment models are likely to imply that "cure" has been achieved in animals.

Apart from the difficulty inherent in extrapolating from animal to human tests, further difficulty arises in assessing experimental procedures designed to alleviate parkinsonism because of the nature of the tests on which clinical assessment of patients with this condition is based. Whereas a condition such as diabetes (for the relief of which foetal tissue transplantation has also been trialled) can be monitored accurately, there are no comparable quantitative measurements which could serve to provide a reproducible and reliable guide to the progress of parkinsonism. When translated to experimental animals, in which the capacity to interrogate the subject about possible remission of symptoms is lacking, the means of assessing the severity of experimental "parkinsonism" are notably lacking in precision and reproducibility. An additional, major complication when comparing animal models for treatment, for instance, of diabetes and parkinsonism, is that the manner in which the disease process affects normal function is well understood in diabetes but remains the subject of speculation in the case of parkinsonism. As a result, diabetes produced in experimental animals is likely to resemble the equivalent human disease much more closely than does any animal model of parkinsonism. This likely dissimilarity between experimental and clinical situations serves to introduce doubt into any inferences about human treatment of parkinsonism drawn from animal models of treatment.

Difficulty in interpreting the response of animals with experimentally produced brain lesions to transplantation of foetal brain cells in a way that has any relevance to human disease is not confined to models of parkinsonism. For example, the animal model that is thought to be closest to Alzheimer's disease entails surgical damage to the fimbria–fornix region of the rat's brain. Partial reversal of the resulting impairment in learning and memory by the transfer of foetal brain cells capable of producing the chemical neurotransmitter acetylcholine is assessed by a "water-maze" test in which the animal's ability to locate a submerged platform is tested. Without disparaging the value of this test, as a means of measuring rodent ability to negotiate a water maze, its relevance to the complex and subtle intellectual changes that characterize human Alzheimer's disease could legitimately be seriously questioned.

Technical aspects of foetal brain transplantation in experimental animals which have implications for human application

The results of animal experimentation are frequently simplified in the course of explaining the manner in which their clinical application may be achieved. Whilst this can be a very reasonable means of explaining to others the underlying concepts, the omission of technical detail that it requires can prejudice subsequent understanding of significant aspects of that clinical application. For example, if experimentation suggests that factors such as selection of donors, preparation of tissue to be transplanted or preliminary treatment of the prospective recipient, consistently exert a major influence on the outcome of foetal brain transplantation in animals, this can not readily be ignored in projecting human application of the technique. If the proposed clinical procedures are likely to differ substantially from those which experimentation suggests would be optimal, because of the circumstances obtaining in the human situation, then this divergence should be disclosed.

One of the commonest features of experimental protocols for transplantation of dopamine-producing foetal brain cells to animals suffering from "parkinsonism" is the surgical production, several weeks before transplantation, of a cavity in that part of the recipient's brain that is to receive the transplant. However, this preliminary operation is a most difficult technical aspect to accommodate within any extrapolation from the experimental model to clinical medicine. One reason for the advantage afforded by a two-stage experimental procedure, with cavity production as the first stage, may be the increased likelihood which this brings that blood vessels will grow into the graft. Thus, it was found at an early stage of research that "consistent survival of transplanted central and peripheral neurons was obtained only when the transplant was placed in contact with a vessel-rich tissue".[58] A suitable bed for graft placement could be provided, either by the highly vascular membrane, the pia mater, surrounding the brain or, alternatively, by the recently developed vascular bed lining the artificial cavity.

A typical experimental protocol to facilitate the reversal of Parkinson-like lesions in rats might entail the induction of the model disease by local injection of the chemical 6-hydroxydopamine (6-OHDA), followed 2 months later by the production of a cavity in the appropriate part of the brain. The implantation of foetal brain tissue into this cavity would then be undertaken after a further 6 weeks.[59, 60] Apart from providing a suitably vascularized bed for the implant, it has been suggested that some of the success of such experimental protocols may be attributable to coincidence between the time of maximum release of nerve cell growth-stimulating factors by brain tissue damaged during cavity formation and implantation of the graft.[61] In addition to the likely contribution made by the vascularized cavity to the success of transplantation, it is also probable that reversibility of the experimental lesion, 2 or 3 months after its infliction, is inherently much more attainable than is reversal of a disease of a decade or more duration in a human patient. A third feature of the experimental model, which is unlikely to have clinical equivalence, concerns the most common age of recipient animals. It has generally been found that brain-cell grafts develop much better in younger rats than in adults. Although the relative success of foetal brain-cell implants in restoring function has not been extensively studied in recipient rats of a range of ages, there are indications that many of the therapeutic model systems may be effective only if very young animals are used as recipients. For example, *20-month-old* rats with bilateral experimental lesions of the frontal cortex have been reported *not* to benefit from foetal brain implants.[62] This contrasts with experience in young recipients treated in an identical manner.[63] Once again, it raises the question of the applicability to human parkinsonism of an animal model, which is dependent upon the use of immature rats as recipients. As already indicated, Parkinson's disease commonly afflicts individuals in late middle age.

Apart from considerations relating to operative procedure and age of recipient, some of the optimal donor characteristics that have been suggested by experimentation appear difficult to match clinically. For example, experimental protocols for foetal brain-cell transplantation in rats have highlighted the critical importance of using donors within a precise gestational age range. This requirement is likely to have major procedural and ethical implications for any human application of the procedure to Parkinson's disease. Valid extrapolation from the optimal age for foetal rat brain tissue to a corresponding stage of development of human tissue is difficult, if not impossible to achieve. However, the demonstration that major limitations to the usefulness of foetal-rat brain grafts are introduced by minor changes in donor age suggests that similar restrictions may also to apply to the use of human foetal tissue. Experimental observations in rats suggest that foetal brain tissue remains for a very limited period at the developmental stage optimal for transplantation. For instance, tissue from 15-day donors grew much better after transplantation than did similar material removed from 18-day foetal rats.[64] The capacity of suspensions of cells from foetal rat brain to survive in tissue culture declined markedly even if donors were only 1 day in excess of the optimal age.[65] Tissue from foetal donors slightly over this age survived very poorly.[66]

On the basis of the limited evidence available, the importance of foetal donor age in influencing the capacity of tissue to survive transplantation, which was demonstrated by experiments with rats, appears also to extend to human tissues. Whereas brain tissue from 9-week-old human foetuses has been reported to survive, and even to reverse lesions, after transplantation to the brain of 6-OHDA-exposed rats, similar tissue from foetuses of 11 weeks and older had minimal, if any, effect.[67] An incidental, but interesting, "technical" aspect of the preparation of dopamine-producing cells from human foetuses was that the number of cells processed in a single experiment was 1600,[68] whereas the content of these cells in the normal adult human is estimated to be about 450 000.[69] This could legitimately lead to questions about both the logistics and efficiency of foetal brain-cell transplantation in reversing parkinsonism.

Another critical aspect of donor age when foetal brain cells are to be transplanted arises from the possibility of introduction of serious hazard for the recipient. The hypothetical risk identified by one of the pioneers of experimental brain cell transplantation is that collection of tissue from rat embryos *too early* in development may lead to the development of a teratoma, that is a type of tumor, rather than nervous tissue in the recipient.[70]

A third aspect of the techniques presently used in experimental transplantation that could reasonably be expected to carry some implications for any attempts to transfer the procedure to a human situation is the physiological condition of the transplanted tissue. For example. in one experimental study, which entailed the transplantation of human foetal brain tissue to rats, the method of termination of the pregnancy was altered specifically in order to improve survival of the grafts:

> "To obtain less damaged foetal tissue, the routine vacuum aspiration was slightly modified. After dilatation of the cervical canal, but prior to suction, foetal tissue was removed by forceps."[71]

As modification of the abortion technique was acknowledged in this Swedish study as a means of improving the viability of the brain cells to be transplanted to experimental rats, it would be realistic to expect that pressure could also be experienced for appropriate modifications when similar tissue is to be harvested for transfer to human patients. Judging from the literature, the technical details of harvesting human foetal brain tissue in condition optimal for subsequent transplantation do not appear to have been extensively researched. Never-the-less, it seems quite likely that close attention to these details would have considerable influence on the outcome of any clinical application.

Finally, a property of any tissue or organ which is under consideration for transplantation is its state of preservation at the time that it becomes available. The considerations which apply are similar to those discussed in relation to removal of organs from brain-dead and anencephalic subjects. The most important of these is the "warm ischaemia" time, i.e. the interval elapsing after cessation of blood circulation during which the organ is subject to rapid deterioration because it remains at body temperature. Considering the analogy between experimental animals and the aborted foetus to be used as a source of brain cells, the question of timing of intervention if the foetus is delivered intact becomes a question. As already noted, the validity of any attempts made to diagnose brain-stem death in the foetus *ex utero* has been questioned.[2] Certainly, in the case of foetuses that are sufficiently young to be pre-viable (which would include any foetus under consideration as a brain-cell donor), some authorities have suggested that intervention is permissible irrespective of the presence of vital signs. This was certainly the judgement of the UK Peel Report.[27] A similar position was argued recently by a bioethicist: "it is morally defensible" to remove organs or tissues from pre-viable foetuses, even if they are still alive "if dead fetuses are not available or are not conducive to successful transplants".[73] The writer recognized that there could be "added" concerns regarding the use of non-viable living fetuses because of their possible sensitivity to pain and the fact that such donors are not legally "brain-dead". Nevertheless, she considered that the first of these concerns "may be satisfactorily addressed on a practical level by using anaesthesia". An example of earlier practice in relation to collection of foetal brain tissue in the freshest possible state for microscopic examination has been cited in Chapter 2, when the problem of identifying post-mortem changes in brain cell structure was considered. Foetuses removed by caesarean section (and, therefore, likely to be delivered alive) were dissected in order to provide brain tissue for cryopreservation soon after.[74] The co-author of this 1973 report was Anders Bjorklund who has subsequently become one of the pioneers of foetal brain-cell transplantation.

Immunological limitations to foetal brain-cell transplantation

The majority of animal experiments intended to develop models for human brain-cell transplantation have been undertaken utilizing transfer between inbred or closely related animals in which immunological rejection of grafts is unlikely. In contrast, any human application of the procedures would occur in totally unrelated, outbred donor–recipient combinations. This inevitable introduction of tissue incompatibility when human transplantation is initiated carries substantial implications for any extrapolations from experimental to clinical situations. Although foetal tissues in general have often been claimed to be less liable than grafts from older donors to rejection by an immune response, this proposition has failed to receive experimental support in recent years.[75]

An argument that has been advanced in favour of the survival of grafts of tissue from *any* source within the brain is that host immune responses against tissue transplanted there appear to be less vigorous compared with those which are directed against grafts in other locations. This observation has led to the brain being categorized as an "immunologically privileged site". The original connotation of this term was that foreign tissues transplanted to the brain would survive indefinitely. However, it has become increasingly clear that, whilst immune reactions against tissue transplanted into the brain are delayed, they are not prevented. For instance, grafts placed in the brain of rats have been reported to survive for as long as 100 days before the appearance of the first signs of rejection.[76] While 100 days may represent a substantial fraction of the life-span of a rat, it is certainly not legitimate to deduce that the process of rejection of a graft in the brain of a human recipient would extend over a proportionally similar period of the recipient's life. In all probability, the course of rejection of transplanted brain cells in an otherwise untreated human recipient would not be likely to occupy much more time, in absolute terms, than the rodent equivalent.

As already indicated, the majority of studies involving transfer of foetal brain tissue to rats have utilized *young* recipients. As the capacity of animals to reject intracerebral grafts of foreign tumor cells has been shown to increase with the age of the recipient,[77] the duration of survival of therapeutic grafts in mature humans may be less than predicted from some of the animal experiments. That "immunological privilege" reflects only a *relative* lessening of capacity of the immune system to operate in the brain has been emphasised by the demonstration that it is feasible to immunize the entire immune system of an animal by introducing foreign tissue into the brain.[78] Some recent studies of the effects of transplanting foetal neurons between species, such as the mouse and rat, have suggested that long-term survival of these grafts is possible.[79] However. it seems more likely that the long-term use of powerful immunosuppressive drugs, such as cyclosporin A with its attendant side-effects. would be required to obtain extended acceptance of a graft.

The mechanism of action of foetal brain grafts placed in animals with experimental Parkinson's disease

Superficially it might appear to be of little importance whether one understands the detailed mechanism of action of a procedure such as transplanting foetal brain cells, provided that this is effective in alleviating experimental models of parkinsonism. For instance, antibiotics such as penicillin were of great use in clinical practice for decades before their mechanism of action was precisely understood. However, there are several compelling reasons for seeking to understand possible mechanisms of action of the transplanted tissue as fully as possible *before* adapting experimental procedures as complex as intracerebral transplantation of foetal brain tissue for clinical use. As there are undoubtedly major differences between the process of development of human parkinsonism and of chemically or surgically produced "parkinsonian" lesions in animals, it would be reassuring to know that the experimental therapy produced its effect by modifying an abnormality that was equally important in producing both human and animal disease. Seemingly similar end results may be produced by pathological processes that are significantly different. It would be difficult to predict either the likelihood of short-term clinical success or of the longer term persistence of any success obtained in the absence of reliable information about the manner in which the experimental transplants were achieving their effects. Equally important, the possibility of longer term adverse effects of a new form of transplant therapy, such as this, will remain a matter of guesswork so long as little is understood of the mechanism by which grafts produce their effect.

Proposed mechanisms to explain the actions of foetal brain grafts in experimental animals include the release by graft cells of neurotransmitters lacking in the recipient's brain, the formation of highly specific connections capable of transmitting nerve impulses between graft and host neurons, and the provision by the graft of an environment conducive to the repair of damaged host brain cells.[80-84] The operation of some combination of all of these mechanisms, together with a non-specific component, is also possible.[85, 86] There have also been reports that the transplantation of non-neuronal cells (which are themselves incapable of transmitting nervous impulses) from the brain can reverse experimental lesions of neurons.[86, 87] The non-neuronal cells producing this effect normally perform the function of supporting the neurons and facilitating their functioning. Chemical extracts from some of these cells may also assist brain repair.[88]

As the references mentioned in the preceding paragraph document, substantial doubt remains concerning the mechanism of action of experimental brain grafts. Especially disquieting are reports such as that from Brundin *et al.* indicating that the extent of behavioural improvements in 6-OHDA-treated rats that had subsequently received a foetal brain-cell implant failed to correlate with the extent of survival of the transplanted cells.[89] This result suggests that the mechanism of action of the transplant remains completely unclear. It raises serious doubts about the extent to which reproducible responses to the procedure could be anticipated in a clinical setting.

Confusion about possible mechanisms by which cells implanted in the *human* brain could relieve parkinsonian symptoms appears to be as prevalent in the limited clinical information published as it is in published interpretations of the corresponding animal experiments. In summarizing the results of human adrenal autotransplantation reported up until mid-1988, Marsden remarked that both radiological scanning techniques applied to surviving recipients and autopsies undertaken on those who had died indicated that irrespective of any relief of symptoms, the transplanted tissue had *not* survived.[19] A dissociation of this type between the quantity of implanted tissue surviving (i.e. the "dose") and the clinical outcome (the "response") is disquieting. It is axiomatic in any scientific proof that a causal connection exists between a form of therapy and its presumed results that some reproducible association between dose and response be demonstrated.

Predictions of potential adverse effects of foetal brain transplantation from experimentation

Experimental models of human disease, and of its treatment, that are based on animals not only provide a means of assessing possible benefits of the new therapy but may also serve as warning of potential hazardous side-effects. One of the most interesting possible complications of the therapeutic transplantation of foetal brain tissues derives from the disturbance of the "blood–brain barrier" which appears to follow this procedure. Normal brain tissue in man and other animals is, to a large extent, excluded from the degree of contact experienced by other tissues with blood cells and molecules, such as hormones, antibodies and drugs, which are present in the circulating blood. Separation of the normal brain from these cells and molecules is achieved by a mechanism referred to as the blood–brain barrier. The effective operation of this barrier is likely to be necessary for some of the normal functional characteristics of the nervous system. However, it has now been shown that transplants of both adrenal gland[90] and foetal brain tissue[91] to the brain of the rat result in substantial dysfunction in the local blood–brain barrier. As a result, the transplant and surrounding recipient brain will become exposed to the contents of the circulating blood in a relatively indiscriminate manner. It will be surprising if long-term effects on function are not discovered as a consequence.

The possibility of immunological reactions against foetal brain-tissue transplants has already been raised (on pp. 202–203). When these occur, they are likely to lead to progressive curtailment of both growth and function of the implant. The possibility also exists of an alternative, but equally adverse, consequence if excessive growth and expansion of an implant eventuates. For instance, the hypothetical possibility has already been raised that the transfer of tissue from donors at too early a developmental stage might lead to the subsequent growth of teratoma tumors from primitive cells in the implant.[70] This might occur if cells were transplanted prematurely, i.e. before their capacity to differentiate in other directions, apart from into nervous tissue, had been lost as a consequence of their specialization. The occurrence of excessive growth of an experimental implant with consequent compression and damage of surrounding tissues in the recipient animal's brain has already been reported. For instance, in a study of the transplantation of foetal brain grafts to rats which had been subjected to lesions which selectively compromised their learning capacity, it was found that the transplanted tissue often "grew to a considerable size in the host brain and produced moderate to extreme damage".[92] This was evident symptomatically in a worsening of the recipient rat's performance in neurological testing. Attention was also drawn to the potential hazard of excessive growth of foetal tissue implanted in the brain by a report of the production of a large mass in the brain of a monkey in receipt of foetal monkey brain. It was concluded that:

> "In evaluating foetal neuronal transplantation as a treatment for neurodegenerate diseases the possibility of serious deleterious effects on the host should be considered."[93]

It is interesting to recall that in their early trials of implanting adrenal tissue into patients with Parkinson's disease, a Swedish group had taken the precaution of including with the graft a marker, visible on X-ray. The purpose of this inclusion was to facilitate localization of the graft and its destruction should this become necessary because of damage to surrounding tissues.[94] Use of a similar procedure was also reported by a group from New York.[95]

Experimental alternatives to foetal brain as a source of grafts for Parkinson's disease patients

Of its nature, research that is directed towards a specific, well-defined clinical goal, such as developing a cure for parkinsonism, tends to be notable for steadily increasing concentration of effort on a narrowing aspect of the subject. This is not surprising when one reflects that what is sought is a detailed, reproducible protocol that can be safely applied in clinical practice, rather than a mass of generalized, but incomplete information about a variety of options. However, a disadvantage of this tendency to narrowing of focus is that the effort expended on the most apparently promising approach in comparison with alternatives may be out of proportion to the relative advantage which it offers. Preoccupation with one potential solution may prejudice the thorough examination of others.

If transplantation is to be used as an experimental treatment for parkinsonism, the principal alternative to using foetal brain cells appears at present to be the transfer of lines of cells, cultivated *in vitro*. Such cell lines may have the capacity to substitute for damaged brain cells when introduced into the appropriate location. The major deterrent to the use of *any* cell line in any variety of clinical transplantation is the risk that malignant transformation may occur in the transferred cells with the production of a tumor in the recipient. There seem to be at least two influences which might render tumor development a hazard after transplantation of cell lines. In the first place, it is conceivable that the modifications, which have occurred *in vitro* as the cell line acquired "immortality", may have included transformations which also conferred malignant potential. Secondly, the probable use of immunosuppressive drugs to prevent rejection of the transplanted cells as a foreign graft by the patient's immune system could effectively allow a cell line with potential for low-grade malignancy to behave as a highly malignant tumor once it was introduced into the recipient.

The experimental transplantation of cell lines to treat models of parkinsonism in animals has utilized cells that were originally derived from malignant tumors. In an earlier report of this approach, a malignant cell line derived from the rat adrenal gland and producing dopamine was exposed to conditions during tissue culture which were intended to halt its proliferation. Following transplantation to rats with parkinsonian-like symptoms, produced by exposure to 6-OHDA, a short-lived improvement in the neurological abnormalities of these animals was observed.[96] A second report from another laboratory was slightly more optimistic as regards the survival of the transplanted cells.[97] In a related approach, a human cell line derived from a malignant neuroblastoma was treated to prevent further cell division and then transplanted to monkeys that had sustained surgical lesions to the brain, which were designed to induce parkinsonian symptoms.[98] It was demonstrated microscopically that the implanted cells could survive for prolonged periods (up to 9 months), although no indication was given of whether the cells continued to produce dopamine during that time. Another study in which rodent and human cell lines, the multiplication of which had been chemically arrested, were transplanted to rats with surgical lesions, demonstrated both symptomatic improvement in the recipients and extended implant survival.[99] In a variant of this procedure, presented at the 1991 annual meeting of the Society for Neuroscience in New Orleans, improvement was observed in rats with Parkinson-like lesions following the implantation of bovine cells enclosed within plastic capsules.[100] The purpose of the capsule was to prevent rejection of the grafted cells by the cells of the recipient's immune system.

In summary, it appears that it may be possible to arrest cell division in malignant cell lines, capable of producing dopamine, in such a way that malignant characteristics do not re-emerge after transplantation of these cells. The extent to which these cells can alleviate symptoms in recipient animals with Parkinson-like conditions is less clear. The duration of any benefits produced by transplanted cells incapable of further division also remains to be established. Thus, the transplantation of cell lines for relief of parkinsonism is not likely to be of early application but may ultimately prove to have value. It is certainly an approach worth further effort.

Apart from the use of cell lines, several other alternative applications of tissue transplantation to the treatment of Parkinson's disease could, at least theoretically, be possible and could certainly justify experimentation. Sladek and Shoulson[55] suggested that the transplantation of tissue from the patient's carotid body to the brain might improve parkinsonian symptoms (the carotid body is a small organ close to the artery of the same name, containing cells which produce neurotransmitters). They noted also the possibility of cross-species transplantation of tissue from the brain of foetal animals, as well as emphasizing the potential for producing cells suitable for implantation by applying genetic engineering techniques to cells previously isolated from the patient's body. An intriguing discovery, which may have long-term implications for the use of transplantation in the treatment of brain disease, has been the demonstration that the brain of the adult mouse contains cells which retain the potential to transform into new neurons.[101] This could raise the possibility of activating such cells in the patient's brain to replace neurons damaged by disease. It may be recalled that one hypothetical mechanism previously suggested to explain the restorative effects of foetal brain-cell grafts in some experimental animals related to stimulation of the transplant recipient's own neurons (pp. 203–204).

THE IMPLICATIONS OF EXPERIMENTAL TRANSPLANTATION OF FOETAL BRAIN CELLS TO ANIMALS FOR TREATMENT OF HUMAN PARKINSON'S DISEASE

To what extent is it possible to predict the ideal conditions for transplantation of foetal brain cells to patients with parkinsonism from present knowledge obtained in animal experimentation? To what extent is it possible to anticipate any difficulties that may be encountered when the techniques that have been utilized in the laboratory are applied clinically?

Several aspects of the investigations in animals seem likely to raise difficulties if attempts are to be made to adapt them to the treatment of human parkinsonism. A majority of the experiments undertaken in animals have involved two stage procedures. As indicated on p. 199, it was common practice to produce a cavity in the brain 1 or 2 months before transfer of foetal brain cells. Trials in which this preliminary stage was omitted have generally given inferior results as assessed by the success of the implant in reversing the signs of the experimental disease. Whilst the inclusion of this preliminary operation into the protocol provides an ingenious means of facilitating experimental study of the functional capacity of brain grafts, it also introduces a confounding factor into extrapolation from animal to human procedures. It is improbable that the procedure of brain-cell transplantation for parkinsonism would become an acceptable form of treatment of human patients if it included a preliminary operation to produce damage to that area of the brain which was subsequently to receive the graft. On the other hand, the omission of such a clinical equivalent to the experimental procedure may constitute a significant impediment to transfer of the procedure. Parenthetically, it is interesting to speculate whether such a preliminary operation, which would resemble the neurosurgery performed in some parkinsonian patients in the 1940s (see pp. 193–194), might not *itself* produce the immediate improvements reported at that time and so preclude the second stage of transplantation.

A second aspect concerns the possible implications, for any form of treatment entailing transplantation of brain tissue, of the ongoing nature of the pathological process in spontaneously occurring human Parkinson's disease. It is clear that all of the animal models of parkinsonism, even including that produced by the increasingly used administration of the chemical MPTP, differ fundamentally, in being based on single episodes of acute injury, from the disease that occurs in man. With the exception of that small group of patients who have developed parkinsonism after exposure to MPTP, human patients invariably have a disease that progresses over a prolonged period. Whilst the continuing worsening of symptoms does not indicate with absolute certainty that the pathological process of unknown cause must be continuing, this certainly remains the most reasonable interpretation. If this interpretation is accurate, there is a considerable likelihood that, in the absence of additional therapy to arrest the pathological process, the implanted cells, may in due course, also succumb to it. In an analogous situation, it has been speculated that continuation of the abnormal process responsible for the original damage to the pancreatic islets in patients with juvenile diabetes may have contributed to the failure of transplants of foetal islet cells to reverse the disease. Certainly, if the disease has not gone into remission, other organ grafts may be susceptible to the pathological process which produced the need for transplantation. Consequently, it is reasonable to anticipate that damage to the transplanted cells by the original disease process may render extrapolations from lesioned animals to diseased patients inaccurate.

Another feature that could impair extrapolation from experimental animals to human patients concerns the length of time which should be allowed for evaluation. The adequacy of observation of animals, undertaken for relatively limited periods after brain-cell implantation, as a guide to the extended post-operative course to be predicted in human patients remains questionable. Apart from damage to the implant as a result of an ongoing disease, the possibility of chronic graft rejection if the patient's immune system has not been permanently suppressed should be a cause for substantial concern. Other possible complications (noted on p. 205), which animal experimentation suggests cannot be ignored, include failure of the implanted tissue to function or, alternatively, its overgrowth. Overgrowth of an implant (irrespective of its functional performance) may result in the production of symptoms as a result of pressure on surrounding structures in the brain. It is not legitimate to infer that a period of, say, 6 months post-operative survival with maintained improvement in the rat (with a life span of 3 years) is equivalent to a prognosis of sustained improvement over 16% of normal human life span in a recipient patient. On the contrary, there is little to suggest that processes such as immune recognition and chronic graft rejection of a foreign graft would not occur at a similar pace in man and the rat. Recognition of the prolonged period that is likely to be required before it would be possible to be confident of sustained and reproducible improvement in human recipients of brain-cell grafts prompted an Editorial in the *Lancet* calling for a halt to the use of the procedure until those patients already treated could be adequately observed.[26] A similar call came from two neuroscientists who, having noted the inadequacy of animal experimentation as a basis for the stage of human application that had already been attained (in June 1988) concluded, "we could benefit from more patience rather than more patients".[55]

An interesting aspect of foetal brain-cell transplantation, in relation to which animal studies may provide some guide to likely constraints on human therapy, concerns the nature of the tissue donor. Abundant evidence has accumulated from experimentation to indicate that donor age is of paramount importance in determining the outcome of transplantation. It should be self-evident that factors such as donor age, the state of preservation of the tissue available for transplantation and its freedom from contamination by other types of cell will be closely related to the termination technique that has been used. Experimentation has convincingly established the importance of donor age (with differences of 1 or 2 days in the gestational age of foetal rat donors radically altering the usefulness of the transplanted tissue). Furthermore, experiments in which human foetal brain cells were implanted in rats with brain lesions suggested that it was critical that the foetal source of tissue should be of a gestational age of 9 weeks. Even allowing for the (very considerable) qualification that this age has been identified from studies of the effect of implanted human cells in a 6-OHDA-treated rat, this information retains considerable potential relevance to human therapy. In particular, it is noteworthy that termination of pregnancy at 9 weeks would customarily be effected by the use of suction. While ensuring that foetal tissues are likely to be recovered in a much better state of preservation than is the case with prostaglandin termination, the use of suction will invariably yield a severely disrupted foetal brain. This introduces considerable difficulty both in identification of the tissue required from the substantia nigra and in ensuring the exclusion of contaminating tissues of other types from the specimen to be transplanted.

The retrieval of one specific portion of the brain from the tissues recovered in the course of suction termination is likely to raise substantial logistic questions about clinical application. Identification of substantia nigra from disrupted foetal remains has been achieved as a research procedure. However, the extent to which it could reproducibly be accomplished as a clinical routine remains questionable. Could it be "scaled up" sufficiently to underpin substantial clinical transplantation programmes? In answer to this question, it is interesting that the group at the Midlands Centre for Neurosurgery and Neurology, which has made the running on foetal brain cell transplantation in the UK, was compelled, on account of this difficulty, to alter the gestational age of foetal brain cells to be transplanted: 12 months after commencing their program, it was reported that the group had "experienced difficulty in gathering and identifying donor tissue for transplantation" following suction termination. In order to circumvent this difficulty, the report indicated that:

"rather than first trimester abortion material we now use older fetuses from 12–18 weeks gestation. These larger fetuses are delivered intact and dissection results in bigger cell blocks." [96]

This disclosure of detailed attention to the source of tissue to be transplanted contrasts with an earlier statement by the group's leader. When the procedure was first introduced, Professor Hitchcock, seeking to distance the transplantation from the termination, affirmed that:

"The tissue I used was collected routinely. It was not obtained specially for me. I do not know what method was used but it was obtained in the usual way." [103]

An alternative to altering the gestational age of donor tissue from first to second trimester (with the attendant likelihood of substantially compromising the chances of effecting improvement in the recipient's parkinsonism) would have been be to adjust the method of termination to achieve the best fit with the interests of prospective recipients. This course was actually followed, and reported, by a Swedish group. Gustavi noted that:

"with the techniques for first trimester abortion then in use, damage to the foetal brain cells rendered them unsuitable for transplantation." [104]

Faced with a demand for first trimester foetal brain tissue linked to a requirement that such tissue be fresh and uncontaminated by other tissues, he opted for the solution of varying the procurement technique. Accordingly, following the induction of general anaesthesia of the pregnant woman, limited suction under guidance of ultrasound was used to deliver portions of the foetal body free from placental fragments. Another Swedish solution to the problem of obtaining foetal tissue in accord with the requirements of transplantation was explained to an Australian newspaper:

> "According to Professor Lars Hamburger who has participated in experiments using foetal tissue in Gothenburg, Sweden, laws now forbid doctors from varying the method of abortion in any way to suit the convenience of the people who want to use the tissue. But this is a new law. Before it was enacted, Dr Hamburger told the *Herald*, the preferred method was to dilate the cervix to the point where the foetus could be extracted whole and alive."[30]

In discussing the resolution of the divergent aims of obtaining brain tissue from foetuses in the first trimester without the hindrance likely to be imposed by its retrieval from the remnants of suction termination, Professor Hitchcock stressed that modification of abortion technique in order to accommodate subsequent use of foetal tissue ran contrary to the recommendations of the Peel Report.[102] (This was an enquiry into the use of the foetus in research, undertaken in the UK in 1972.)[72] Predictably, a less inhibited correspondent of the *Lancet* called for the formal modification of existing abortion practice in order to improve the suitability of harvested tissue for subsequent transplantation.[105]

TIME FOR REVIEW

The necessity for some form of government-initiated review of foetal brain-cell transplantation as a treatment for Parkinson's disease was recognized in both the UK and USA within a few months of each other. The initiating events, in the case of the British Government, were the series of widely publicized operations undertaken at the Midland Centre for Neurosurgery and Neurology at Smethwick already described on pp. 182–192. Government involvement in the USA preceded any acknowledged trial of the procedure in a parkinsonian patient. It was triggered by a formal request to the Assistant Secretary for Health from the National Institutes of Health for permission to undertake a clinical trial of the procedure. There had been earlier review of the subject of foetal usage, including by implication that relating to tissue transplantation, in both countries. Consideration of the subject had been undertaken by the US Department of Health, Education and Welfare (1975) and the UK Peel Committee (1972). However, since these exercises there had been little beyond recapitulation of the earlier conclusions. For instance, the British Medical Association guidelines, mentioned on p. 188, which were released in 1988, provided little more than a restatement of the Peel Committee recommendations.

The contrasting form of the two inquiries bore considerable resemblance to that of their respective precursors. The USA exercise published its background materials and submissions in their entirety.[106] However, the UK committee noted the sources of submissions but did not release their content.[107] The terms

of the enquiries differed significantly. The USA operation was especially concerned with the acceptability of allocating Federal Government funding for
research on foetal tissue transplantation. The UK exercise was directed to review
of the Peel Report and to consider whether modifications or additions to the
code of practice contained in it were required.

Reading of the UK and USA reports reveals a number of considerations, additional to those already discussed in this chapter, which are likely to influence the
practice of foetal brain-cell transplantation. The subjects from the reports that
I wish to comment upon in concluding this chapter are:

- the nature of scientific input to examination of ethical aspects
- the relationship of foetal brain-cell transplantation to embryo experimentation and abortion
- the relevance of vital signs in the non-viable foetus
- the place of agents intermediate between supplier and end-user of foetal cells.

Scientific input to ethical analysis

Because of the differing form of the USA and UK enquiries, it is possible to examine the data provided to committee members and their responses to specific
points only in the case of the USA report. Reading of the scientific information
provided to the committee and of the attitudes of committee members following their receipt of it indicate the potential which exists for such information
to influence the outcome of committee deliberations. This is especially so in
relation to Question 9:

> "For those diseases for which transplantation using foetal tissue has been proposed,
> have enough animal studies been performed to justify proceeding to human trans-
> plants? Because induced abortions during the first trimester are less risky to the
> woman, have there been enough animal studies for each of these diseases to justify
> the reliance on the equivalent of the second trimester human fetus?."[106]

On the subject of the optimal age of foetal donors, it is disconcerting to find
statements by the Human Fetal Tissue Transplantation Research Panel
(reporting to the Advisory Committee) such as:

> "Research in diabetes, Parkinson's disease and neural regeneration has found that
> first trimester fetal tissue is not only more apt, but optimal for transplantation."[106]

However, the majority of published reports of attempts to use foetal pancreatic
islets in the control of diabetes have disclosed an absolute preference for more
mature, *second* trimester tissues. The significance of this inaccurate input to the
committee is, I suggest, that the specific donor age believed to be associated with
the most favorable results could be of critical importance in assessing both the

ethical acceptability of foetal cell transplantation and its practicality. For example, part of Question 6 enquired:

> "Is there any way to ensure that induced abortions are not intentionally delayed in order to have a second trimester fetus for research and transplantation?"[106]

Another misleading input in the background to the USA report related to the current (1988) status of research and clinical trial of foetal pancreas transplantation. It was asserted that:

> "Since experimental studies have reached the stage of demonstrating that human fetal pancreas can grow, differentiate and function in animals, it now seems scientifically justified to move to experimental studies in men, while continuing with research in animals."[106]

A more accurate statement would have indicated that well in excess of a hundred instances of foetal pancreas transplantation to diabetic patients had been *reported* by the mid-1980s and that, because of the lack of success of these, the procedure had been abandoned in most clinics and laboratories. (It is highly likely that an additional, considerably greater number of trials with negative outcomes had remained unreported.) An unchallenged contention about foetal pancreas transplantation provided in testimony to the Panel by Robin Chandler Duke of the Population Crisis Committee was:

> "Although the research is still in the early stages, the preliminary results indicate that patients in whom the transplants have been attempted have been able to either decrease, or completely eliminate, their insulin intake."[106]

(The scientific literature remains unaware of these achievements. As indicated above, the results are far from preliminary and equally far from successful.) Nevertheless, the impact of these submissions was reflected in the Panel's conclusion that "human clinical trials were timely and appropriate".

The preceding history of trial of foetal pancreas transplantation in human patients with an almost total lack of success had clearly not been appreciated by at least one panellist, John A. Robertson, J.D. He identified the burden of proof as being a neglected issue, in the consideration of foetal tissue transplanation:

> "Given the likely benefits of foetal tissue transplant research, the burden of showing that such research should not occur falls...and should fall...on its opponents."[106]

His contention ignores the question of whether any burden of proof is incurred by those using purported, but entirely unsubstantiated, scientific achievements as grounds for argument. As if recognizing this deficiency in his opening statement and wishing to insulate his argument from the likely consequences of its recognition by others, Robertson continued:

> "the assumption of widespread success, on which the opponent's claims of influence on abortion decisions rests, is itself highly questionable at this early stage of clinical research. As you well know, there is no certainty or guarantee that fetal tissue transplants will work for any disease, much less that they will be successful for all diseases for which they offer hope."[106]

The two arguments hardly sit easily together in one statement.

Implications for foetal brain-cell transplantation of attitudes towards embryo experimentation and abortion

The subject, which both UK and USA enquiries together with the media and community group alike, identified as linked to foetal brain-cell transplantation was that of the preceding induced abortion. However, another issue, namely that of human embryo experimentation. was also clearly perceived as highly important by the UK committee of inquiry:

> "It seems to us totally illogical to propose stringent legislative controls on the use of very early human embryos for research, while there is a less formal mechanism governing the research use of whole live embryos and fetuses of more advanced gestation."

This excerpt from the Warnock Report[108] was cited by the Polkinghorne committee. Of particular concern was the Warnock recommendation that:

> "no live human embryo derived from *in vitro* fertilisation...may be used as a research subject beyond 14 days after fertilisation."

The Polkinghorne committee read this recommendation as indicating that any special status accorded the human embryo should also extend to the foetus. The potential inconsistencies for society inherent in maintaining separate codes of treatment for subjects who are otherwise biologically identical, except in the matter of technique of conception, was apparent to the committee. This inconsistency had been adeptly identified much earlier:

> "If our society accepts that abortions are permissible until life is considered to be viable on its own, at 28 weeks gestation, then logically it would seem possible to devise a code of practice under which test-tube embryos could be experimented upon up to 28 weeks. Logic apart, this still seems repugnant."[109]

A further comment on the difference perceived to exist in using IVF, as distinct from free-range, embryos was provided by Professor Hitchcock:

> "I would not take part in any experiment where there was test tube fertilisation. It would be grossly unethical and immoral."[33]

The relationship of foetal brain-cell transplantation to induced abortion was a major factor influencing the establishment of both of the USA and UK 1988 inquiries. In the case of the USA inquiry, it was undoubtedly the major factor. The responses of the two committees were remarkably similar in that tacit distinctions were drawn between ethical and legal issues with transplantation being accorded a clean bill of health on the latter by both. This decision was expressed by the USA report as follows in response to the first question presented to it:

> "Is an induced abortion of moral relevance to the decision to use human fetal tissue for research? Would the answer to this question provide any insight on whether this research should proceed?"[106]

The committee's response was:

> "It is of moral relevance that human fetal tissue for research has been obtained from induced abortions. However, in light of the fact that abortion is legal and that the research in question is intended to achieve significant medical goals, the panel concludes that the use of such tissue is acceptable public policy."[106]

The Polkinghorne report's response to a similar question raised legal status as a major consideration but, perhaps unintentionally, introduced an additional aspect with wider implications. In deciding that association with induced abortion did not render foetal usage unacceptable:

> "the Committee does not rely solely on the legality of abortion performed under the 1967 Act, for the legal and moral are distinct and only partially overlapping categories."[108]

In the following paragraph, this argument is extended:

> "We do not believe that in circumstances of such moral complexity it is right to regard the termination of pregnancy as inevitably so heinous that any subsequent use of the fetal tissue thereby made available is morally disqualified."[108]

The argument concludes that:

> "it does not follow that morally there is an absolute prohibition on the ethical use of fetuses or fetal tissue from lawful abortion."[108]

It appears to me that inclusion of the terms "inevitably" and "absolute" indicates the committee's decision effectively became that association with induced abortion *does not invariably carry* negative connotations for subsequent use of the products of the event. There is a categorical difference between this argument and the contention that induced abortion *invariably does not carry* negative connotations. That a particular association does *not necessarily always* arise falls well short of validating the conclusion that it *never* does.

I suggest that the Polkinghorne committee inevitably raises the question of whether the association between induced abortion and foetal usage should properly be examined case by case rather than being considered once and for all as a class of association. I am far from convinced that this was the intention of the committee. Nevertheless, I suggest that the manner in which its report has been written leaves little scope for alternative interpretations. This solution of dealing with the problem of association between the two events by seeking to establish that it is not sustainable as a universal proposition recurs in reference to the 1967 legislation "in the circumstances envisaged by the 1967 Act, this grave step is permitted only in situations where there are also other serious moral issues to be considered such as those arising from concern for the health of the mother". As the 1967 Act has patently operated subsequently as a *de facto* authorization for abortion "on demand", such an argument that is based on the declared intent of the Act 23 years previously lacks strength. In summary, if one is to accept the committee's argument at face value, it would be necessary to examine the circumstances of each individual case in order to decide on the legitimacy of subsequent foetal usage. This would effectively require a much closer juxtaposition of consideration of the specific circumstances surrounding the termination and the validation of subsequent use of the foetus than is likely ever to have been undertaken.

The relevance of vital signs in the non-viable foetus

The Polkinghorne committee recommended a substantial shift in position away from the recommendations of the earlier Peel report. After noting its "profound respect for the living human fetus", the committee concluded:

> "We are unable to accept the implication of the Peel Report that there is a category of pre-viable fetus, of less than 20 weeks gestational age whose early stage of development would permit its being used for research or other purposes, without the requirement that it lacks the signs of life."[108]

This position has certainly not been universally accepted. For example, Mahowald, writing in the Hastings Center Report of February 1987 suggested that it may be "morally defensible" to harvest tissues from live aborted foetuses" if dead fetuses are not available or are not conducive to successful transplants".[73]

In adopting its position on the use of live, albeit pre-viable, foetuses the

Polkinghorne report has inescapably placed the question of the diagnosis of death of the previable foetus *ex utero* on the agenda of any protocol for foetal usage, which entails the collection of specific tissues from the whole foetus at the earliest acceptable time. The report recommended that foetal death be diagnosed by the absence of spontaneous respiration and heartbeat, in the absence of hypothermia. This recommendation falls far short of the conditions considered necessary for diagnosis of death in the perinatal subject as already discussed in Chapter 4. The supporting statement that "presence or absence of heart beat is already used as a test for determining death in the fetus *in utero*" is superficial and unconvincing given the major physiological differences applying to foetal condition in the two situations under comparison. Thus, the foetus *ex utero* is no longer in closely regulated maternal environmental conditions and foetal heart rate becomes subject to potentially reversible changes attributable to changes in environment. The comment quoted at the beginning of the chapter, namely that it was most unlikely that criteria of brain death, prerequisite before *other* categories of subject were used as organ sources, would be satisfied is relevant. [2]

Intermediation between supplier and user of foetal tissue

In dealing with the difficult subject of regulating communication between the end-user of foetal tissue and its original supplier, the Polkinghorne report placed considerable reliance on the introduction of an intermediary agent to whom requests for foetal tissue of a particular gestational age might be made. The report was on the extent to which communication between the intermediary and the supplier, which was intended to ensure provision of tissue in condition most suited to the proposed use, would be acceptable.

Whilst the Polkinghorne report did not examine the subject of the possible identity of suitable intermediaries, this featured prominently in the National Institutes of Health (NIH) inquiry because of the active participation in it of organizations which had been established to fulfil this need. One such entity, Hana Biologics, a publicly-held biotechnology company, was represented by its Vice President for Research and Development, Fred Voss. He outlined the company philosophy:

"Four years ago, Hana recognized that what we had learned about growth, differentiation and replication of cells could be put to use in a new and potentially very significant area: providing proliferated cells for transplantation into humans to restore normal functions lost to diseases." [106]

Touching on the mechanics of tissue supply, he indicated that "the actual procurement is usually done by non-profit organizations". In relation to supply, he noted that tissue from spontaneous abortions was not collected because it was less likely to be viable and because immediate processing was impossible.

Additional background on Hana Biologics was provided by a 1988 article in *Chemical Week*.[110] It was pointed out that Hana's mainstay business was supplying the biotechnology industry with growth media needed to culture cells for research and manufacturing. In the early 1980s:

"Hana decided to use its expertise in cell culture to grow fetal cells—and enter the new field of fetal cell implants. A great need exists for such cells."[110]

The article indicated that the company "hopes to have islet cell therapy [for diabetes] on the market by 1991". Other research in progress, or intended, included the transplantation of foetal brain cells for Parkinson's, Huntington's and Alzheimer's disease, and of foetal liver cells for haemophilia. The primary objective of the company in all of these activities appeared to be to devise and develop uses for foetal tissue as one would prepare any product for a specific market niche.

One of the non-profit organizations fulfilling the role identified by Fred Voss was the International Institute for the Advancement of Medicine. Its executive director, James S. Bardsley Jr. summarized its role as follows:

"The issue of human foetal cadaver tissue acquisitions can and must be removed from the abortion controversy. IIAM has demonstrated the feasibility of this task."[106]

The Institute was said to possess "the largest procurement network of its kind in the U.S.". Its collection network included free-standing abortion clinics, but not hospitals or doctor's offices.

Whilst the possible regulatory mechanisms considered in the Polkinghorne and NIH reports related to current practices, the inquiries provided indications that these restrictions should not necessarily be regarded as immutable. For example, a concurring statement contributed to the NIH report by a group of panel members headed by Professor J. A. Robertson speculated that:

"if the situation changes so that the supply of fetal tissue from family planning abortions proves inadequate, the ban on donor designation of recipients and aborting for transplant purposes should be re-examined. The ethical and legal arguments in favour of and against such a policy would then need careful scrutiny to determine whether such a policy remains justified."[106]

The potential exists for the ethics to match the novelty of the science in the near future.

REFERENCES

1. Phillips, M. A matter of life and death, as medical ethics go plunging down the slippery slope. *The Guardian*, (London), April 22, 1988.

2. Sealey, M. *Hospital Doctor*, July 28, 1988.
3. Boultbee, P. J. Unanswered questions about transplants. *The Daily Telegraph* (London), April 22, 1988.
4. White, R. J., Wolin, L. R., Massopust, L. C., Taslitz, N. and Verdura, J. (1971) Cephalic exchange transplantation in the monkey. *Surgery*, **70**, 135–139.
5. Hamblin, T. J. (1988) Nipping in the bud. *British Medical Journal*, **297**, 629.
6. Fleming, C. (1988) If we can keep a severed head alive... *British Medical Journal*, **297**, 1048.
7. Gillie, O. BMA ban on transplant of complete foetal brains. *The Independent* (London), May 7, 1988.
8. Anscombe, G. E. M. A modest proposal with frightening potential. *Catholic Herald* (London), June 3, 1988.
9. Bailey, E. Brain transplants. How and when. *Telegraph Sunday Magazine*, (London), March 27, 1988.
10. Christian, C. Why foetal brain implants stir such controversy. *Doctor* (London), June 2, 1988.
11. My story, by brain transplant wife. *The Sunday Times* (London), April 17, 1988.
12. I watched mother come out of hell. *The Sunday Times* (London), May 1, 1988.
13. New life plan by brain op. woman. *The Sunday Mercury* (Birmingham) June 26, 1988.
14. Editorial: Brain Problems, *New Scientist*, p. 24, April 28, 1988.
15. Backlund, E. O., Granberg, P. O., Hamberger, B., Knutsson, E., Martensson, A., Sedvall, G., Seiger, A. and Olsen, L. (1985) Transplantation of adrenal medullary tissue to striatum in parkinsonism. First clinical trials. *Journal of Neurosurgery*, **62**, 169–173.
16. Olsen, L., Backlund, E. O., Gerhardt, G., Hoffer, B., Lindvall, O., Rose, G., Seiger, A. and Stromberg, I. (1986) Nigral and adrenal grafts in parkinsonism: recent basic and clinical studies. *Advances in Neurology*, **45**, 85–94.
17. Lindvall, O., Backlund, E. O., Farde, L., Sedvall, G., Freedman, R., Hoffer, B., Nobin, A., Seiger, A. and Olson, L. (1987) Transplantation in Parkinson's disease: two cases of adrenal medullary grafts to the putamen. *Annals of Neurology*, **22**, 457–468.
18. Madrazo, I., Drucker-Colin, R., Diaz, V., Martinez-Mata, J., Torres, C. and Becerril, J. J. (1987) Open microsurgical autograft of adrenal medulla to the right caudate nucleus in two patients with intractable Parkinson's disease. *New England Journal of Medicine*, **316**, 831–834.
19. Marsden, C. D. (1988) Parkinson's disease as a pathfinder. An overview of neural transplants. *The Parkinson Newsletter*, (Parkinson's Disease Society, London) **66**, 4–7.
20. Lewin, R. (1988) Cloud over Parkinson's therapy. *Science*, **240**, 390–392.
21. Madrazo, I., Leon, V., Torres, C., Aguilera, M. C., Varela, G., Alvarez, F. and Fraga, A. (1988) Transplantation of fetal substantia nigra and adrenal medulla to the caudate nucleus in two patients with Parkinson's disease. *New England Journal of Medicine*, **318**, 51.
22. Lewin, R. (1988) Brain graft puzzles. *Science*, **240**, 879.
23. Freed, C. R. (1988) Transplantation of fetal substantia nigra and adrenal medulla to the caudate nucleus in two patients with Parkinson's disease. *New England Journal of Medicine*, **319**, 370.
24. Dwork, A. J., Pezzoli, G., Silani, V., Fahn, S. and Hill, R. (1988) Transplantation of fetal substantia nigra and adrenal medulla to the caudate nucleus in two patients with Parkinson's disease. *New England Journal of Medicine*, **319**, 370–371.

25. Pearce, J. M. (1988) Adrenal and nigral transplants for Parkinson's disease. *British Medical Journal*, **296**, 1211–1212.
26. Editorial (1988) Embryos and Parkinson's disease. *Lancet*, **i**, 1087.
27. O'Brien, J. Brain transplants 'not first' says professor. *The Sunday Telegraph* (London), May 17, 1988.
28. Shrimsley, A. I've got a new brain and a new life. *The News of the World* (London), November 13, 1988.
29. Schoon, N. Brain transplants expose need for new guidelines. *The Independent* (London), April 18, 1988.
30. Rodell, S. The brain cell dilemma. *The Herald* (Melbourne), May 4, 1988.
31. Implant scheme could help other nervous disorders. *The Huddersfield Daily Examiner*, June 2, 1988.
32. Prentice, T. Experts to question Yacoub. *The Times* (London), May 7, 1988.
33. Pallot, P. and O'Brien, J. BMA to give its backing to brain cell transplants. *The Daily Telegraph* (London), April 18, 1988.
34. Prentice, T. and Seton, C. BMA approves brain cell transplants. *The Sunday Times* (London), June 5, 1988.
35. Hitchcock, E. R., Clough, C., Hughes, R. and Kenny, B. (1988) Embryos and Parkinson's disease. *Lancet*, **i**, 1274.
36. Goetz, C. G. *et al.* (1989) Multicenter study of autologous adrenal medullary transplantation to the corpus striatum in patients with advanced Parkinson's disease. *New England Journal of Medicine*, **320**, 337–341.
37. Parkin, P. Newton orders inquiry into brain cell ops. *The Daily News* (London), June 2, 1988.
38. Pallot, P. More brain cell grafts planned. *The Daily Telegraph* (London), April 19, 1988.
39. Stuttaford, T. Early days for brain cell implants. *The Times* (London), April 21, 1988.
40. Heartbreak of brain-op queue, *The Sunday Mercury* (Birmingham), November 20, 1988.
41. Lindvall, O. *et al.* (1988) Fetal dopamine-rich mesencephalic grafts in Parkinson's Disease. *Lancet*, **ii**, 1483–1484.
42. U.S. surgeons in brain ops. *The Birmingham Express and Star*, November 12, 1988.
43. Lyall, J. Brave new world. *The Nursing Times and Nursing Mirror*, June 25, 1988.
44. Spalding, S. and Broadfield, D. Brain cell cure plea by patient. *The Observer*, (London), June 5, 1988.
45. Sherman, J. and Prentice, T. New medical treatments face 'value for money' check. *The Times*, (London), May 3, 1988.
46. Editorial comment (1988) *The Parkinson Newsletter*, **66**, 9.
47. Blakeslee, S. (1991) Fetal cell transplants show early promise in Parkinson patients. *The New York Times*, November 12, C3-4.
48. Pallis, C. A. (1971) Parkinsonism: natural history and clinical features. *British Medical Journal*, **iii**, 683–690.
49. Marsden, C. D. and Parkes, J. D. (1976) "On-off" effects in patients with Parkinson's disease on chronic levodopa therapy. *Lancet*, **ii**, 292–296.
50. Pearce, J. M. (1984) Drug treatment in Parkinson's disease. *British Medical Journal*, **288**, 1777–1778.
51. Marsden, C. D. (1987) Movement disorders. In D. J. Weatherall, J. G. G. Ledingham and D. A. Warrell, (Eds.) *Oxford Textbook of Medicine*, 2nd edn, pp. 21.218–21.225. Oxford University Press, Oxford.
52. Cooper, I. S. (1965) Surgical treatment of Parkinsonism. *Annual Reviews of Medicine*, **16**, 309–330.

53. Meyers, H. R. (1940) Surgical procedure for postencephalitic tremor with notes on the physiology of premotor fibres. *Archives of Neurology and Psychiatry*, **144**, 455–459.

54. Meyers, R. H. (1940) The modification of alternating tremors, rigidity and festination by surgery of the basal ganglia. *Research Publications of the Association for Research in Nervous and Mental Disease*, **21**, 602–665.

55. Sladek, J. R. and Shoulson, I. (1988) Neural transplantation: a call for patience rather than patients. *Science*, **240**, 1386–1388.

56. Dunnett, S. B., Whishaw, I. Q., Rogers, D. C. and Jones, G. H. (1987) Dopamine-rich grafts ameliorate whole body motor asymmetry and sensory neglect but not independent limb use in rats with 6-hydroxydopamine lesions. *Brain Research*, **415**, 63–78.

57. Bjorklund, A., Dunnet, S. B., Stenevi, U., Lewis, M. E., and Iversen, S. D. (1980) Reinnervation of the denervated striatum by substantia nigra transplants: functional consequences as revealed by pharmacological and sensorimotor testing. *Brain Research*, **199**, 307–333.

58. Stenevi, U., Bjorklund, A. and Svendgaard, N. A. (1976) Transplantations of central and peripheral monoamine neurons to the adult rat brain: techniques and conditions for survival. *Brain Research*, **114**, 1–20.

59. Mahalik, T. J., Finger, T. E., Stomberg, I. and Olson, L. (1985) Substantia nigra transplants into denervated striatum of the rat: ultrastructure of graft and host interconnections. *The Journal of Comparative Neurology*, **240**, 60–70.

60. Dunnett, S. B., Bjorklund, A., Gage, F. H. and Stenevi, U. (1985) Transplantation of mesencephalic dopamine neurons to the striatum of adult rats. In A. Bjorklund and U. Stenevi, (Eds.) *Neural Grafting in the Mammalian CNS*, pp. 451–469. Elsevier Science Publishers, Amsterdam.

61. Nieto-Sampedro, M., Manthrope, M., Barbin, G., Varon, S. and Cotman, C. W. (1983) Injury-induced neuronotrophic activity in adult rat brain: correlation with survival of delayed implants in the wound cavity. *Journal of Neuroscience*, **3**, 2219–2229.

62. Stein, D. G., Labbe, R., Firl, A. and Mufson, E. (1985) Behavioural recovery following implantation of fetal brain tissue into mature rats with bilateral cortical lesions. In A. Bjorklund and U. Stenevi, (Eds.) *Neural Grafting in the Mammalian CNS*, pp. 605–614. Elsevier Science Publishers, Amsterdam.

63. Bjorklund, A. and Stenevi, U. (1984) Intracerebral neural implants: neuronal replacement and reconstruction of damaged circuitries. *Annual Review of Neuroscience*, **7**, 279–308.

64. Hallas, B. H., Das, G. D. and Das, K. G. (1980) Transplantation of brain tissue in the brain of rat. II. Growth characteristics of neocortical transplants in hosts of different ages. *American Journal of Anatomy*, **158**, 147–159.

65. Brundin, P., Isacson, O. and Bjorklund, A. (1985) Monitoring of cell viaibility in suspensions of embryonic CNS tissue and its use as a criterion for intracerebral graft survival. *Brain Research*, **331**, 251–259.

66. Brundin, P., Barbin, G., Isacson, O., Mallat, M., Chamak, B., Prochiantz, A., Gage, F. H. and Bjorklund, A. (1985) Survival of intracerebrally grafted rat dopamine neurons previously cultured *in vitro*. *Neuroscience Letters*, **61**, 79–84.

67. Brundin, P., Nilsson, O. G., Strecker, R. E., Lindvall, O., Astedt, B. and Bjorklund, A. (1986) Behavioural effects of human fetal dopamine neurons grafted in a rat model of Parkinson's disease. *Experimental Brain Research*, **65**, 235–240.

68. Brundin, P., Strecker, R. E., Widner, H., Clarke, D. J., Nilsson, O. G., Astedt, B., Lindvall, O. and Bjorklund, A. (1988) Human fetal dopamine neurons

grafted in a rat model of Parkinson's disease: immunological aspects, spontaneous and drug-induced behaviour, and dopamine release. *Experimental Brain Research*, **70**, 192–208.

69. German, D. C., Schlusselberg, D. S. and Woodward, D. J. (1983) Three-dimensional computer reconstruction of midbrain dopaminergic neuronal populations: from mouse to man. *Journal of Neural Transmission*, **57**, 243–254.

70. Das, G. D. (1985) Development of neocortical transplants. In A. Bjorklund and U. Stenevi, (Eds.), *Neural Grafting in the Mammalian CNS*, pp. 101–123. Elsevier Science Publishers, Amsterdam.

71. Olson, L., Stromberg, I., Bygdeman, M., Granholm, A. C., Hoffer, B., Freedman, R. and Seiger, A. (1987) Human fetal tissues grafted to rodent hosts: structural and functional observations of brain, adrenal and heart tissues *in oculo*. *Experimental Brain Research*, **67**, 163–178.

72. Report of the Advisory Group to the Department of Health and Social Security, Scottish Home and Health department and the Welsh Office. (1972) *The Use of Fetuses and Fetal Material for Research*, H.M. Stationery Office, London.

73. Mahowald, M. B. (1987) The ethical options in transplanting fetal tissue. *Hastings Center Report*, **17**, 1, 9–15.

74. Nobin, A. and Bjorklund, A. (1973) Topography of the monoamine neuron systems in the human brain as revealed in fetuses. *Acta Physiologica Scandinavia*, (Suppl. 388), 4.

75. McCullagh, P. (1987) In *The Foetus as Transplant Donor: Scientific, Social and Ethical Perspectives*. John Wiley and Sons, Chichester.

76. Raju, S. and Grogan, J. B. (1977) Immunologic study of the brain as a privileged site. *Transplantation Proceedings*, **9**, 1187–1191.

77. Lodin, Z., Hasek, M., Chutna, J., Sladecek, M., and Holan, V. (1977) Transplantation immunity in the brain. *Journal of Neuroscience Research*, **3**, 275–280.

78. Geyer, S. J., Gill, T. J., Kunz, H. W. and Moody, E. (1985) Immunogenetic aspects of transplantation in the rat brain. *Transplantation*, **39**, 244–247.

79. Bjorklund, A., Stenevi, U., Dunnett, S. B. and Gage, F. H. (1982) Cross-species neural grafting in a rat model of Parkinson's disease. *Nature*, **298**, 652–654.

80. Castro, A. J., Tonder, N., Sunde, N. A. and Zimmer, J. (1987) Fetal cortical transplants in the cerebral hemisphere of newborn rats: a retrograde fluorescent analysis of connections. *Experimental Brain Research*, **66**, 533–542.

81. Dunnett, S. B. (1987) Specificity of cerebellar grafts. *Nature*, **327**, 366–367.

82. Connor, J. R. and Bernstein, J. J. (1987) Astrocytes in rat fetal cerebral cortical homografts following implantation into adult rat spinal cord. *Brain Research*, **409**, 62–70.

83. Bray, G. M., Vidal-Sanz, M. and Aguayo, A. J. (1987) Regeneration of axons from the central nervous system of adult rats. *Progress in Brain Research*, **71**, 373–379.

84. Kromer, L. F., Bjorklund, A. and Stenevi, U. (1981) Regeneration of the septohippocampal pathways in adult rats is promoted by utilizing embryonic hippocampal implants as bridges. *Brain Research*, **210**, 173–200.

85. Kesslak, J. P., Nieto-Sampedro, M., Globus, J. and Cotman, C. W. (1986) Transplants of purified astrocytes promote behavioural recovery after frontal cortex ablation. *Experimental Neurology*, **92**, 377–390.

86. Mickley, G. A., Teitelbaum, H. and Reier, P. J. (1987) Fetal hypothalamic brain grafts reduce the obesity produced by ventromedial hypothalamic lesions. *Brain Research*, **424**, 239–248.

87. Smith, G. M., Miller, R. H. and Silver, J. (1986) Changing role of forebrain

astrocytes during development, regenerative failure, and induced regeneration upon transplantation. *The Journal of Comparative Neurology*, **251**, 23–43.

88. Sabel, B. A., Dunbar, G. L. and Stein, D. G. (1984) Gangliosides minimize behavioural deficits and enhance structural repair after brain injury. *Journal of Neuroscience Research*, **12**, 429–443.

89. Brundin, P., Strecker, R. E., Londos, E. and Bjorklund, A. (1987) Dopamine neurons grafted unilaterally to the nucleus accumbens affect drug-induced circling and locomotion. *Experimental Brain Research*, **69**, 183–194.

90. Rosenstein, J. M. (1987) Adrenal medulla grafts produce blood-brain barrier dysfunction. *Brain Research*, **414**, 192–196.

91. Rosenstein, J. M. (1987) Neocortical transplants in the mammalian brain lack a blood–brain barrier to macromolecules. *Science*, **235**, 772–774.

92. Dalrymple-Alford, J. C., Kelche, C., Cassel, J. C., Toniolo, G., Pallage, V. and Will, B. E. (1988) Behavioural deficits after intrahippocampal fetal septal grafts in rats with selective fimbria–fornix lesions. *Experimental Brain Research*, **69**, 545–558.

93. Ridley, R. M., Baker, H. F. and Fine, A. (1988) Transplantation of fetal tissues. *British Medical Journal*, **296**, 1469.

94. Backlund, E. O., Granberg, P.-O., Hamberger, B., Knutsson, E., Martensson, A., Sedvall, G., Seiger, A. and Olson, L. (1985) Transplantation of adrenal medullary tissue to striatum in parkinsonism. *Journal of Neurosurgery*, **62**, 169–173.

95. Fazzini, E., Burke, R., Cote, L., Goodman, R., Naini, A. B., Pezzoli, G., Pullman, S., Solomon, R., Stern, Y., Weber, C. and Fahn, S. (1989) Stereotoxic implantation of autologous adrenal medulla into caudate nucleus in Parkinson's disease. *Neurology*, 39 (Suppl. 1), 125.

96. Hefti, F., Hartikka, J. and Schlumpf, M. (1985) Implantation of PC12 cells into the corpus striatum of rats with lesions of the dopaminergic nigrostriatal neurons. *Brain Research*, **348**, 283–288.

97. Jaeger, C. B. (1985) Immunocytochemical study of PC12 cells grafted to the brain of immature rats. *Experimental Brain Research*, **59**, 615–624.

98. Gash, D. M., Notter, M. F. D., Okawara, S. H., Kraus, A. L. and Joynt, R. J. (1986) Amitotic neuroblastoma cells used for neural implants in monkeys. *Science*, **233**, 1420–1422.

99. Kordower, J. H., Notter, M. F. and Gash, D. M. (1987) Neuroblastoma cells in neural transplants: a neuroanatomical and behavioural analysis. *Brain Research*, **417**, 85–98.

100. *Washington Times*, November 13, 1991.

101. Reynolds, B. A. and Weiss, S. (1992) Generation of neurons and astrocytes from isolated cells of the adult mammalian central nervous system. *Science*, **255**, 1707–1710.

102. Hitchcock, E. R., Clough, C. G., Hughes, R. C. and Kenny, B. (1989) Fetal brain tissue. *Lancet*, i, 839.

103. McKie and Ferriman, A. Major doubts over brain transplants. *The Observer* (London), May 1, 1988.

104. Gustavii, B. (1989) Fetal brain transplantation for Parkinson's disease: technique for obtaining donor tissue. *Lancet*, i, 565.

105. Blunt, S. B. (1989) Fetal brain tissue and Parkinson's disease. *Lancet*, i, 1021.

106. Report of the Advsiory Committee to the Director, National Institutes of Health (1988) *Human Fetal Tissue Transplantation Research*, December 14. Bethesda, Maryland.

107. *Review of the Guidance on the Research Use of Fetuses and Fetal Material*, July (1989) Her Majesty's Stationery Office, London.
108. *Report of the Committee of Inquiry into Human Fertilisation and Embryology* (1984). Her Majesty's Stationery Office, London.
109. *The Guardian Weekly* (London), February 7, 1982.
110. Spalding, R. J. (1988) Salvaging fetal cells to cure. *Chemical Week*, October 12.

7 Human Subjects and Human Objects

The preceding five chapters have considered several specific situations in which it has been proposed that individuals who are assessed as having no further interest in being considered as alive, or who are deemed never to have acquired such an interest, are identified as available for use. In each case, the condition of the specific class of individuals has been held to be equivalent to death: in no case, however, are the individuals described as "dead". In discussing the various classes of subject—brain dead, cerebrally dead, anencephalic or foetus *ex utero*—the specific arguments that have been presented in support of their reification, or classification as objects, were outlined and some of the implications of them were considered. This chapter seeks to identify, and to explore in a more general context, some of the points raised in discussion of the specific situations. Whilst each of the clinical situations covered in the earlier chapters arose more or less as an isolated issue, I believe that there exists considerable common ground between them.

WHAT'S IN A NAME? THE SHAPING OF AN ISSUE BY TERMINOLOGY

The terminology which is selected to introduce a new concept or a newly observed phenomenon may fulfil more than one function. In the first instance, it serves to identify the subject so that the individual drawing attention to it can indicate to others what he or she wishes to discuss. Secondly, it can provide an indication of the nature of the subject and define some of its features. In some instances, it may provide an indication of preceding events, which are believed to be causatively associated. Yet another function of terminology can be to strengthen the case for the very *existence* of the subject to which it refers. An entity which has a name, especially if this becomes accepted into common use, is more likely to be popularly considered to exist than will another entity which can be characterized only by using several sentences. A title that is succinct and easily remembered may serve not only to entrench the concept to which it refers but also to convey presumptions about associated features: it may also impede proposals for alternative concepts. The perception of three of the issues examined in earlier chapters has been enhanced by succinct descriptions—brain dead, brain absent and brain donor. To some extent, the titles have assumed an existence in their own right without further questioning of their accuracy as a description of the states to which they refer. I believe it would be legitimate to retain substantial reservations in relation to each term. Selection of the term "brain death" achieved both identification of the concept and considerable characterization of its features. Both the term and the concept have survived and achieved almost complete acceptance, notwithstanding a succession of observations which have called into question the precise nature of the state to which the term refers. As indicated in Chapter 2, I believe that introduction of the term was largely superfluous when used in its original context of providing a guide to the discontinuation of resuscitation. The decision to cease resuscitation could legitimately be made, if it was clearly in the best interests of the patient, irrespective of whether "brain death" was considered to have occurred. The clinical criteria employed to diagnose the state provide a reliable indication that recovery will not occur. For this reason, irrespective of the state that one proposed to account for them, these criteria would certainly provide adequate grounds to cease resuscitation. Since its introduction, as a basis for discontinuing resuscitation, the justification that "brain death" provides for use as an organ donor has not been generally accepted as also sanctioning use of an individual in experimentation. The reason for this discrepancy is not immediately clear to me. Perhaps it reflects the general lack of understanding of the nature of the state identified by the term "brain death". If so, the comment of Pallis to the effect that "a currently uninformed public will sooner or later discover how misleading this simple formulation really is"[1], referred to in Chapter 3, may be close to the mark.

The term "anencephaly" has been quite misleading, as also has corresponding lay terminology such as "born without brains" to describe anencephalic infants. Both the etymological basis of the term itself and the common equivalent expression "brain absent" provide incorrect descriptions of the pathological condition. Nevertheless, both terms have been very influential. Otherwise serious attempts to analyse the status of anencephalic infants by non-medical commentators have often assumed the absence of the brain. Popular descriptions of the condition in press releases emanating from medical sources such as the Harefield Hospital have explicitly referred to an anencephalic as being "born without a brain".[2] Presumably, the use of such inaccurate descriptions in presentations to a *medical* audience would be eschewed.

Reference to "donors" in relation to any of the categories of individual discussed in Chapters 2–6 exemplifies another use of terminology to achieve something more than the identification of a type of individual. General acceptance of the term "donor" has effectively compromised any argument as to whether subjects such as anencephalic infants or the foetus *ex utero* can legitimately be considered to be *donating*. Attempts to question this presumption have been rare and clearly start at a substantial disadvantage. One example, the review by Shewmon *et al.* that was considered in Chapter 5, indicated its non-acceptance of the validity of use of the term "donation" in relation to the anencephalic infant by substituting "organ source" and placing the word "donor" between inverted commas.[3] The need to resort to such devices by anyone wishing to present alternative views illustrates most effectively the power which the opportunity to select the terminology confers in the subsequent argument. Depending upon the background of the user, use of terminology in the ways referred to above could be understood, and excused. Nevertheless, the influence that it can exert to support a position in the face of solid conflicting evidence should be recognized.

There exist other examples of the purposeful use of terminology to skew arguments in relation to the categories of individuals we have been considering. Thus, particular advocacy positions have been advanced. One of the most obvious ways in which terminology has been misused in order to advance some arguments relating to reification of individuals has been by the introduction of euphemism. Of the three principal subjects discussed in earlier chapters, anencephalic infants have been the occasion of some of the most florid examples of euphemism to be found in medical literature. Examples of this have been given in Chapter 5. For instance, the reference to recognizing "the contribution of this doomed foetus to mankind" by a physician and to anencephalics as "human materials" by an ethicist both appear to me to be blatant attempts to obscure the issue. Similarly, the allusion to organ removal as "hastening death" rather than describing it as a highly effective means of rapidly causing death of an anencephalic by exsanguination represents a major euphemistic achievement. Another instance of the use of terminology to put down opposing views has been the forceful presentation of the brain-death concept to discount the personal experience of paramedical personnel "swayed by the evidence of their senses into regarding brain-dead individuals as still alive".

Apart from its use in relation to anencephalics, appropriate selection of reinforcing technology has been a feature of some advocacy for the general acceptance of "cerebral death" as an updated version of "brain death". Thus, one of the most persistent advocates of the substitution of "cerebral death" for "brain death", Dr Ronald Cranford, has regularly referred to anyone opposing his own views as "putrefactionists".

Yet another way in which terminology can be employed to influence an argument is by utilizing it in analogies constructed around issues under discussion. A common example of such an analogy, which I consider to be quite dishonest, equates the brain-dead subject with a freshly guillotined individual. The substantial inaccuracy inherent in this comparison has been discussed in Chapter 3. Another use of a very inaccurate analogy, discussed in Chapter 4, equates the anencephalic infant with a parasitic twin in the condition of acephaly in which the head is lacking. As with all of the examples noted in this section, the conclusion remains that terminology cannot be assumed to be a neutral input into consideration of an issue.

THE RESPECTIVE ROLES OF HYPOTHESIS AND OBSERVATION IN DETERMINING THE STATUS OF AN INDIVIDUAL

There are no clearcut and generally accepted guidelines for making decisions concerning the status of an individual in relation to attributes such as person-hood. Similarly, the related question of how one determines that a human indi-vidual is, or has become, an object rather than a subject is not readily answered. The development of the brain-death concept affords an example of the manner in which such problems have been addressed. This may be relevant to each of the types of clinical situations considered in previous chapters. A major issue is the extent to which emphasis is to be apportioned between hypothesis or con-cept and reproducible observation in determining an individual's status. As a first approach, scientific or clinical data derived from observation is likely to be required for the process of *recognition* of a particular state, such as irrecoverable loss of brain function. On the other hand, *definition* of a state of brain death or of cerebral death can only be made as a philosophical exercise. The hypothesis or concept that is developed in this exercise may take note of scientific or clinical data but it is also likely to be strongly influenced by social and legal considera-tions. The two processes of recognition and definition, both of which are essen-tial if questions about the status of any individual are to be answered, involve quite different approaches.

The notion of brain death was derived, and has been sustained, as a philosophical exercise and not as a result of analysis of data collected from sub-jects entering this state. Observation and experimental investigation of individuals satisfying the criteria for brain death have not disclosed what is the essential nature of the brain-dead state. This was conceived as, and remains, a theoretical subject. However, it appears from much of what has been written about brain death by non-medical commentators that this point has been over-looked. One reason for this may be a failure to distinguish between "brain death" as a conceptualized state and "brain death" as a diagnosis, carrying a reliable prognosis, which is attached to individual patients meeting certain criteria. A patient who is "brain dead" in the second sense may or may not also conform to the theoretical conception of brain death.

The basic premise underlying the derivation of the concept of brain death was that if brain function had been irrevocably lost, then death had occurred. The continuation of functioning in other organ systems, such as the cardiovascular system, was not considered to be an impediment to the diagnosis of brain death. To derive a concept in this way seems legitimate. Nevertheless, it could be pointed out that a derivation in this form could not guarantee that such a state actually occurs in real patients. Nor could it guarantee that patients meeting the criteria for diagnosis as "brain dead" were actually examples of the state postulated by the concept.

There have been two manifestations of cessation of brain function which have been included, both in the reasoning underlying the conceptual state and in the criteria required for a clinical diagnosis of brain death in patients in the ward. The original single function, the loss of which can be readily diagnosed clinically, is spontaneous respiration. Loss of respiration, in the absence of medical intervention, will reliably lead to cessation of all other brain functions. More recently, analyses of what is intended by the concept of brain death have tended to place more emphasis on the permanent loss of consciousness than on loss of respiration. The justification for identifying this as the crucial feature of the brain-death concept has generally been that, with loss of consciousness and self-awareness, those attributes which are believed to be distinctively human have ceased. However at a clinical rather than a conceptual level, this becomes decidedly an arbitrary choice. If permanent loss of qualities such as consciousness and cognition is admitted as the key feature in the concept of brain death, then death in the human species is thereby envisaged as being different from death in any other species. Furthermore, it is not easy to envisage ways in which an observer could be assured that subconscious functions had ceased solely on the basis of failure to evince conscious awareness of the external environment.

In order to identify conceptual brain death with conventional death, it would be possible to argue that loss of brain function is, after all, what conventional death is about or, alternatively, that brain death inevitably presages the early onset of conventional death. The alternative does not strictly equate brain death with death but would maintain that there is a sufficiently close linkage.

As mentioned above, development of the philosophical concept of brain death was not dependent upon, nor could it be proven by, observational data. The stimuli to development of the concept were not items of scientific data. They included a perception that there existed a requirement for some form of diagnosis of death in order to discontinue resuscitation. The advantage that a diagnosis of brain death could afford indemnity for a physician from legal action after discontinuation of resuscitation was probably influential in some countries. Additionally, development of the concept of brain death was increasingly indicated as a prerequisite to organ transplantation—both to legitimize organ removal and to reassure the general population as to the probity of transplantation practice.

The concept of brain death has not been static since its first enunciation. Even though the concept was philosophically, rather than experimentally or observationally, based it has been subject to progressive modification as a result of the recognition in patients diagnosed as brain dead of a number of features (discussed on pp. 39–40) inconsistent with the original concept.

There has been considerable discussion of whether brain death, as clinically diagnosed, constitutes a concept or only provides a set of criteria which permit the recognition of irrecoverable loss of brain function. I suggest that the term "brain death" has, in fact, acquired both connotations. To some commentators, this term conveys a concept: to others it represents the observable features of patients in whom the diagnosis has been made. The confusion between brain death as a concept and as a criterion of death appears to have persisted. Concerning the *concept* of brain death, I believe that it is entirely legitimate to develop such a notion in isolation from clinical or laboratory data. A concept that has been developed by reasoning alone rather than as an interpretation of data will not be subject to subsequent disproof on the basis that the supporting data has been subject to re-interpretation. On the other hand, a concept that is not derived from a substantial body of reproducible data, obtained in this case from examination of patients independently shown to have sustained brain death, cannot be claimed as proven to be an accurate representation of reality.

The nature of the brain-death concept is such that it is unlikely that scientific observation to test it will ever be feasible. An observer cannot measure subjective modalities like sentience to determine whether they are being experienced in any class of non-communicating patients. Subconscious activity is not amenable to observation. It is probably impracticable to establish the consistent and simultaneous occurrence of destructive changes in the brain, which accompany and account for functional loss. The unknowability of most of the information which the brain death concept might predict as applying to individuals in this state seems to guarantee the impossibility of confident demonstration of whether brain death, as conceived, exists in any individual.

There are effectively two questions which are not always distinguished: What is brain death? and, How is it to be recognized? To the first, there can only be a response based on philosophy. Scientific data will never define the essence or nature of brain death. On the other hand recognition of a state that is *termed* brain death (whatever its nature) can be achieved with considerable accuracy by observation. It is not possible to know the extent to which the accurately and reproducibly diagnosable clinical state corresponds with brain death. As it is conceptualized it could be always or frequently: it could be rarely or never. Perhaps the extent of correspondence between concept and reality varies with the interval that has elapsed since the clinical diagnosis was made. In passing, it is worth noting that, although the brain-death concept has not been, and cannot be, confirmed or refuted by scientific observation, the fact that the concept has been framed has probably influenced the types of investigations which have been undertaken and also those that have been omitted.

The preceding discussion has attempted to draw to attention the seemingly contradictory interpretation of an individual's status that may arise from consideration of conceptual and observable perspectives. Whilst the discussion has been restricted to the example of brain death, the issue is likely to arise, to some extent, in the case of all of the categories of individual under consideration in earlier chapters. In each instance, medical attendants, commentators or the community at large are attempting to classify individuals into abstract states on the basis of concrete observations. The contradictory outcome of attempting to grade individuals in this way is again exemplified when the status of the anencephalic is considered.

One issue which, I believe, has not been addressed in attempts to classify anencephalics as "human materials", "non-persons" or objects which should be available for the use of others, is the nature of the human "norm" with which they should be compared. Anencephalics have commonly been compared with non-anencephalic *children* rather than with the newborn. As discussed in Chapter 4, the latter comparison reveals many similarities in neurological function. These similarities, however, rapidly disappear as the non-anencephalic infant matures and cerebral function supplants the operation of lower brain centres that is characteristic of the normal neonate. In contrast, the anencephalic has no capacity or potential for further development of cerebral function.

The anencephalic provides perhaps the best example of the complications that may be introduced into attempts to classify individuals who manifest any of the conditions discussed in preceding chapters. Are human potential and such distinctions as that between human subjects and objects to be based on the anatomical structure of the individual's nervous system, on its functional capacity, on the impression which its functioning produces on others or on some other parameters? The functional capacity that is predicted for the anencephalic by applying current understanding of relationships between structure and function to the pathological anatomy characteristic of the condition is substantially at variance with what is commonly observed in practice on the part of such infants. As discussed in Chapter 4, observation of the functional capacity of anencephalic infants has led to a re-appraisal of the relative contributions of cerebral cortex and lower brain centres to behavioural patterns in *normal* infants. It should follow that attempts to assign status as a human subject on the basis of either the extent of deviation from anatomical normality or of restriction of brain function are likely to be as flawed scientifically as they would have been traditionally considered to be on moral grounds.

A final point that arises out of considering the relative place of conceptual systems and verifiable data in classification of individuals is the necessity for distinguishing between processes that are irreversibly in train and those which have passed to completion. Concepts of brain death appear to me conveniently to ignore the probability that a finite interval may elapse between the "point of no return" (a description sometimes used to describe the occurrence of brain death) and the completion of the process. Whilst consideration of the brain death concept may comfortably proceed without undue concern for this distinction, the same cannot necessarily be said for analysis of observation of subjects who have met the requirements for clinical diagnosis of brain death. As implied by the range of brain functions that can still be retained (detailed on pp. 39–40), the point of diagnosis of brain death might be placed anywhere along the pathway of an irreversible transition from life to death. This is not to question in any way the reliability of the prediction that an individual who has been identified by the correct application of brain-death criteria is in an irrecoverable state the only outcome of which is conventional death. It is, however, to register apprehension at a growing tendency to accord completely reliable predictions the status of fulfilment. This issue, and the reasons for apprehension on account of it, will be considered in the following section.

WHEN THE FUTURE BECOMES THE PRESENT: RECLASSIFICATION OF INDIVIDUALS ON THE BASIS OF PROGNOSIS

A medical prognosis is a forecast of the likely course of a patient's condition. The traditional reason for formulating a prognosis has been that of assisting a patient, and his or her family, to anticipate the probable outcome of the current disease and to guide the medical attendant in planning further treatment. Both of these reasons are clearly directed primarily, if not exclusively, to the benefit of the patient. Prognostication has also been undertaken as a means of assisting a *community*, including that individual to whom it directly relates. This extended role of prognosis arises in the course of triage when the outlook for a number of individuals is examined collectively as a basis for making decisions on the best distribution of finite medical resources among them. In effect, this process is an attempt to decide which of a number of alternative patterns of disbursement of limited resources among different individuals, none of whom has an exclusive claim to them, is likely to lead to the maximum benefit for the group. The recent trend to using a patient's prognosis as a means of identifying individuals who are likely to be of potential use to others, as discussed in earlier chapters, represents a radical departure from this precedent. In effect, *the individual has become the finite resource*.

Prognosis may be concerned primarily with the capacity of an individual to survive. Alternatively, survival may not be in question and prognosis could then relate exclusively to the probability of recovery towards a normal state. Being a forecast, a prognosis is concerned with an individual's *future* condition rather than with the current status. Obviously, if an accurate prognosis is being fulfilled, the patient's current status will increasingly approximate to it. Current management of any patient, for example, whether to initiate or continue intensive treatment or, alternatively, to cease it, is likely to be substantially influenced by the prognosis that has been formulated. However, it is reasonable to anticipate that this influence will be exerted within a framework of seeking that outcome considered to be in the best interests of the subject to whom it relates.

It is an interesting paradox that the pattern of using a patient's prognosis to identify those individuals who may be usable for the benefit of others is often notable for its inversion of the "conventional" management pattern that is likely to have been followed for the benefit of that patient. One example of this paradoxical response, referred to in Chapter 2, relates to the management of the brain-dead patient. As discussed at that stage, a diagnosis of brain death provides a highly reliable forecast that recovery of consciousness will never occur. (The reliability with which such a diagnosis guarantees that all function of the brain has *already* ceased has, I believe, been called into question by observations of such patients reported over more than two decades.) The response that medical principles would traditionally suggest to a reliable prognosis of irrecoverability from a deeply comatose state would be to desist from any further vigorous attempts to resuscitate the patient. These would be unjustifiable and might even be potentially burdensome. However, the revised approach to this situation, when the individual is assessed as a suitable source of organs for transplantation, is to undertake the most vigorous resuscitation with no holds barred. I suggest that it is not necessary for one to question the reliability of brain death as a fore-cast of irrecoverability of brain function in order to recognize the paradox inherent in completely reversing the response that diagnosis of brain death was primarily intended to achieve.

Another example of acknowledging the implications of prognosis for manage-ment in the interests of the patient, but then proceeding to employ that prognosis to justify a totally different management in the interests of others, has been provided by some recent examples of the use of anencephalic infants. Having argued that the prognosis of such patients is so poor as to suggest that the shortest life would be the best, some physicians have proceeded to enter anencephalic infants into programmes of intensive resuscitation. The paradox in this situation, as outlined in Chapter 5, is inherent in juxtaposition of the con-tention, based on "a principle of beneficence", that termination of an anen-cephalic pregnancy in the third trimester was justifiable in order to spare the infant from worthless existence with the subsequent infliction of the most inten-sive resuscitation preparatory to organ removal. In the case of both the brain dead and the anencephalic, the formulation of a particular prognosis has led to embarkation on a course of treatment utterly opposed to that which would have been suggested by the prognosis to be in the patients' interest.

A possible response to my contention might be that, whilst these reactions to the prognosis of irrecoverability are paradoxical, no harm has been done. Such a response could make the following points:

1. The two classes of individual are already either "brain dead" or "brain absent".
2. There is no question of recovery of either class of patient in any circumstances.
3. Adverse effects cannot be experienced by the subject following resuscitation and organ removal.
4. There is an excellent possibility that another patient may receive the benefit of an organ transplant.

I could readily acknowledge the irrecoverability of patients who are brain dead or anencephalic (2), and the strong possibility of benefit to other patients who become organ recipients (4). However, I believe that objection should be raised to the use of the first and third points.

In relation to the question of whether brain-dead and anencephalic subjects could experience any adverse consequences in the course of resuscitation and organ removal, I suggest that this remains quite unknowable in either case. As indicated in Chapter 2, some parts of the brain are likely to remain viable and possibly functioning to some extent, after clinical diagnosis of brain death. The question of the significance of any functions mediated by such residual brain cells is unassessable. As also indicated in Chapter 2, the identity of the parts of the brain involved in *subconscious* activity and their capacity to function in an unconscious subject is not accessible to investigation. Current understanding of brain function fails to attribute specific functional roles to large parts of the organ. As for the possibility of anencephalic infants experiencing adverse effects as a result of extended resuscitation and organ removal, the case for their not doing so appears to rest very heavily on the present, incomplete understanding of the status of pain-conducting pathways within the nervous system.

When one considers the question of whether brain-dead and anencephalic subjects can have an interest in not being used as organ sources, I believe that the possibility of an adverse experience by the individual in the course of this is only one of a number of components in such a judgement. The remaining point (1) in the rejoinder suggested above to my position, namely that the individuals under discussion are *already* in a certain state, raises some general implications that require a response. My particular concern is with the attitude which endorses management of patients *for the benefit of others* as though a prognosis has already been fulfilled. This attitude seems to open the possibility of the intrusion of similar influences into the management of categories of patient other than the brain dead and anencephalic. As indicated above, the anticipation that a carefully considered prognosis is extremely likely to be fulfilled might well lead one, *in the interests of the patient*, to adopt measures which assumed that this had occurred. Withholding of intensive therapy from individuals in irreversible states of coma is an example of such an approach.

The relevant point with respect to both brain dead and anencephalic patients is that neither class of subject is dead. A brain-dead subject, correctly diagnosed, is certain to satisfy the conventional requirements for death within minutes of disconnection of respiratory support. Nevertheless, he or she is not already dead. Despite adoption of brain-death criteria as grounds for organ removal for some two decades, notwithstanding the continuation of other physiological systems, including blood circulation, it is notable that "death" has not replaced "brain death" as the diagnosis. I have little doubt that, given the existing short-fall in organ supply for transplantation and the consequent efforts to augment procurement (as outlined in Chapter 3), this substitution in terminology would have been introduced if it had been considered that this change would be acceptable, especially to the medical and paramedical personnel responsible for the care of these patients.

Without forming a judgement on the legitimacy of organ removal from either beating-heart, brain-dead or anencephalic subjects, I submit that support for present practice must be based on acceptance of at least one of the following two propositions. (As the arguments in the two situations are not identical, I will develop these propositions only in relation to brain-dead subjects, whilst recognizing that a similar approach is possible in the case of the anencephalic.)

1. The forecast for the subject meeting the clinical criteria of "brain death" is certain, namely an early transition to "conventional" death. This outlook is then considered to be sufficient to warrant intervention in anticipation of its fulfilment.
2. Brain-dead subjects have already attained such a state of impoverished existence ("non-person", "human material", etc.) that they cannot retain any interest in not being subjected to organ removal. (Interestingly, this lack of interest does not seem to extend so far as to validate their incorporation in experimentation.)

Both of these propositions in relation to the brain dead introduce implications for other classes of subjects. The first implies that it is permissible, because of its certainty and imminence, to *anticipate* the achievement of the predicted outcome of death, which is accepted as a prerequisite for the removal of vital organs. On the other hand, the second proposition effectively relocates the prerequisite state for organ removal forward to something preceding conventional death. The distinction between the two propositions may not usually be drawn: I believe that it should be. Whereas the first proposition might be construed as bending the rules by acting in anticipation of the occurrence of the legitimizing event, the second could only be interpreted as creating new rules to suit the requirements of the situation. Both propositions effectively modify the treatment of the subject in the interests of others thereby converting that subject from an end in him or herself into a means to some other end.

If anticipation that the forecast course of the patient's condition has already occurred is to be accepted as grounds for use in the case of a brain-dead subject, then a consistent approach would permit extensions of the practice of anticipating that a prognosis has been fulfilled to other cases. The prognosis need not be for early and certain death: the use need not be as a source of transplantable organs. An example of a case in which the prognosis was for early death but the use was to serve as an experimental subject in receipt of an organ transplant has been mentioned in Chapter 5. Baby Fae, an infant facing the prospect of certain death from a congenital deformity of the heart, received a cardiac transplant from a baboon in a procedure which attracted widespread criticism on the basis that it represented the use of a human subject in an unjustified experiment.[4]

IMPLICATIONS FOR OTHER CLASSES OF DISABLED INDIVIDUALS OF REIFICATION OF THE BRAIN DEAD, BRAIN ABSENT AND BRAIN DONORS

The individuals we have been considering would usually be considered to be beyond the common understanding of the term "disability". Even the most severe examples of progressive, degenerative brain disease or of quadriplegia with a high lesion would be unlikely to be considered in a common class with a brain-dead individual. Nevertheless the likelihood that there are shared causative processes and the tendency, noted by the US Task Force on anencephaly (Chapter 4), for a continuum to exist between the most severe cases of spina bifida and the least complete manifestations of anencephaly could facilitate perception of infants with these two conditions as falling in a common category. Similarly, the physical and biological similarity between the aborted second-trimester foetus, as used in the UK as a brain donor, and the hopelessly premature 22-week neonate could lead to a strong association in the mind of the observer. In relation to cessation of brain function in older subjects, the point has been made that distinctions between "brain death" and "cerebral death" or "persistent vegetative state" appear increasingly likely to be quantitative rather than qualitative. Coupled with this, diagnosis of the latter condition can require prolonged observation and still lack complete certainty. Are there ways in which conversion of any of these patients to "object" status could influence the management of other classes of patient?

It is reasonable to question whether the lack of a close physical similarity between patients with the types of condition we have been considering in this monograph and most conventional categories of the disabled could be guaranteed to preclude the possibility of transfer of attitudes, developed towards the former, to the latter. Logically, one might assume that the differences are so great as to preclude transfer. However, attitudes towards others are rarely shaped by logic alone. It is appropriate to recall the previously discussed reports of reticence on the part of many medical and paramedical personnel to become involved in organ harvesting from brain-dead subjects. The strongly positive attitudes of some nursing staff towards anencephalic infants should also be noted. These represent instances of the transfer to brain-dead and anencephalic patients of attitudes held towards other patients not affected by these conditions. It does not appear to be unreasonable to suspect that transfer of attitudes may also occur in the *other* direction, namely from brain-dead and anencephalic subjects to others not affected by either of these conditions. Is it possible, for instance, that concerted attempts to inculcate acceptance of reification of some categories of individual among staff responsible for intensive care units (in order to facilitate "donor recruitment") may influence the way in which other classes of patient are perceived by these staff?

The possibility may not be fanciful that uncomfortable similarities between a number of the groups of patients mentioned above, who share physical similarities, may influence the attending medical staff. Such similarities have unquestionably already exerted an impact. Thus the resemblance between brain-dead subjects under maintenance, preparatory to organ removal, and "conventional" patients has led to resistance on the part of some doctors and nurses to participation in that maintenance. What is the likelihood that these or other medical personnel will have their attitude towards the permanently comatose, the severe case of spina bifida or the extremely premature infant coloured by experience of brain-dead, anencephalic or foetal subjects used as sources of organ transplants? In considering the possibility that management of the first group of patients will be influenced by experience of management of the second, I am not referring to decisions taken *in the best interests* of the comatose, those with spina bifida or the extremely premature that the most appropriate form of treatment is the provision of no more than basic support. Depending upon individual circumstances, such a course of management may well be entirely appropriate on those grounds. What *should* be of concern, however, is the possibility that, having introduced into medical practice the attitude that evaluation of some individuals as human objects to be used as means to other ends is permissible, it may not prove feasible to quarantine attitudes towards other patients from that influence. If a "principle of beneficence" can be advanced and apparently accepted as grounds for terminating an anencephalic pregnancy in the third trimester and then proceeding to submit the infant to intensive resuscitation and organ removal, could a similar argument be successfully sustained in relation to a category of severely disabled individuals unable to communicate (or to formulate) their wishes for management? Whilst the use of classifying terms such as "brain dead" or "brain absent" may enable one to recommend specific forms of management, it is probable that a significant number of those responsible for implementing that management may be more influenced by the evidence of their senses than by the description on the treatment sheet.

Even superficial consideration of potentially corresponding classes of patient might suggest that a requirement for consistency necessitates comparable approaches. For example, the imputed similarities between the consequences of the brain lesions in anencephalics and those in a "persistent vegetative state" have been held to be grounds for comparable approaches to management. Reinforcement of any tendency for transference of attitudes from "human objects" to other patients might be provided by further dissemination of the trend, discussed on pp. 232–235, for prognosis to be accorded a status equivalent to that of current condition. For example, the respective prognoses relating to cognitive function of a brain-dead individual and of another patient who is permanently comatose but spontaneously breathing, are likely to be very similar. If one is prepared to act in relation to one prognosis as though it has already been fulfilled, is it inconsistent *not* to do so in the case of the other? The comments of Dr Joyce Peabody of the Loma Linda Clinic (already mentioned in Chapter 5) are particularly interesting. Having been responsible for the medical management of a dozen anencephalic infants during what was intended to be a preparatory period before organ removal, she was first reported to be "sequestered" whilst considering the episode.[3] Subsequently, the *Los Angeles Times* reported her as saying that "The slippery slope is real".[5]

In considering the possibility that use as a means will be extended to new categories of patient, the point already raised on p. 235, namely that "use" need not automatically be construed as requiring procedures as drastic as organ removal, deserves re-emphasis. If many of those responsible for providing medical care come to perceive, rightly or wrongly, that the difference between "human objects" and some categories of the severely disabled is only a quantitative one, i.e. a matter of degree rather than a difference in their basic nature, it may not require major attitudinal modification on their part to accept that the question of use of the two groups becomes no more than one of establishing an appropriate proportionality between degrees of disability and permissible use. That is, the extent of use of individuals as a means that the medical community is prepared to tolerate will be specified in accord with the severity of their medical condition.

I suspect that it is not reading too much into some changes in attitude towards use of "human objects" and the placement of increasing emphasis on prognosis, together with the readiness to formulate substituted judgements on behalf of the incommunicative permanently disabled, to identify a more fundamental change in approach. Perhaps it is symptomatic of this that there appears to have been an increasing tendency among some sections of the medical community to adopt a concept of ownership rather than guardianship in relation to some categories of individuals. This concept probably appeared first in relation to "traditional" cadaveric organ donors. Considerable discussion about the legal status and ownership of organs and tissues from this source has occurred during the last three decades.

The question of ownership as it relates to the body of a deceased individual would appear to be as legitimate a subject as that of discussion of ownership of *any* property formerly held by the deceased. The conventional cadaver can hardly be represented ever to have been the subject of guardianship. However, with the general transition from the practice of organ removal from "cardiac-arrest, cadaveric" subjects to the use of "beating-heart, brain dead" and of anencephalic sources in the late 1950s, the notion of ownership has undergone a similar transference. The completed transfer is now reflected very clearly in the terminology selected in discussion of the subject. To recall some of the examples provided in Chapter 5, one published discussion of the use of anencephalics as a potential source of organs canvassed the situation of parents "wishing to donate" their anencephalic children. Use of the term "donor" itself has already been identified on pp. 226–227 as an example of selection of terminology to determine the issue to be argued.

Introduction of the question of ownership in relation to the cadaver could be seen as applying concepts developed in the legal context of succession to fill a pre-existing void. Before the 1960s, any notion of property rights in the case of the human body, insofar as they existed at all, could probably be derived only from relatively archaic legislation relating to body-snatching. However, in the case of the various categories of hopelessly and irreversibly disabled individuals, such as the anencephalic, the foetus *ex utero*, the persistently comatose and the brain dead, I believe that there was a well defined precedent of guardianship. This concept now appears to be giving way, to an increasing extent, to that of ownership.

This change in attitude towards disabled individuals has not been restricted to those categories of patients suitable as organ sources for transplantation. It appears to me to be underway primarily in response to the perceived opportunity for making use of some categories of human subject who were previously considered to be appropriate for the exercise of guardianship. One of the areas in which this change has been most explicitly recognized is that of human embryo experimentation. The question of whether the embryo that is to be generated by IVF, to be experimented upon or to be frozen for later transfer is to be afforded guardianship and protection has been addressed by a number of enquiries and a range of answers has emerged. Nevertheless, formal consideration of the question of ownership versus guardianship appears not to have occurred in the case of "human objects" and the extremely disabled. Perhaps, prevailing practice and the choice of terminology have pre-empted this.

ISSUES FOR THE COMMUNITY

I believe that the time has come when the community at large should close the gap created by the progress of medical technology and address the question of whether some classes of patients are to be designated as "human objects" rather than subjects. In doing so, it may be able to regain the initiative in setting the principles which are to shape attitudes towards such individuals. At present, this has been assumed on a *de facto* basis by the medical personnel responsible for their management and any subsequent use. Community re-entry into this process will require, in the first instance, that an informed awareness develops in relation to existing medical practice.

Informed awareness in the case of brain death and organ collection from the brain dead, for instance, would entail some understanding of the condition of such patients and of current practice in relation to the clinical transplantation procedures in which they are used. The dangers inherent in the widening gap between clinical practice and community comprehension of it were recognized by Christopher Pallis, a British neurologist. In calling for a spread of knowledge concerning brain death, he commented that "a currently uninformed public will sooner or later discover how misleading this simple formulation really is". A more accurate level of community knowledge of anencephaly would also be desirable before the community is required to make decisions on the possible use of such infants. In the interests of informed decision-making, it is necessary that the popular media description of "born without brains" be replaced by some less facile description. In the same way, if vocal support for adoption of the term, and the concept of "cerebral death" continues, it is to be hoped that better information about patients in persistent comatose states will become more widely available. As discussed on pp. 226–227, the impact of any terminology which includes the word "death" should not be underestimated. I have little doubt that the attitudes of others towards any patient manifesting "cerebral death" would be likely to be coloured by the term itself. The responsibility to inform the wider community about the manner in which "cerebral death" differs from "brain death" (and, incidentally, how both differ from the community's present perception of "death") should be accepted by medical and paramedical personnel.

If a community, or its representatives, has addressed the general question of possible designation of individuals as objects to become available for the use of others and decides that existing practices should be modified to facilitate this, the identity of candidate classes becomes an issue. Decisions will be required on which groups of subjects should be so designated, how they are to be identified and which uses are to be regarded as appropriate for each group. Undoubtedly, considerable input from medical and paramedical personnel with different fields of expertise and a range of outlooks will be required to achieve this. On the other hand, if the community baulks at extending such recognition to existing practice, it may wish to press for modification of that practice the better to reflect its attitudes. Whatever the form of enquiry into this subject and the nature of the resolution achieved between community and medical positions, I believe that the ultimate decisions should be seen to rest with the community. This would not preclude their being taken by community representatives after adequate technical briefing.

A number of topics can be readily identified for consideration whenever the issue of community recognition of medical practice, as it relates to the use of specifically identified classes of individuals, is examined. Of these topics, one of the earliest might be the question of *existence of imperatives*. An example which comes readily to mind, and which has been presented during advocacy of extended usage of some groups of individuals, is the question of whether the community should recognize an imperative not to waste valuable resources in the form of reified humans who could be employed as transplant sources or as experimental and training material. It is beyond question that beating-heart, brain dead individuals (as, incidentally, "cardiac-arrest" cadavers before them) have afforded the opportunity to many patients for greatly extended lives of higher quality. As will be discussed below, the extent of the requirement for a supply of organs from this source continues to increase and there is little doubt that the benefit which could be conferred upon the community would match any increased availability. The strength of the argument for an increased availability of organs for transplantation from anencephalic infants is dubious. Minimal success has been achieved with transplantation of hearts or kidneys from anencephalics.

The usefulness of these organs has not been established and, as previously remarked, there appear to have been instances of "organs in search of a recipient". The benefit available from use of transplantation of foetal brain tissue remains completely speculative. It seems clear that considerable time will be required for the assessment of the extent and duration of any remissions of Parkinson's disease produced in this way. At present, the lead is being given by a Swedish neurosurgical group which, by and large, has shown responsibility in its release of information about patients, and a British group, which has not.

One imperative that a reasonable community is likely to accept without debate is that of acting consistently in its dealings with patients likely to be considered as sources of transplants. A consistent and fair approach has been recognized as indicated both on moral grounds and as a "public relations" measure to engender community confidence in the process of organ acquisition. Recognition of this imperative for consistency in any classification of individuals as "non-persons", and in their subsequent use, would require consideration of codes of practice in relation to other categories of subject sharing features in common with the group in question. As mentioned earlier, any guidelines to regulate the use of the foetus *ex utero* should be consistent with existing codes of practice both for disposition of IVF embryos and for management of extremely low birth weight neonates. Recommendations for dealing with anencephalic infants should take into account their substantial similarities to patients in a persistent vegetative state. Finally, it should be clear that a practice does not become an imperative merely because the community agrees that it is permissible.

A second issue which would need to be aired at some stage during development of community policies on the use of designated classes of subject concerns the logistic aspects of the proposals. Consideration of logistics necessarily accompanies that of possible imperatives to the extent that some of the arguments for the acceptance of a proposed imperative for use are likely to be dependent upon quantification of the likely benefits. Many people may concede that an imperative exists in relation to a particular course of action if, for example, it is likely to advantage large numbers. They may be less sure if it is seen to have only a restricted application. This point might be illustrated by reference to the use of anencephalics as transplant sources. Much of the superficial discussion of this subject has raised the prospect that very substantial numbers of potential paediatric organ recipients will be assisted by this measure. I suspect that this has often been an effective "selling point". However, in reality, the detailed study of Shewmon *et al.*, discussed in Chapter 5, implies that only a handful of such patients could hold any reasonable expectation of being helped by the supply of organs available from anencephalics.[3] When the existing supply of such organs is discounted to take account of the spontaneously decreasing frequency of anencephaly, and the impact on this of diagnosis and termination of pregnancy, as well as the effect of dietary improvement among susceptible women during pregnancy, the likely benefit appears even thinner. It may be concluded that acceptance of the use of anencephalics as organ sources is unlikely to have more than a marginal impact on existing shortages of organs.

The major logistic question in relation to classifying individuals as suitable organ sources undoubtedly arises from the widening gap between availability of the class of "beating-heart donors" currently used for this purpose and the increasing numbers of patients who are recognized as potential beneficiaries of transplantation. Measures to decrease the frequency of motor vehicle accidents, if successful, will predictably accentuate the deficiency. The two responses possible to this situation are to increase the extent of recruitment of organ donors from the existing "beating-heart" pool or to increase the size of the pool potentially available for recruitment. The limitations to increased recruitment and the limited success so far achieved have been considered on pp. 84–92. As regards increasing the size of the pool from which donors may be drawn, the two possibilities are a widening of the definition of brain death and re-introduction of the original practice of harvesting organs from individuals who have sustained cardiac arrest. The step which has been advocated to widen the definition of brain death entails its extension to patients with "cerebral death". In view of the considerable reticence that exists among medical personnel to recruit donors actively from among "beating-heart", brain-dead subjects, the acceptability (let alone the morality) of removal of organs from spontaneously breathing patients seems very doubtful to me.

Reverting to the use of "non-beating-heart" or "cardiac-arrest" donors appears to be a more promising option than that of extending the boundaries of brain death. "Non-beating-heart" donors may be considered in two categories according to whether cardiac arrest occurred despite maintenance of artificial ventilation or as an early consequence of its deliberate cessation. In general, it is likely that many organs from the first group may have sustained damage as a result of progressively impaired circulation before cardiac arrest occurred. Whilst not an optimal type of donor for this reason, such patients have been successfully used as a source of transplantable kidneys. On the other hand, the use of organs from individuals in whom cardiac arrest has followed disconnection from a ventilator, was the original practice when cadaveric kidney transplantation was introduced and kidneys and livers from such patients have been successfully transplanted. Abandonment of this group of patients occurred in response to the anticipation that organs from "beating-heart" donors would better survive transplantation. Interestingly, this change occurred without any formal alterations to regulations for organ harvesting. However, recent reports of several series of transplants in which "non-beating-heart" donors were used suggest that excellent results can be obtained following this procedure. It appears that much of the organ damage previously observed in organs removed *after* cardiac arrest resulted from the inadequacy of the earlier methods of preservation employed *after* organ removal. Consequently, the only valid comparison to be used in assessing the relative merits of "beating-heart" versus "non-beating-heart" donors is that based on recent use of current methods of organ preservation as applied to both types of organ.

Apart from the substantial increase in availability of organs that would occur if "non-beating-heart" donors were used to supplement, or even to replace "beating-heart" donors, doubts about the real status of brain-dead patients would become irrelevant. Furthermore, reservations of some medical personnel about participation in the removal of organs from patients whose heart continued to beat would be overcome. Likewise, the discrepancy between what the community believes about organ removal from brain-dead donors and what is actually practised would be lessened.

Another issue that is likely to receive increasing attention in framing policies both on the use of various classes of individual as organ sources, and on the protocols for such use, is the question of the extent to which a duty of care is owed to potential recipients. It should be readily apparent that any surgeon offering to treat a patient by transplantation of an organ or tissue will require that the transplant be in optimal condition. This is essential if the opportunity of benefit to the recipient is to be maximized. In consequence, the surgeon's duty of care will necessitate the use of procedures for organ or tissue acquisition that are likely to preserve it in the best condition. As recognized by Shumway at an early stage of development of cardiac transplantation, it was not justifiable (at least with the technology for organ preservation available in the early 1970s) to transplant a heart which had not been removed until after spontaneous cessation of the heartbeat.[6] An alternative view presented at that time by Calne was that, as livers had been successfully transplanted from "non-beating-heart" donors, any other organ could also be obtained from this source.[7] The number of recent reports of successful renal transplantation from donors who had already experienced cardiac arrest suggests that there no longer exists serious doubt, on the issue of fairness to the recipient, about using kidneys from "non-beating-heart" donors. Re-introduction of this class of donor in the case of liver and heart transplantation would require the establishment of a reasonable likelihood that potential recipients of organs from this source would not be significantly disadvantaged in comparison with recipients of these organs collected under existing protocols from "beating-heart" donors. There appears to be a good possibility that the advances which have been achieved recently in the technology for organ preservation after removal could provide this assurance.

The issue of duty of care to the recipient remains a substantial one in any programme to utilize organs from anencephalic infants. It appears to be increasingly clear that an inverse relationship effectively exists between the likelihood that an anencephalic infant will meet brain-death criteria consistently applicable to other classes of subject and the likelihood that his or her organs will remain in suitable condition to justify transplantation. Similarly, in the case of foetal brain transplantation for Parkinson's disease, even if one assumes that this procedure is shown at some future date to be worthwhile for the recipient, it is likely that the optimal requirements from the recipient's viewpoint will increasingly diverge from those that are met by the procedures otherwise likely to be employed to terminate the pregnancy. The possibility of failure of the brain implant, or of significant deleterious effects from it, in the longer term also remains quite open.

An issue which seems to have become increasingly more prominent with extension in the clinical use of transplantation is the impact, potential and realized, of organ procurement procedures on certain groups within the community. Subjective effects do not readily lend themselves to measurement and, for this reason are readily, and unreasonably, discounted when arguments are weighed up. Nevertheless, there has been a steady stream of reports and of individual incidents in which some of the medical and paramedical personnel involved in the maintenance of individuals to be used as a source of organs for transplantation, and in the collection of those organs, have experienced distress. This has taken the form of unwillingness to be further involved, sometimes of relocation to a different field of medicine and, in some cases, of retirement. The occasion most frequently producing negative responses has been the removal of organs from "beating-heart", brain-dead donors. Reaction to these negative responses has included calls for the education of participating staff not to be "confused by the evidence of their senses" into mistaking such patients as being individuals. Another reaction has been to provide counselling for affected staff. Similar negative responses have been observed, albeit on a numerically much smaller scale, among staff when anencephalic infants have been submitted to extended resuscitation in order that they may be used as an organ source. For example, the paediatric cardiac surgeon, Leonard Bailey, has referred to the "tolerance" of nursing staff towards maintenance of anencephalics preparatory to organ removal as a major limitation to this procedure. Reservations about the principle of using and managing patients for the benefit of others appear still to be widely distributed among medical personnel.

The responses of staff to procedures associated with organ collection are, I suggest, a most important issue for the community to take into account when it considers its attitudes towards designation of some groups of patients as human objects and their subsequent use. These medical personnel act as agents for the community in implementing the measures required by transplantation programmes which the community supports. It is possible that some of the projected expansions in the classification of usable human objects, if sponsored by the community, would impose considerably greater stresses on the personnel involved. The example of "pre-donation" maintenance of persistently comatose patients if they are classified as "cerebrally dead" comes to mind. Thus, in writing of the treatment of "cerebral death" subjects, Puccetti referred to the necessity for "active intervention to stop the breathing prior to preparation for burial".[8] A related current issue concerns withholding hydration and nutrition from such patients. Irrespective of one's assessment of the rights and wrongs of this complicated question, it is necessary, again, that the community recognize that some of the medical and nursing staff responsible for implementing such a policy may be adversely affected by it. Failure to address the issue of ambivalent responses of medical personnel to participation in organ procurement programmes, together with the discrepancies which exist between medical and community comprehension of procurement procedures, has the potential to erode the relationship of trust between patient and doctor.

When considering the impact of organ procurement procedures in the community, it should be recognized that this impact can extend forcefully to some categories of donor. The most prominent, albeit relatively small, group of "donors" whose lives, or deaths, may be influenced by organ procurement are prisoners scheduled for execution. Whilst policies for mandatory acquisition of organs from executed individuals apply only in a few countries, the question of fulfilment of previously expressed wishes for use of organs from those executed in other jurisdictions remains a very difficult issue, however it is expressed. Capital punishment and termination of pregnancy share the common features that the legally sanctioned ending of life, by reason of the deliberative precision with which procedures may be controlled, is ideally suited to provide transplantable organs exactly as required.

A community that elects to consider the issue of classifying some classes of individuals as usable will be required to determine the grounds that are to be admissible in making the classification. Should an individual be assessed on "purely scientific" grounds, for example, pathological anatomy? Should an anencephalic infant be assessed as subject or object on the basis of inferred brain structure or on such subjective factors as the perception of the infant by others? Is the impression that family and nursing staff have of such an infant to receive attention? It will be necessary for those deliberating on these subjects on behalf of the community to recognize that interpretations of scientific data can change and, with time and further research, they almost invariably do so. As discussed in Chapter 4, this has happened in the case of anencephaly. If anatomical pathology is accorded precedence in making the subject/object distinction, its reevaluation may produce the situation in which identical patients may be classified as objects in one decade and subjects in the next, or vice versa.

As discussed in Chapter 3, re-evaluation of the status of individuals in the groups we have been discussing is always a possibility. A current example is the frequent call for alteration of brain-death criteria in order to shift the primary emphasis to retention of consciousness rather than to spontaneous respiration. This could entail a community electing to classify "cerebral death" patients as equivalent to the brain dead, and using them accordingly. I would strongly emphasize the possibility that community-influenced re-evaluation of what constitutes brain death may not automatically imply *broadening* of the category. It is possible that the outcome of such re-evaluation might result in restriction of the scope of application of the term. Whilst dealing with evaluation or re-evaluation of the status of various classes of subject, it is highly desirable that those undertaking the exercise on behalf of the community eschew adoption of very generalized approaches. Generalization can be a desirable and useful process. However, in this case it carries the risk of concealing specific points, which could have vitiated the thrust of the general argument. A good illustration of this effect has been identified by Shewmon *et al.* and discussed in Chapter 5. These authors drew attention to the likelihood of a negative correlation between the probability of a single anencephalic infant satisfying the criteria for brain death and, at the same time, also being an appropriate organ source. As emphasized by Shewmon, the organs of those infants with the most severe forms of the malformation, who would therefore be most likely to come close to satisfying the criteria, were unlikely to be suitable for transplantation.[3] However, general consideration of anencephalics as organ sources may bracket compliance with brain-death criteria and suitability of organs—a combination that would rarely occur in practice.

Formulation of any decisions on behalf of the community in relation to classification as human objects may require collection of information about the earlier impact within the community of use of individuals. As noted in Chapter 3, the total number of published studies on the consequences of organ donation from one member of a family on the surviving members remains very small. Furthermore, the power of these surveys may have been limited because they were completed within 1 or 2 years of the event. The long-term consequences of organ donation on the grieving process in surviving family members remains unknown. Until much more information is collected, it is difficult to draw reliable conclusions about all forms of impact of organ donation.

Another aspect which, I suggest, would require further enquiry concerns the existence and nature of alternative organ sources for transplantation. The breadth of alternatives may extend to novel methods of organ removal, for instance partial hepatectomy to provide transplantable liver from a living, related donor. It may encompass novel methods of presentation of a graft as, for example, in the introduction of cell lines enclosed within a capsule, into the recipient. Alternatives may include procedures that do not involve transplantation such as the technically more difficult reconstruction of defective hearts in neonates or even *in utero*. The existence of less acceptable alternatives to use of brain-dead and anencephalic subjects has been noted earlier. The use of paid, unrelated "donors" (with a strong risk of their exploitation) and of animals (with the high risk of graft rejection) have been identified as unacceptable. As discussed above, alternatives such as the use of "cardiac-arrest" rather than "beating-heart", brain-dead donors, if they were to become technically adequate, could reduce some of the existing problems associated with transplantation.

Whenever a community resolves to set its guidelines relating to designating categories of patient for use, there is likely to arise need for regulatory decisions for some types of individual and of proposed use. Examples of specific aspects of human use, which could require regulation, include the existing tourist trade to Third World countries in search of transplantable organs and the use of brain-dead subjects in experimentation. All of these subjects have attracted attention recently. A likely conclusion to any community enquiry into the use of humans as objects could be legislation. In earlier chapters, reference was made to suggestions for the use of legal mechanisms to adjust the timing of death for tax mitigation purposes. There have also been calls for increased penalties for causing "cerebral death" and, on the other hand, for reduced penalties for killing those already in that state. There have been several legislative attempts in the USA to re-define brain death so as to include anencephalics within its orbit. Whilst the nature of any proposals for future legislative changes in order to certify individuals as "not alive" or "not persons" is likely to reflect the local circumstances at the time, it may be worth noting that some legislation in the past seems to have been influenced by factors other than the apparent primary cause. For instance, a perceived need to provide legal indemnity to those responsible for organ removal appears to have provided considerable impetus for much of the USA brain-death legislation. The lesson for the future which might be drawn from this is that legislative measures are best directed to a specific problem rather than to attempt to achieve multiple ends.

REFERENCES

1. Pallis, C. (1985) Defining death. *British Medical Journal*, **291**, 666–667.
2. Fraser, L. Storm over 'kept alive' donor baby. *The Mail on Sunday* (London), December 14, 1986.
3. Shewmon, D. A., Capron, A. M., Peacock, W. J. and Schulman, B. L. (1989) The use of anencephalic infants as organ sources. A critique. *Journal of the American Medical Association*, **261**, 1772–1781.
4. Knoll, E. and Lundberg, G. D. (1985) Informed consent and baby Fae. *Journal of the American Medical Association*, **254**, 3359–3360.
5. Goldsmith, M. F. (1988) Anencephalic organ donor program suspended: Loma Linda report expected to detail findings. *Journal of the American Medical Association*, **260**, 1671–1672.
6. Griepp, R. B., Stinson, E. B., Clark, D. A., Dong, E. and Shumway, N. E. (1971) The cardiac donor. *Surgery, Gynecology and Obstetrics*, **133**, 792–798.
7. Calne, R. Y. (1971) Ethics, the law and the future. In R. Y. Calne, (Ed.) *Clinical Organ Transplantation*, pp. 517–524. Blackwell, Oxford.
8. Puccetti, R. (1988) Does anyone survive neocortical death? In R. M. Zaner (Ed.) *Death: Beyond Whole-Brain Criteria*, pp. 75–95. Kluwer Academic Publishers, Dordrecht.

Index

Index compiled by Jill Halliday